SIMPLE & EASY

PEDIATRIC CARDIOLOGY

The Basics for Everyone Caring for Children

II

SIMPLE & EASY

PEDIATRIC CARDIOLOGY

The Basics for Everyone Caring for Children

Editors

William Evans

Professor of Pediatrics
University of Nevada School of Medicine
Childrens Heart Center Nevada

Ruben Acherman

Professor of Pediatrics
University of Nevada School of Medicine
Childrens Heart Center Nevada

Carlos Luna

Associate Professor of Pediatrics
University of Nevada School of Medicine
Childrens Heart Center Nevada

Childrens Heart Center Nevada Press

Childrens Heart Center Nevada Press

childrensheartcenternevadapress.org

3006 S Maryland Parkway
Suite 690
Las Vegas, NV 89109

Simple and Easy Pediatric Cardiology: The Basics for Everyone Caring for Children

ISBN: 978-0-9887047-0-1

Copyright © 2013 All rights reserved

Note

Medical knowledge is not static. New information and discoveries bring constant change. We have diligently checked our text and each reference; nonetheless, errors are always possible. Thus, we disclaim all responsibility for inaccuracies, and we do not warranty any of the information contained herein. Readers should confirm all information with other sources, especially medication indications, interactions, complications, and dosing.

No part of this book may be reproduced or transmitted in any form or by any means currently available or by any means that may become available anytime in the future without written permission from the publisher. We have made every effort to trace copyright holders for borrowed material. If we have inadvertently overlooked any, we will make the necessary arrangements at the the earliest opportunity. To purchase additional copies call 702-732-1290 or 866-732-1290 or visit childrensheartcenternevadapress.org.

First Edition

Dedication

To our patients

To our mentors

To our families

VI

Foreword

This is no ordinary textbook. It is simple without being oversimplified, multi-authored with unified editing that avoids conflicting statements, easy to handle yet covering an encyclopedic range of subject matter.

It was conceived as a substitute for the massive textbooks of pediatric cardiology for a reader in a hurry to arrive at the knowledge necessary to handle a clinical situation. Such a reader might be a pediatrician, family physician, nurse, or medical student. But it is authoritative enough to be a useful source for the pediatric or adult cardiologist or a fellow in training for one of those subspecialties.

The book is not just illustrated; it is decorated by one of the contributors who is both a cardiologist and an artist. The prose avoids dryness, is unpredictably interspersed with outlines that help the flow, and is unusually almost entertaining, attesting to the enthusiasm of the writers.

As I said earlier, it is no ordinary textbook, but it is one that the world should find useful.

p a u l   r   l u r i e

From the editors

To the best of our knowledge, Paul Raymond Lurie, born in 1917, is the oldest living pediatric cardiologist. Following World War II, Paul and his colleagues, Ruth Whittemore and Frank Gray, launched pediatric cardiology at Yale in the late 1940s. Later, Paul founded the program at Riley Children's Hospital in 1950. Paul was the first to adapt the Seldinger technique for cardiac catheterization in children, and later he was the first to introduce myocardial biopsy in pediatrics. After retiring from heading the Division of Pediatric Cardiology at Childrens Hospital of Los Angeles, Paul has remained academically active by spearheading the cardiomyopathy registry and recently contributing valuable perspectives on endocardial fibroelastosis and ventricular noncompaction. He is a mentor, a scholar, and a friend.

Evans WN. Paul Raymond Lurie: an innovator and founder of paediatric cardiology. Cardiol Young 2010; 20: 402-409

VIII

Preface

Studying heart disease can be difficult. However, this book presents an instructional approach that is straightforward. We divide the text into 3 Parts, and we supplement these sections with an extensive Appendix and a comprehensive Index. Part 1 describes clinical problems and how to evaluate patients at presentation, details specific cardiovascular abnormalities, and discusses a variety of cardiovascular-related disorders. Parts 2 and 3 succinctly describe normal and abnormal embryological, anatomical, and physiological concepts; explain diagnostic testing; and discuss interventional catheter and surgical procedures. The Appendix includes current endocarditis prophylaxis guidelines; a clearance form for hyperactivity-disorder medications and competitive sports; a brief formulary; a compendium of laboratory tests; a glossary of eponyms; and a list of defined abbreviations.

Each chapter begins with a brief background statement. Additional subsections expand topics. Bullet points emphasize symptoms, signs, laboratory tests, anatomy, physiology, diagnostic procedures, and treatment methods. Black-arrow (➤) bullets highlight key points. The text includes more than 350 full-color figures and tables that help clarify difficult concepts. This work also includes some medical history, as an acquaintance with the past can help explain the evolution to current management. Chapter references serve as sources for further study. The problem chapters conclude with clinical vignettes and multiple-choice questions (an answer key precedes the index).

This book can benefit everyone who cares for children including medical and surgical technicians, medical students, nurses, physician extenders, residents, fellows, and physicians in practice. The contents conform to most residency programs' curricula for pediatric cardiology rotations. The clinical vignettes and questions also help prepare residents for similar questions found on the American Board of Pediatrics certification exam. This is not, however, a guide for when to refer patients to pediatric cardiology; rather, primary care providers should feel free to refer any patient they deem needs evaluation.

Caring for children with heart disease encompasses more than clinical facts, imaging, and treatment. As we look into the eyes of a frightened child, we must never let a fascination with cold, gleaming technology replace the power of a warm, reassuring smile. Please enjoy this book.

x

Table of Contents

Part 1 — Problems

1 Heart Murmurs	1
2 Failure-to-Thrive	15
3 Dysmorphic Features	25
4 Abnormal Heart Rates & Rhythms	47
5 Heart Failure	69
6 Patent Ductus Arteriosus & the Premature Infant	83
7 Oxygen Desaturation	93
8 Extremis	109
9 Aborted or Sudden Cardiac Death	121
10 Late Post-Procedure Problems	131
11 Prolonged Fever	139
12 Chest Pain	155
13 Syncope	165
14 Hypertension	175
15 Obesity & Lipid Disorders	187

Part 2 — Anatomy & Physiology

16 Cardiovascular Embryology	203
17 Situs & Cardiac Position	217
18 Fetal & Neonatal Cardiovascular Physiology	229
19 Cardiovascular Malformations	239

Part 3 — Diagnostic & ℞ Methods

20 Chest X-Ray	307
21 Electrocardiogram	321
22 Echocardiogram	349
23 Fetal Echocardiogram	367
24 MRI & CT	389
25 Cardiac Catheterization & Intervention	395
26 Electrophysiology Pacemakers & ICDs	415
27 Cardiovascular surgery	427

Appendix

A Endocarditis Prophylaxis — 457

B ADD Medications & Sports Clearance Form — 461

C Formulary — 463

D Laboratory Values — 489

E Eponyms — 505

F Abbreviations — 515

Index — 519

XIV

Contributors

RUBEN ACHERMAN
Professor of Pediatrics
University of Nevada School of Medicine
Childrens Heart Center Nevada

DEAN BERTHOTY
Radiologist
Sunrise Children's Hospital
Las Vegas, Nevada

KATHLEEN CASS
Associate Professor of Pediatrics
University of Nevada School of Medicine
Childrens Heart Center Nevada

WILLIAM CASTILLO
Associate Professor of Pediatrics
University of Nevada School of Medicine
Childrens Heart Center Nevada

MICHAEL CICCOLO
Chief
Congenital Cardiovascular Surgery
Childrens Heart Center Nevada

WILLIAM EVANS
Professor of Pediatrics
University of Nevada School of Medicine
Childrens Heart Center Nevada

ALVARO GALINDO
Professor of Pediatrics
University of Nevada School of Medicine
Childrens Heart Center Nevada

KATRINKA KIP
Associate Professor of Pediatrics
University of Nevada School of Medicine
Childrens Heart Center Nevada

IAN LAW
Clinical Associate Professor of Pediatrics
University of Iowa
Carver College of Medicine

JOSEPH LUDWICK
Associate Professor of Pediatrics
University of Nevada School of Medicine
Childrens Heart Center Nevada

CARLOS LUNA
Associate Professor of Pediatrics
University of Nevada School of Medicine
Childrens Heart Center Nevada

GARY MAYMAN
Professor of Pediatrics
University of Nevada School of Medicine
Childrens Heart Center Nevada

ROBERT ROLLINS
Assistant Professor of Pediatrics
University of Nevada School of Medicine
Childrens Heart Center Nevada

ABRAHAM ROTHMAN
Professor of Pediatrics
University of Nevada School of Medicine
Childrens Heart Center Nevada

VINCENT THOMAS
Assistant Professor of Pediatrics
University of Nevada School of Medicine
Childrens Heart Center Nevada

NICHOLAS VON BERGEN
Clinical Assistant Professor of Pediatrics
University of Iowa
Carver College of Medicine

XVI

Part 1

Problems

XVIII

1 Heart Murmurs

Contents

Background	3
Cardiovascular Exam	4
Innocent murmurs	8
Pathological Murmurs	8
Special Circumstances	12
Clinical Vignettes	13

1 Heart Murmurs

william evans

BACKGROUND

Heart murmurs have fascinated physicians and frightened parents since Laënnec invented the stethoscope in 1816. Innocent murmurs are the sounds of blood flow through a normal heart and great vessels. Pathological murmurs are the sounds of abnormal, turbulent blood flow across intracardiac defects, great artery malformations, or acquired cardiovascular abnormalities. Lack of symptoms does not distinguish innocent from pathological murmurs; thus, we avoid the term "asymptomatic murmur."

The following is not a guide for consistently differentiating innocent from pathological murmurs. Even experienced clinicians encounter difficulty when deciding if a murmur is innocent or not. Also, some malformations have minimal or no murmur findings; therefore, a murmur's absence does not eliminate the possibility of heart disease. Some stress innocent murmurs may change or disappear with a patient's position, but examples exist for both pathological and innocent murmurs changing with position. Others suggest fixed-splitting of the 2nd heart sound (S_2) can differentiate an innocent pulmonary flow murmur in a normal heart from a pulmonary flow murmur associated with an atrial septal defect (see the following "Auscultation" section). Yet auscultating fixed or variable splitting of S_2 is difficult in the young with high heart rates. Furthermore, accurate auscultation is a skill difficult to acquire. Studies show poor correlation between a noncardiologist's auscultatory impressions and individual cardiovascular defects. Accordingly, primary care providers are not responsible for differentiating pathological murmurs from innocent murmurs in every case.

An electrocardiogram (EKG) is a weak aid for discriminating a pathological murmur from an innocent murmur. Also, a computer-interpreted EKG may suggest heart disease even when a followup echocardiogram (Echo) reveals none. The principal indications for an EKG include abnormal heart rate and rhythm evaluation, ruling out preexcitation (Wolff-Parkinson-White syndrome), or ruling out long QT syndrome (LQTS). Another EKG indication is to check for ST-T wave changes that may result from serious cardiovascular malformations, myopericarditis, or other causes of myocardial stress. For more on pediatric EKG interpretation, see Chapter 21.

Following physical examination, Echo is the principal testing method for murmur evaluation. Even pediatric cardiologists cannot always determine the complete cardiovascular diagnosis without an Echo. Nonetheless, every caregiver should attempt to diagnose the cause of a cardiac murmur. Such an attempt is challenging, but the exercise is rewarding when an Echo confirms one's auscultatory impressions. [1-5]

CARDIOVASCULAR EXAM

Although the presenting problem may be a "murmur," the cardiovascular physical examination begins before auscultation. Following vital signs, the cardiovascular exam includes growth parameters (see also Chapter 2), inspection, palpation, and lastly auscultation.

Growth Parameters
• Normal height & weight

Normal growth does not rule out heart disease. Pulmonic stenosis (PS), aortic stenosis (AS), some atrial septal defects (ASD), some ventricular septal defects (VSD), and isolated coarctations (CoA) may have no effect on growth parameters.

• Weight below the height percentile

A moderate to large VSD, patent ductus arteriosus (PDA), or other malformations may cause congestive heart failure (CHF). CHF increases the work of breathing. An increased work of breathing uses calories and hinders weight gain. As most caloric expenditure goes to weight gain, the effect on height is less.

• Height & weight both impaired

If the height and weight curves both plot below the 5th percentile, then an endocrine problem or a syndrome is possible. Also, cardiovascular malformations may further impact growth parameters in patients with syndromes or endocrine abnormalities.

Inspection
• Note dysmorphic features
• Comfortable or in respiratory distress
• Check for pallor, cyanosis, or mottling
• The precordium may be visually hyperdynamic
• Check for edema or jugular venous distention in older patients

Palpation
• Precordial activity

With some cardiovascular malformations, precordial overactivity may be the solitary cardiac exam finding.

• Thrill

Turbulent blood flow, through conditions such as a VSD and semilunar valve stenosis, may produce palpable precordial thrills. A suprasternal notch thrill is usually from valvular aortic stenosis, and a thrill may be present even with mild stenosis.

• Pulses

Check upper and lower extremity pulses, as pulses can be weak in low cardiac output, bounding in a PDA or aortic regurgitation, and discrepant in a CoA. A CoA causes strong pulses in the upper extremities and weak or absent femoral pulses. A CoA is easy to miss if an examiner fails to check pulses.

• Abdomen

With congestive heart failure, hepatomegaly and ascites may be present.

Auscultation
Normal heart sounds

Normal heart tones include the 1st and 2nd heart sounds (S_1 and S_2). S_1 arises during the onset of ventricular systole with mitral and tricuspid valve closure. S_2 occurs at the beginning of diastole and includes 2 distinct sounds, aortic valve closure (A_2) and pulmonary valve closure (P_2). In young infants and children, with high heart rates and poor cooperation, even the most experienced practitioner may be unable to auscultate heart sounds beyond recognizing S_1 and S_2. A split S_1 is often inaudible in infants or children, but it can be normal or accompany right bundle branch block (RBBB also increases S_2 splitting). Normal splitting of S_2 into its A_2 and P_2 components is audible in quiet, cooperative children with low heart rates.

The relative closure times for the pulmonary and aortic valves cause S_2 to split into 2 components. Usually, the A_2 component arises slightly earlier than the P_2 component because the higher diastolic pressure in the aorta results in a more rapid closure of the aortic valve than the pulmonary valve. As the figure below shows, deep inspiration accentuates normal splitting of S_2 into its A_2 and P_2 components. Deep inspiration creates negative intrathoracic pressure. Negative intrathoracic pressure causes more right ventricle (RV) filling, momentarily augmenting pulmonary blood flow and delaying pulmonary valve closure.

Expiration increases intrathoracic pressure, momentarily decreasing right-heart filling. Decreased right-heart filling results in a quicker pulmonary valve closure, bringing the time for A_2 and P_2 closer together and reducing the audible splitting of S_2. If the pulmonary arterial pressure is high, then P_2 occurs quicker than normal and fuses with A_2, resulting in a "single" loud S_2 (figure below).

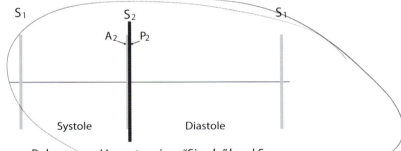

Pulmonary Hypertension. "Single" loud S_2

ASDs cause a delay in the pulmonary valve closure time. In an ASD, more blood than normal enters the RV, and the RV pumps extra blood through the pulmonary valve. The pulmonary valve stays open longer and closes later. Contrary to the effects of inspiration, which momentarily prolongs the time to P_2, an ASD causes extra blood to flow continuously through the right heart. Consequently, the widened, audible splitting of S_2 becomes "fixed" and varies little with respiration, as the figure below displays. The figure also includes a representation of a typical soft systolic ejection murmur from increased pulmonary flow.

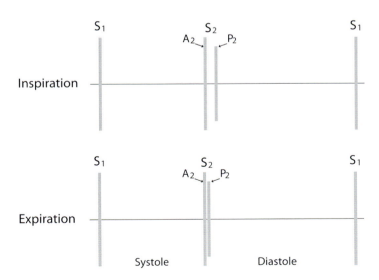

Normal Heart Sounds. Inspiration accentuates S_2 split.

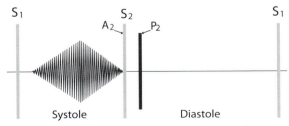

ASD. Ejection murmur, fixed wide S_2 split

1 Heart Murmurs

Heart murmurs

Murmur descriptions

On the facing page, murmur pictorial depictions accompany the following written descriptions: (1) Systolic ejection murmur, (2) Early systolic murmur, (3) Holosystolic murmur, (4) Continuous murmur, (5) Early diastolic murmur, and (6) Mid-diastolic murmur.

- **Vibratory systolic (innocent murmur)**

In the following "Innocent murmur" section, we quote the early 20th-century physician George Still's classic description.

- **Systolic ejection murmur (figure 1)**

The murmur begins with or slightly after S_1, peaking in mid-systole, and ending slightly before or with S_2, as from AS or PS. Systolic ejection murmurs radiate upwards towards the neck.

- **Early systolic murmur (figure 2)**

A uniform murmur beginning with S_1, ending before S_2, as from a small muscular VSD. VSD murmurs usually do not radiate to the neck.

- **Holosystolic murmur (figure 3)**

A uniform murmur existing throughout systole from a VSD or in mitral or tricuspid valve regurgitation (MR, TR). Murmurs from VSDs, MR, or TR tend not to radiate towards the neck. Small VSDs and mild to moderate MR produce high frequency holosystolic murmurs from high velocity blood flow jets. As the blood flow velocities are lower across moderate to large-sized VSDs or the tricuspid valve, these conditions produce lower frequency murmurs.

- **Continuous murmur (figure 4)**

A continuous waxing and waning murmur (machinery quality) audible in systole and diastole as in a PDA.

- **Diastolic murmurs (figures 5 & 6)**

Diastolic murmurs are rare in children. Diastolic murmurs may be audible with aortic or pulmonary regurgitation (AR or PR); with mitral or tricuspid valve inflow turbulence from mitral or tricuspid stenosis (MS or TS); or with excessive inflow (rumble) across the mitral valve (MV) or the tricuspid valve (TV) from a moderate to large VSD (for the MV) and a large ASD (for the TV). AR and PR are early high-frequency diastolic murmurs (figure 5). In contrast, MS, TS, or the murmurs from increased flows across the mitral or tricuspid valves all occur in mid to late diastole and are lower frequency sounds (figure 6).

Systolic grades

Systolic murmur grades

I	Barely audible
II	Easily audible but not loud
III	Moderately loud but no thrill
IV	Loud with palpable thrill from high velocity turbulent flow
V	Loud with thrill and heard with stethoscope's chest piece in contact with the precordium but slightly tilted
VI	Very loud with thrill and still audible with the stethoscope just off the chest

Diastolic grades

Diastolic murmurs grade descriptions are the same, but clinicians often limit diastolic murmur grades to I-IV.

Murmur types & locations

During auscultation, note a murmur's location of maximal loudness, assign a loudness grade, and then characterize the sound. A murmur's description begins with the grade, followed by its characterization and location best heard. Refer to the

1 Heart Murmurs

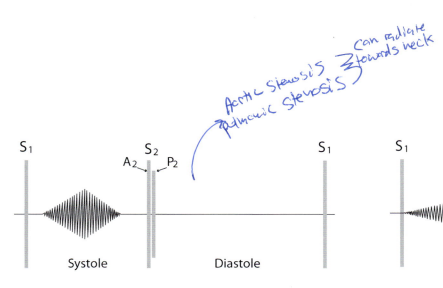

1 Systolic Ejection Murmur

Aortic stenosis — can radiate towards neck
Pulmonic stenosis

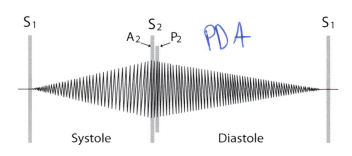

4 Continuous Murmur — PDA

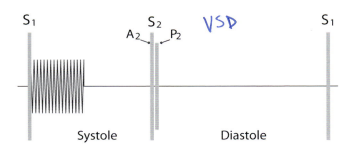

2 Early Systolic Murmur — VSD

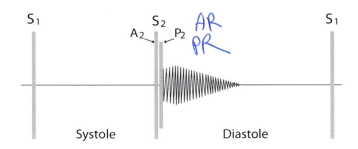

5 Early Diastolic Murmur — AR, PR

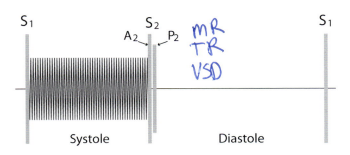

3 Holosystolic Murmur — MR, TR, VSD

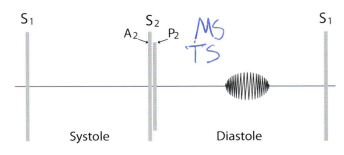

6 Mid-Diastolic Murmur — MS, TS

figure on the top of the facing page for innocent and pathological murmur locations.

➤ Example description: A grade II systolic ejection murmur best heard at the right upper sternal border (as in AS).

Innocent murmurs

The most common heart murmur is an innocent vibratory systolic murmur, or Still's murmur, best described by the English physician George Frederic Still. In his 1909 textbook, *Common Disorders and Diseases of Childhood*, Still wrote, "I should like to draw attention to a particular bruit which has somewhat of a musical character, but is neither of sinister omen nor does it indicate endocarditis of any sort…its characteristic feature is a twangy sound, very like that made by twanging a piece of tense string…. [Whatever] may be its origin, I think it is clearly functional, that is to say, not due to any organic disease of the heart either congenital or acquired." [6] Still's 100-year-old narrative is still a superb description of a vibratory or musical innocent systolic murmur.

Nonvibratory or "flow-type" innocent systolic ejection murmurs are difficult to distinguish from pathological systolic ejection murmurs. Previously, we noted the challenge in determining if a pulmonary-flow systolic ejection murmur is innocent or from an ASD's increased pulmonary flow. A systolic murmur from physiological peripheral pulmonic stenosis (physiological PPS) can sound similar to the systolic murmur from pathological PPS; the former disappears over time from the newborn to later infancy, and the latter persists. For practical reasons, clinicians may not have the opportunity to follow a patient over time; therefore, a primary care provider may correctly seek a pediatric cardiology consultation to distinguish the two. A venous hum results from normal venous blood flow in the neck. A venous hum usually disappears upon lying down. Further, increased blood flow velocity in a normal heart may simply accentuate innocent systolic murmurs, as with fever, anemia, hyperthyroidism, and other conditions causing elevated heart rates or increased cardiac output.

Pathological murmurs

Consider all newborn heart murmurs as pathological until proven otherwise, even when the murmur sounds vibratory. In newborns, murmurs may occur from physiological transitions like a closing PDA. Persistent pulmonary hypertension of the newborn or myocardial depression from perinatal asphyxia may produce transitory audible tricuspid valve or mitral valve regurgitations. However, most newborn pathological murmurs arise from the same defects found in older infants and children including VSDs, ASDs PS, AS, CoA, or a pathological PDA. In patients with normal oxygen saturation, most pathological murmurs are from the conditions listed in the table on the bottom of the facing page. For descriptions and illustrations of cardiovascular malformations that we describe throughout this and other chapters, see Chapter 19.

There may be no correlation between a pathological murmur's loudness and the severity of a cardiac abnormality, especially in newborns. The short systolic or holosystolic murmurs from small VSDs may be loud at birth, but a moderate to large VSD may produce no murmur until days or weeks later. Nevertheless, a moderate to large VSD does produce a hyperdynamic precordium.

The murmur findings in small VSDs occur because the pressure in the left ventricle is significantly higher than the right ventricle, even shortly after birth. This pressure difference produces a high velocity systolic jet across the ventricular septum from the left ventricle to the right

1 Heart Murmurs

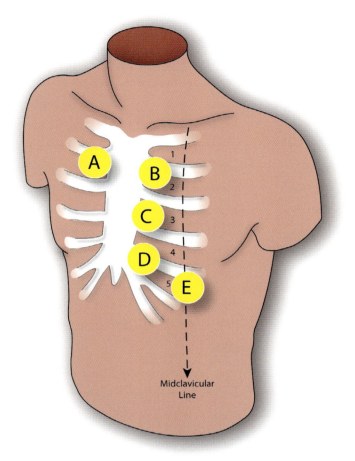

Systolic Murmurs

A
Aortic stenosis
Pulmonic stenosis

B
ASD
Pulmonic stenosis
PDA
Coarctation of aorta
Outlet VSD
Still's

C
Still's
VSD
Aortic stenosis

D
VSD
Tricuspid regurgitation
Still's

E
VSD
Mitral regurgitation
Still's

Congenital Heart Disease Pathological Murmur Ranking

Rank	Condition	Occurrence
1	VSD	± 40%
2	ASD	± 15%
3	PS	± 10%
4	AS	± 5%
5	CoA	± 5%
6	PDA	± 5%

ventricle. However, if a VSD is moderate to large, then ventricular pressures are nearly equal at birth.

In newborns with moderate to large VSDs, right ventricular pressure decreases more slowly because of a delay in the normal fall in pulmonary arterial pressure and vascular resistance. Eventually, the left ventricular pressure usually exceeds the right ventricular pressure, especially with a moderate-sized VSD. The pressure difference between the left and right ventricle causes turbulent flow across the VSD, resulting in an audible systolic heart murmur. This is the physiological reason for minimal murmur findings in a moderate to large VSD at birth but an audible murmur a few weeks later. Keep this in mind when explaining to parents why a murmur was absent at birth but present at the 4-week exam. For more on the changes in cardiovascular physiology with birth, see Chapter 18. Contrary to VSDs, however, the severity of PS and AS usually equates to the murmur's loudness—louder usually equals worse.

Regardless of age, in oxygen-desaturated patients with heart disease, a loud systolic ejection murmur is frequently from PS as in tetralogy of Fallot (ToF), critical valvular PS, or PS with 1-functional ventricles. Rather than single ventricle or univentricle, we use the term "1-functional ventricle"; see Chapter 19 for more information.

Many cyanotic cardiovascular malformations, however, generate no murmurs or soft nonspecific murmurs. Yet the same defects often produce hyperdynamic precordiums. One detects a hyperdynamic precordium through palpation not auscultation. Conditions with hyperdynamic precordiums and minimal murmur findings include transposition of the great arteries (TGA), total anomalous pulmonary venous return (TAPVR), pulmonary atresia, truncus arteriosus without truncal valve stenosis, or tricuspid atresia without a restrictive VSD or PS.

All pathological murmurs need pediatric cardiology evaluation. A disservice may result if a noncardiologist diagnoses a "small VSD" without a confirmatory Echo, as the murmur may actually originate from another condition. Further, an Echo-determined location of a small VSD, not discernible by auscultation alone, may have significant, long-term effects. A small VSD in the muscular septum often closes. However, even a small VSD in the outlet septum may develop aortic regurgitation, and the onset of an early diastolic murmur of AR may portend a poor clinical outcome. For more on Echo, see Chapter 22.

Other heart sounds

- Rubs

Friction rubs occur with pericarditis and pericardial effusions. However, a friction rub is often absent in moderate to large pericardial effusions.

- Extra heart sounds

"Gallop sounds" (S_3 or S_4 gallops) may be audible. Recognizing an extra sound is more valuable than distinguishing whether a gallop is an S_3 or S_4 sound, which is difficult even for expert auscultators.

- Clicks

On occasion, auscultation may also reveal a systolic "click sound." An early systolic ejection click (EC) most commonly occurs with a bicuspid aortic valve without stenosis, as figure A of the facing page shows. An early systolic ejection click may also accompany valvular pulmonic stenosis or aortic valve stenosis. As figure B shows, a midsystolic click (MC) may be audible in mitral valve prolapse. Nevertheless, even the best auscultators cannot always appreciate clicks.

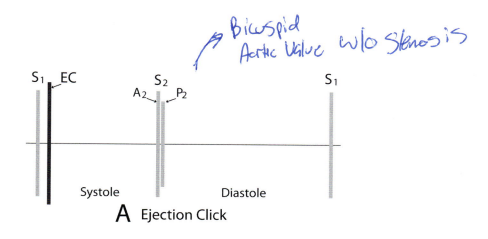

A Ejection Click — Bicuspid Aortic Valve w/o Stenosis

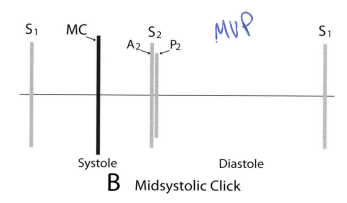

B Midsystolic Click — MVP

CARDIAC EVALUATION FOR SPECIAL CIRCUMSTANCES

Clearance for ADD Drugs

Many clinicians share in treating children with neuropsychiatric disorders. Attention deficit disorder (ADD) is the most common. Pharmacological treatment of ADD may require several medications that have direct and indirect adrenergic effects on the cardiovascular system.

For a well child without a heart murmur, with both negative past medical and family histories, controversy exists over the need for an EKG or pediatric cardiology evaluation before starting medications for ADD. However, children should probably have an EKG and pediatric cardiology evaluation when they have known heart disease, an undiagnosed heart murmur, or a concerning medical history. See Appendix B for a medical and family history screening form, which is also suitable for aiding sports clearance. [7]

Clearance for Sports

Sudden cardiac death occasionally occurs in young athletes. The most frequent causes of sudden cardiac death include unrecognized structural and electrical cardiac problems including cardiomyopathies, coronary artery abnormalities, long QT syndrome, or preexcitation. For more on sudden cardiac death or aborted sudden cardiac death, see Chapter 9.

Possibly, any post grade-school youth who wishes to engage in intensely competitive sports should have an EKG. Nevertheless, an EKG does not rule out all potential causes of sudden cardiac death. Primary care clinicians should consider pediatric cardiology evaluation for a heart murmur before granting competitive sports clearance clearance. [8-10]

Other Issues

For certain issues, pediatric cardiologists, if available, should offer support for primary care colleagues. As pediatric cardiologists, rather than primary care providers, should be the ones to take responsibility for clearing patients with undiagnosed heart murmurs or known heart disease for competitive sports or other exercise activities. Because recommendations may require information from EKG, Echo, Holter monitoring, exercise testing, MRI, CT, electrophysiology procedures, or cardiac catheterization. Similar to sports or other exercise clearance, pediatric cardiologists should also assume responsibility for providing information on insurability for life insurance or disability insurance. Further, pediatric cardiologists should advise noncardiologists on which conditions require endocarditis prophylaxis and for which procedures.

CLINICAL VIGNETTES

1. A 15-year old male presents for sport clearance. On exam, he has normal growth parameters and normal vital signs. His pulses are equal in the upper and lower extremities. He has a quiet precordium. He has a thrill in the suprasternal notch and a grade IV systolic ejection murmur best heard at the right upper sternal border associated with an ejection click. His most likely diagnosis:

a. Tetralogy of Fallot
b. Atrial septal defect
c. Valvular aortic stenosis
d. Valvular pulmonic stenosis

2. A 6-week old female infant presents with poor oral intake. The mother reports normal birth weight and no pre- or postnatal problems, but she notes the child has been breathing fast. On exam, her respiratory rate is > 60 per minute, her weight is below the 5th percentile, and her height is at the 50th percentile. Her pulses are equal throughout, and her liver is palpable 1 cm below the right costal margin. Her precordium is hyperdynamic, and she has a grade III low-frequency holosystolic murmur best heard at the lower left sternal border. Her most likely diagnosis:

a. Valvular pulmonic stenosis
b. Valvular aortic stenosis
c. Large atrial septal defect
d. Moderate-sized ventricular septal defect

1 Heart Murmurs

REFERENCES

1 Laennec RTH. De l'Auscultation Médiate ou Traité du Diagnostic des Maladies des Poumons et du Coeur. Paris, Brosson & Chaudé, 1819

2 Mahnke CB, Nowalk A, Hofkosh D, Zuberbuhler JR, Law YM. Comparison of two educational interventions on pediatrics resident auscultation skills. Pediatrics 2004; 113: 1331-1335

3 Dhuper S, Vashist S, Shah N, Sokal M. Improvement of cardiac auscultation skills in pediatric residents with training. Clin Pediatr 2007; 46: 236-240

4 Mangione S, Nieman LZ. Cardiac auscultatory skills of internal medicine and family practice trainees. A comparison of diagnostic proficiency. JAMA 1997; 278: 717-722

5 Gaskin PRA, Owens SE, Talner NS, Sanders SP, Li JS. Clinical auscultation skills in pediatric residents. Pediatrics 2000; 105: 1184-1187

6 Still GF. Common Disorders and Diseases of Childhood. London, Henry Frowde, 1909

7 Vetter VL, Elia J, Erickson C, Berger S, Blum N, Uzark K, Webb CL. A scientific statement from the American Heart Association Council on Cardiovascular Disease in the Young Congenital Cardiac Defects Committee and the Council on Cardiovascular Nursing. Circulation 2008; 117: 2407-2423

8 Wyman RA, Chiu RY, Rahko PS. The 5-minute screening echocardiogram for athletes. J Am Soc Echocardiogr 2008; 21: 786-788

9 McLeod CJ, Ackerman MJ, Nishimura RA, Tajik AJ, Gersh BJ, Ommen SR. Outcome of patients with hypertrophic cardiomyopathy and a normal electrocardiogram. J Am Coll Cardiol 2009; 54: 229-233

10 Corrado D, Migliore F, Bevilacqua M, Basso C, Thiene G. Sudden cardiac death in athletes: can it be prevented by screening? Herz 2009; 34: 259-266

2 Failure-to-Thrive

Contents

Background	17
Classification	18
Evaluation	19
Cardiovascular Problems	21
Clinical Vignettes	22

2 Failure-to-Thrive

william evans

BACKGROUND

Children's healthcare includes monitoring growth. During each office visit, plot a child's height and weight on standard growth charts developed by the National Center for Health Statistics. Current charts derive from data compiled by the National Health and Nutrition Examination Survey III (NHANES III). Growth charts are available from the Centers for Disease Control and Prevention's website. Plot growth parameters for Down syndrome patients on a Down syndrome growth chart, which are available online. Chapter references include growth-chart websites for both Down syndrome and non-Down syndrome children.

The term "failure-to-thrive" (FTT) usually means suboptimal weight gain in infants and young children. Definitions for FTT vary and include a weight < the 5th or even the 3rd percentile, weights falling 2 standard deviations on a growth curve over time, or a weight < 80% of ideal.

With significant cardiovascular malformations, inadequate weight gain often occurs with less effect on height. Nonetheless, most dysmorphic syndromes have abnormal height and weight curves, whether a cardiovascular malformation is present or not. On occasion, a clinician struggles to determine whether growth failure arises from congenital heart disease, a syndrome, or from both. [1-6]

FTT CLASSIFICATION

We divide factors contributing to poor growth into those mainly extrinsic (some call nonorganic) and to those mainly intrinsic (some call organic). We stress the cardiac causes of failure-to-thrive.

Extrinsic

- **Caregiver inexperience**

Poor parenting skills, primarily from lack of knowledge, may underlie FTT.

- **Caregiver intent**

Consider child neglect; unfortunately, neglect may cause FTT.

- **Caregiver impairments**

Impairments can include psychological conditions, problems with maternal milk production in breast-fed babies, socioeconomical factors, and others.

Intrinsic

General conditions

- Cardiovascular malformations
- Gastrointestinal disease
- Lung disease & cor pulmonale
- Renal disease
- Malignancy

Specific noncardiac problems

- **Cystic fibrosis**

Patients have pulmonary and gastrointestinal problems.

- **Dysmorphic syndromes**

See Chapter 3.

- **Endocrine, metabolic, renal problems**

Type-1 diabetes, thyroid disorders, inborn errors of metabolism, and renal tubular acidosis.

- **Gastrointestinal problems**

Gastroesophageal reflux, milk allergies, celiac disease, esophageal compression (including vascular rings), oral defects, other gastrointestinal malformations.

- **Neuromuscular disorders**

Hypotonia, poor suck, and poor appetite.

- **Prematurity or small for gestational age (SGA)**

Early on, SGA infants may have FTT; later, however, SGA infants have a tendency to develop obesity.

FTT EVALUATION

Failure-to-thrive is a complex problem, which may require an inpatient, multidisciplinary workup.

History
- Feeding difficulties
- Calorie count
- Past medical history
- Review of systems
- Social history
- Caregiver issues

Exam
- Growth curves with weight below height common in congestive heart failure (figure below left)
- Growth curves with impaired weight & height common with syndromes or metabolic disorders (figure below)

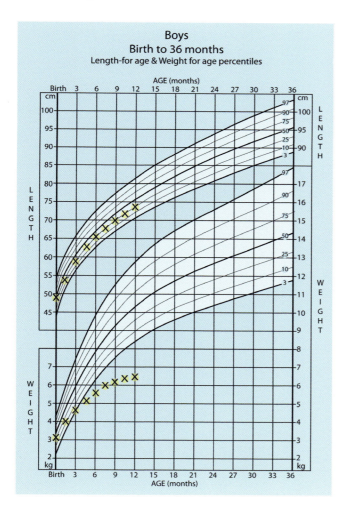

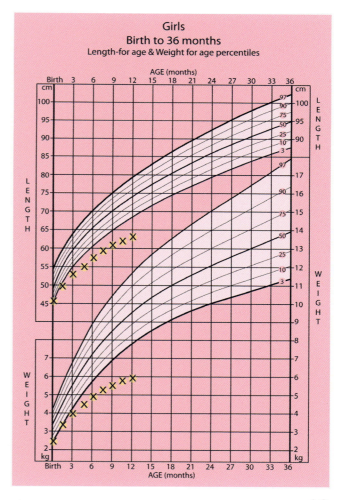

2 Failure-to-Thrive

- Vital signs & oxygen saturation
- Signs of neglect
- Dysmorphic features
- Signs of anemia
- Signs of lung disease
- Murmurs
- Pulses
- Signs of congestive heart failure (CHF)
- Edema suggesting low serum protein or CHF

Noncardiac Testing
- CBC
- Urine analysis
- Chest X-ray
- Blood urea nitrogen (BUN) & creatinine
- Total protein & albumin
- Liver function tests
- Erythrocyte sedimentation rate (ESR)
- C-reactive protein (CRP)
- Thyroid studies
- Stool testing
- Sweat chloride

CARDIOVASCULAR PROBLEMS

Although growth failure may occur with cyanotic heart disease, newborn cyanosis usually leads to early diagnosis and palliative or corrective surgery. Thus, FTT from cardiovascular malformations exists more often in those with CHF than in those with cyanosis. For more on chronic CHF, see Chapter 5.

Congestive heart failure augments the work of breathing and elevates catecholamines that increase caloric expenditure and impair weight gain. Also, CHF-related tachypnea makes eating difficult, compounding the reduction in caloric intake. Cardiovascular problems may accompany dysmorphic syndromes, further complicating inadequate or failing growth.

Conditions

• **Moderate to large VSD or PDA**

Any patient with a moderate to large ventricular septal defect (VSD) or patent ductus arteriosus (PDA) may present with FTT. Those with Down syndrome, chromosome 22q11 deletion, or other syndromes usually have the most significant FTT.

• **Large ASD**

May occasionally cause FTT, especially with a syndrome.

• **Dilated cardiomyopathies**

Ventricular dysfunction, especially with mitral valve regurgitation or pulmonary hypertension, may cause FTT.

• **Cor pulmonale**

History of prematurity and chronic mechanical ventilation suggests chronic lung disease or bronchopulmonary dysplasia (BPD). BPD may cause pulmonary hypertension heart failure, and FTT.

Workup & ℞ Options

Tests

- Electrocardiogram
- Echocardiogram
- B-natriuretic peptide
- Cardiac catheterization
- MRI or CT

℞ options

Following definitive treatment, weight usually normalizes quickly. However, in some patients, no definitive treatment is possible; such patients need chronic medical therapy.

• **Temporizing**

Patients may need anticongestive medications, high caloric formulas, and sometimes gastrostomy tube feedings to improve growth before definitive treatment. In some patients with VSDs, temporizing treatment may be appropriate as some VSDs close spontaneously, eliminating the need for surgery.

• **Definitive**

For more on catheter interventional and surgical procedures, see Chapters 25 and 27.

CLINICAL VIGNETTES

3. A 2-year old male presents with chronically loose stools and recurrent respiratory infections. On exam, his weight is below the 5th percentile and his height is at the 10th percentile. He is thin, pale, and in no distress. His heart rate 100 bpm, and his pulses are normal throughout. He has a normally active precordium with grade I to II systolic ejection murmur heard best at the base of the heart. His CBC shows a hemoglobin of 8 mg/dL and hematocrit of 26%. Before more testing, his most likely diagnosis:

a. An innocent murmur with an upper respiratory infection
b. Cystic fibrosis with an innocent murmur from anemia
c. Valvular pulmonic stenosis
d. A victim of child abuse

4. A 3-month old female infant presents with poor weight gain. On exam, she has physical stigmata of Down syndrome (see Chapter 3). Her weight is well below the 5th percentile and her height is at the 10th percentile. Her respiratory rate is > 50 per minute, but she appears in no significant distress. Her pulses are equal, and her liver is just palpable at the right costal margin. Her precordium is hyperdynamic, the second heart sound is loud, and there is a low frequency grade II holosystolic murmur. Before additional testing, her most likely diagnosis:

a. A large VSD
b. Tetralogy of Fallot
c. Renal tubular acidosis
d. A small ASD

REFERENCES

1 Zenel JA Jr. Failure to thrive: a general pediatrician's perspective. Pediatr Rev 1997; 18: 371-378

2 El-Baba AF, Bassali RW, Benjamin J, Mehta R. Failure to thrive. http://emedicine.medscape.com/article/985007-overview

3 Block RW, Krebs NF. Failure to thrive as a manifestation of child neglect. Pediatrics 2005; 116: 1234-1237

4 Growth charts. www.cdc.gov/growthcharts/clinical_charts.htm

5 Down syndrome growth charts. http://www.growthcharts.com/charts/DS/charts.htm

6 Cronk C, Crocker AC, Pueschel SM, Shea AM, Zackai E, Pickens G, Reed RB. Growth charts for children with Down syndrome: 1 Month to 18 Years of Age. Pediatrics 1988; 81: 102-110

2 Failure-to-Thrive

3 Dysmorphic features

Contents

Background	27	Tuberous Sclerosis	37
Trisomy 21	28	CHARGE	38
Trisomy 18	29	Williams & SVAS	39
Trisomy 13	30	Holt-Oram	40
Fetal Alcohol	31	TAR	41
Noonan	32	Alagille	42
Turner	33	Clinical Vignettes	43
Chromosome 22q11 Deletion	34		
VACTERL	35		
Marfan	36		

3 Dysmorphic Features

william evans

BACKGROUND

In pediatrics, it is relatively common for infants and children to present with dysmorphic features. Frequently, dysmorphic syndromes have associated cardiovascular malformations. Nonetheless, this section is not an exhaustive review of dysmorphic syndromes with cardiovascular defects. We selected conditions with recognizable physical features the reader may encounter more often than myriad rarer conditions. We begin with the chromosomal trisomies (21, 18, and 13) in decreasing order of occurrence. Then, in approximate decreasing order of occurrence, we continue with the following syndromes: Fetal alcohol, Noonan, Turner, Chromosome 22q11 deletion, VACTERL association, Marfan, Tuberous sclerosis, CHARGE, Williams and autosomal dominant supravalvular aortic stenosis, the limb-heart conditions of Holt-Oram and Thrombocytopenia absent radius (TAR), and Alagille.

For each syndrome, we briefly discuss genetic cause if known, incidence, typical noncardiovascular clinical features, and common associated cardiovascular malformations. Whenever possible, we include a patient photograph with the syndrome's description. Ideally, specialists in genetics should direct testing, interpret results, and provide patients and families with the proper post-testing counseling. Syndromes result via abnormal development most often from chromosomal anomalies including trisomies, chromosomal deletions, other gene defects, or multifactorial intrauterine environmental factors including alcohol, infections, or other toxins.

Chromosomal trisomies are among the most common causes of syndromes associated with heart disease. Chromosomal trisomies result from nondisjunction. Disjunction is the normal separation of chromosomes during cell division. During germ cell meiosis, each normal egg or sperm has 1 set of the normal paired chromosomes, so upon fertilization the zygote has a normal, complete set of paired chromosomes. With advanced maternal age, nondisjunction during maternal germ cell meiosis may result in eggs having 2 sets of chromosomes 13, 18, or 21 and eggs without a chromosome 13, 18, or 21. When a typical sperm with 1 chromosome 13, 18, or 21 fertilizes an egg with a pair of 13, 18, or 21 chromosomes, the resulting zygote has 3 (trisomy) chromosomes. Monosomy zygotes are not viable.

See Chapter 19 for more on heart defects that we list in this chapter. Fetal echocardiography can define almost all significant cardiovascular defects. For more on fetal echocardiography, see Chapter 23. [1-4]

TRISOMY 21 • DOWN SYNDROME

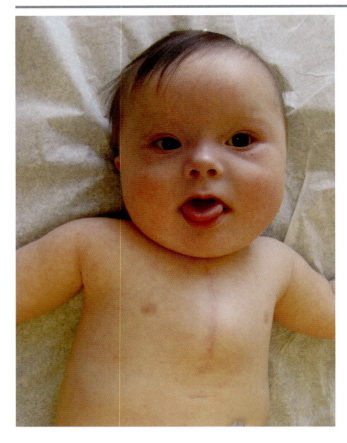

Down syndrome occurs in about 1:800 live births. The risk increases with advancing maternal age, up to 4:1,000 at 35 years and 100:1,000 at 49 years.

Noncardiovascular Features

Neurodevelopmental
- Developmental delay
- Hypotonia, poor feeding
- Seizures

Head & face
- Flat occiput, small chin, & flat nasal bridge
- Small ears & hearing difficulties
- Oblique eye fissures & epicanthal folds
- White spots on iris or Brushfield spots
- Macroglossia
- Short neck

Extremities & skeletal
- A single palmar fold
- Single flexion furrow of the 5th finger
- Additional ulnar loop dermatoglyphs
- Patellar & hip dislocation
- Excessive space between large toe & 2nd toe
- Increased sternal ossification centers
- Atlantoaxial instability

Others
- Leukemia
- Hypothyroidism
- Duodenal atresia
- Cutis marmorata (skin mottling, especially reddish)
- Obesity

Cardiovascular Defects

About 50% of patients have defects.
- Ventricular septal defect (VSD)
- Atrioventricular septal defects (AVSD)
- Patent ductus arteriosus (PDA)
- Atrial septal defect (ASD)
- Tetralogy of Fallot (ToF)
- Rarely coarctation of the aorta (CoA)
- Rarely transposition of the great arteries (TGA)
- Rarely 1-functional ventricles

TRISOMY 18 • EDWARDS SYNDROME

Edwards syndrome or trisomy 18 occurs in about 1:3,000 live births, and the incidence increases with advancing maternal age.

Noncardiovascular Features

Neurodevelopmental

- Severe delay

Head & face

- Microcephaly & prominent occiput
- Narrow palpebral fissures
- Ocular hypertelorism & ptosis
- Upturned nose
- Low-set malformed ears
- Micrognathia, plus cleft lip & palate

Extremities & skeletal

- Clenched hands
- Underdeveloped thumbs & or nails
- Absent radius
- Webbing of 2nd & 3rd toes
- Arthrogryposis (multiple joint contractures)
- Clubfoot or rocker-bottom feet
- Short sternum

Others

- Renal malformations
- Omphalocele
- Undescended testicles
- Choroid plexus cysts

Cardiovascular Defects

More than 90% of patients have defects.

- VSD, ASD, PDA, CoA, & ToF
- Hypoplastic left heart syndrome (HLHS)
- Dextrocardia
- Poly valvular disease

TRISOMY 13 • PATAU SYNDROME

Patau syndrome or Trisomy 13 occurs in about 1:5,000 live births, and the incidence increases with advancing maternal age.

Noncardiovascular Features

Neurodevelopment
- Severe delay

Head & face
- Microcephaly
- Holoprosencephaly & cyclops deformity
- Low-set ears
- Micropthalmia
- Coloboma & cataracts
- Retinal detachment & nystagmus
- Optic nerve hypoplasia & cortical blindness
- Cleft palate

Extremities & skeletal
- Polydactyly
- Overlapping of fingers & thumb
- Rocker-bottom feet

Others
- Areas of aplasia cutis (absence of skin)
- Meningomyelocele
- Omphalocele
- Abnormal genitalia
- Renal abnormalities

Cardiovascular Defects

About 80% of patients have defects.
- VSD, ASD, PDA, ToF, & HLHS
- Double outlet right ventricle (DORV)
- Dextrocardia

FETAL ALCOHOL SYNDROME

David Smith and Kenneth Lyons Jones, at the University of Washington, first described the fetal alcohol syndrome in 1973. Fetal alcohol syndrome (FAS) is a preventable condition. However, in the United States, FAS occurs in about 1:700 live births. No specific genetic test exists, as the condition results from the teratogenic effects of alcohol on the developing embryo. [5]

Noncardiovascular Features
Neurodevelopmental
- Delayed
- Attention deficit disorder

Head & face
- Microcephaly
- Strabismus
- Short palpebral fissures
- Ptosis & epicanthal folds
- Flat midface, upturned nose, & flat nasal bridge
- Underdeveloped ears
- Thin upper lip

Extremities & skeletal
- Hypoplastic toenails
- Clinodactyly of 5th finger (curves towards 4th)
- Cervical vertebral anomalies

Other
- Hirsutism
- Growth retardation

Cardiovascular Defects
Around 30-50% of patients have defects.
- ASDs & VSDs most common

NOONAN SYNDROME

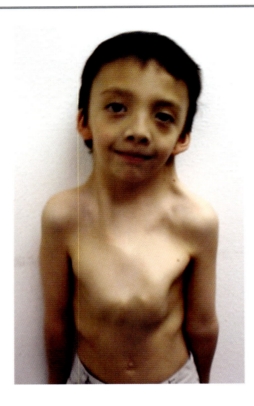

Noonan syndrome is autosomal dominant and occurs in about 1:2,000 live births. Noonan syndrome affects males and females equally. Noonan syndrome stems from mutations in the *PTPN11* (most common), *KRAS*, *RAF1*, and *SOS1* genes. *PTPN11* codes for tyrosine phosphatase, *KRAS* codes for proteins necessary for the propagation of growth factor, *RAF1* codes for proteins that regulate various cellular activities, and *SOS1* codes for proteins involved in pathways that control growth and development. The *PTPN11* and *KRAS* genes reside on chromosome 12, *RAF1* resides on chromosome 3, and *SOS1* resides on chromosome 2. Genetic testing is commercially available. [6]

Noncardiovascular Features

Neurodevelopment
- Mild developmental delay in 30-50% of patients

Head & face
- Macrocephaly
- Hypertelorism, ptosis, proptosis, & nystagmus
- Micrognathia & deeply grooved philtrum
- High arched palate
- Backward-rotated, low-set ears
- Short-webbed neck

Extremities & skeletal
- Short stature
- Scoliosis
- Pectus carinatum or excavatum
- Lymphedema

Others
- Cryptorchidism
- Bleeding disorders
- Hodgkin lymphoma

Cardiovascular Defects

About 50% of patients have defects.
- Dysplastic valvular pulmonic stenosis
- ASD
- Hypertrophic cardiomyopathy (HCM) in about 15-20% of patients
- 95% of Noonan syndrome patients with HCM have a specific type of *RAF1* gene mutation [7]

TURNER SYNDROME

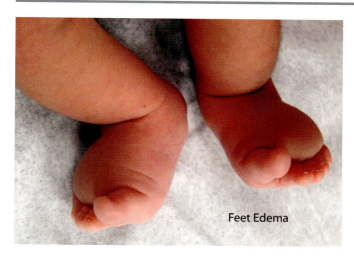
Feet Edema

Turner syndrome is the complete or partial absence of 1 X chromosome. Turner syndrome occurs in about 1:2,500 live female births. Most cases of Turner syndrome do not result from inheritance, as the X chromosome monosomy usually appears as a random event during meiosis of eggs or sperm. Most patients have primary ovarian failure; nonetheless, pregnancy is achievable with donor eggs and in vitro fertilization (IVF). Aortic dissection can occur during pregnancy; thus, obtain an echocardiogram before IVF and during pregnancy.

Noncardiovascular Features

Neurodevelopment
- Usually normal

Head & face
- Low-set ears & hearing impairment
- Visual impairments & glaucoma
- Webbed neck & low hairline

Extremities & skeletal
- Short stature
- Lymphedema of the hands & feet (figure on the left)
- Shortened 4th metacarpal
- Small fingernails
- Shield chest & widely-spaced nipples

Others
- Sterility, rudimentary ovaries, & amenorrhea
- Horseshoe kidney

Cardiovascular Defects

About 20-35% of patients have defects.
- Bicuspid aortic valve, CoA, AS, & HLHS
- Dilated aortic root with occasional dissection

CHROMOSOME 22q11 DELETION

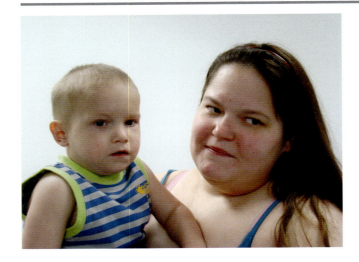

In 1981, Albert De la Chapelle and colleagues in Helsinki, Finland first noted an association between DiGeorge syndrome and a chromosome 22q11 deletion. Chromosome 22q11 deletion syndrome is autosomal dominant and occurs in about 1:4,000 live births, but the incidence may be higher. Because features vary widely, several eponyms remain in use such as DiGeorge syndrome and velocardialfacial or Shprintzen syndrome. The photo above shows a mother and son both with chromosome 22q11 deletion and both with tetralogy of Fallot. Fluorescent in situ hybridization (FISH) can confirm the diagnosis. [8]

Head & face
- Microcephaly & small chin
- Small mouth & asymmetric crying facies
- Hypernasal speech
- Cleft palate
- Hooded eyelids
- Small ears & hearing loss

Extremities & skeletal
- Short stature

Others
- Renal abnormalities
- Hypocalcemia
- Thrombocytopenia
- Immune deficiency
- Autoimmune disorders

Cardiovascular Defects
About 50-75% of patients have defects.
- VSD, ToF, DORV, truncus arteriosus & interrupted aortic arch
- Vascular rings

Noncardiovascular Features
Neurodevelopment
- IQ range 70 to 90
- Learning disabilities
- Attention deficit disorders
- Schizophrenia, bipolar

VACTERL ASSOCIATION

Linda Quan and David Smith, at the University of Washington, first described the association in 1973. VACTERL occurs in about 1:4,000 live births. In 2009, Charles Shaw-Smith of Cambridge, England suggested the VACTERL association may be from microdeletions of the *FOX* gene cluster on chromosome 16q24.1. The principal phenotypical findings are esophageal atresia (usually found at birth when trying to pass nasogastric tube) and anal atresia. The limb abnormalities consisting of radial aplasia or thumb anomalies are inconsistent. No typical facial features exist. However, about 35% of patients have a single umbilical artery. The presence of a single umbilical artery should prompt further evaluation. Genetic testing is not currently commercially available. [9, 10]

Noncardiovascular Features

Neurodevelopment
- Usually normal

VACTERL acronym (diagnosis 3 of 7)
- **V**ertebral anomalies
- **A**nal atresia
- **C**ardiac malformations
- **T**racheoesophageal fistula
- **E**sophageal atresia
- **R**enal malformations
- **L**imb anomalies

Cardiovascular Defects

About 50-75% of patients have malformations.

- VSD, ASD, ToF, & DORV
- Right aortic arch & vascular rings
- Dextrocardia
- Single umbilical artery

MARFAN SYNDROME

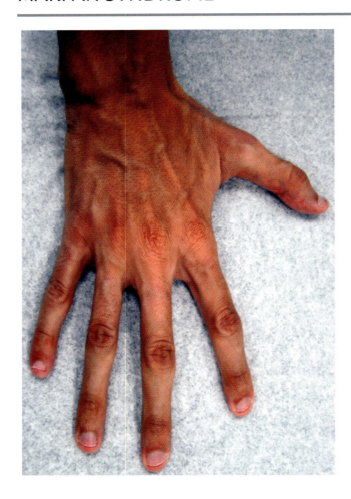

Marfan syndrome is autosomal dominant and occurs in about 1:5,000 live births. Around 60% of patients have a positive family history. Marfan syndrome results from an error in the *FBN1* gene, which codes for the fibrillin protein. As researchers have yet to identify common gene mutations, genetic testing includes screening the entire *FBN1* gene. However, DNA testing cannot rule out Marfan syndrome. The *FBN1* gene resides on chromosome 15q21.1 [11, 12]

Noncardiovascular Features

Neurodevelopmental
- Normal

Head & face
- High arched palate
- Lenticular dislocation

Extremities & skeletal
- Tall
- Wingspan is greater then the height
- Arachnodactyly (figure on left)
- Loose ligaments & increased flexibility
- Steinberg thumb & Walker-Murdoch wrist signs
- Pectus excavatum, pectus carinatum, & scoliosis
- Flat arch

Others
- Spontaneous pneumothorax
- Striae distensae (stretch marks)
- Inguinal hernia
- Lumbosacral meningocele

Cardiovascular Defects

More than 90% of patients have defects.
- Mitral valve prolapse & mitral regurgitation
- Aortic root dilatation, aortic regurgitation, & possible aortic root dissection
- Occasionally pulmonary artery dilation

TUBEROUS SCLEROSIS

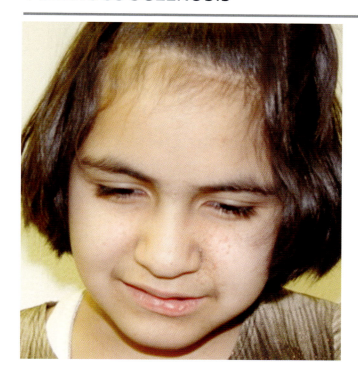

Physicians in the 19th century, or possibly before, had described Tuberous sclerosis (TS). TS is autosomal dominant and occurs in about 1:6,000 live births. Tuberous sclerosis results from mutations in the *TSC1* or *TSC2* genes that code for the tumor-suppressor proteins hamartin and tuberin. The *TSC1* and *TSC2* genes reside on chromosome 9q34. Genetic testing is commercially available. [13, 14]

Noncardiovascular Features

Neurodevelopmental
- Severe delay
- Seizures
- Aggression

Head & face
- Facial adenoma sebaceum (as photo on left demonstrates)
- Tuft of white hair on the scalp or eyelids
- Colobomas & retinal lesions
- Astrocytic hamartomas or phakomas

Skin
- Ash leaf spots, but may need UV light to be visible
- Patchy areas of thick, leathery skin, dimpled like an orange peel
- Molluscum fibrosum or skin tags
- Café au lait spots
- Ungual fibromas

Others
- Brain tumors
- Renal cysts & angiomyolipomas
- Lung cysts

Cardiovascular Defects
- Rhabdomyomas in 50% of patients
- Rhabdomyomas usually regress

CHARGE SYNDROME

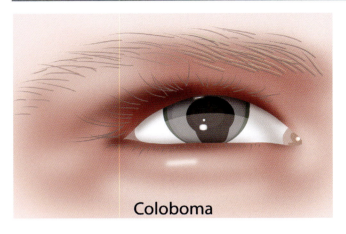
Coloboma

In 1981, Roberta Pagon and colleagues, at the University of Washington, first described the CHARGE association, later classified as a syndrome. CHARGE syndrome mainly results from new mutations; nonetheless, CHARGE can also occasionally be autosomal dominant. CHARGE occurs in about 1:9,000 live births. Patients have mutations in the *CHD7* gene, which is on chromosome 8q12. The *CHD7* gene codes for chromodomain helicase DNA binding protein 7. The CHD7 protein belongs to a family of proteins thought to play a role in chromatin organization. Genetic testing is currently commercially available. [15, 16]

Noncardiovascular Features
Neurodevelopment
- Severe delay

CHARGE acronym (diagnosis 4 of 6)
- **C**oloboma (eye defect as in the figure above)
- **H**eart defect
- **A**tretic choanae
- **R**etarded growth
- **G**enitourinary anomalies
- **E**ar malformations

Cardiovascular Defects
About 60-70% of patients have defects.
- ASD, VSD, & ToF

WILLIAMS SYNDROME & SVAS

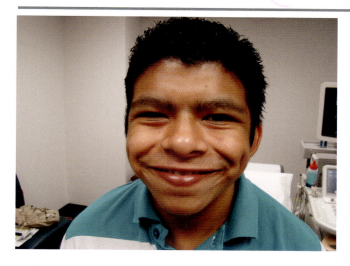

Williams syndrome occurs in about 1:15,000 live births and arises from a deletion of chromosome 7q11.23, which includes the elastin gene. Williams syndrome is autosomal dominant. FISH can confirm Williams syndrome.

Autosomal dominant supravalvular aortic stenosis (SVAS) does not occur with all the classic physical features of Williams syndrome. Amanda Ewart and colleagues, at the University of Utah, and Colleen Morris, at the University of Nevada, described the genetic findings of autosomal dominant SVAS, resulting from a mutation of elastin at 7q11.23. The cardiovascular defects are similar to those found in Williams syndrome. [17]

Noncardiovascular Features

Neurodevelopment
- Development delay
- A "cocktail party" personality
- Lack common sense
- Hyperacusis & phonophobia
- Love of music & may have perfect pitch

Head & face
- Elfin facies
- Widely spaced teeth
- Long philtrum
- Flattened nose

Others
- Hypercalcemia
- Hypothyroidism
- Type I diabetes

Cardiovascular Defects

About 60-80% of patients have defects.
- Supravalvular aortic stenosis AS
- Supravalvular pulmonic stenosis (PS)
- Branch pulmonary artery stenosis
- Coronary artery ostial stenosis
- Aortic arch obstructions
- Renal artery stenosis & systemic hypertension

HOLT-ORAM SYNDROME

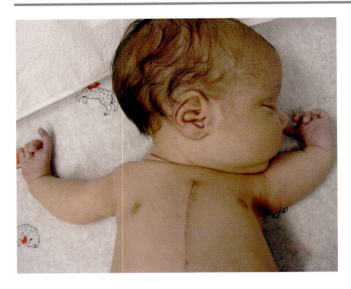

Cardiovascular Defects

About 50-75% of patients have defects.

- ASD & VSD
- Arrhythmias with or without structural defects

Holt-Oram syndrome is autosomal dominant and occurs in about 1:100,000 live births. Researchers have connected Holt-Oram to mutations of the *TBX5* gene, which resides on chromosome 12q24.1. The *TBX5* gene plays a role in heart development, the cardiac conduction system, and the upper limbs. Genetic testing is currently commercially available. [18] The photo above shows a infant after heart surgery with a diminutive left forearm.

Noncardiovascular features

Neurodevelopmental

- Normal

Extremities & skeletal

- Absent or underdeveloped thumbs
- Syndactyly
- Absent radius
- Ulnar defects
- Humerus & shoulder defects

TAR SYNDROME

In 1969, Judith Hall and colleagues at Johns Hopkins first described the Thrombocytopenia-absent radius (TAR) syndrome. TAR appears autosomal recessive and occurs in about 1:100,000 live births. Deletions of chromosome 1q21 may be causative of TAR syndrome, but other yet unknown genetic abnormalities are likely. Genetic testing is not currently commercially available. [19, 20]

Noncardiovascular Features

Neurodevelopment
- Normal

Head & face
- Facial capillary hemangiomata
- Sensorineural hearing loss

Extremities & skeletal
- Bilateral radial aplasia
- Lower limb anomalies
- Scoliosis

Hematological
- Thrombocytopenia

Others
- Cow's milk intolerance
- Renal anomalies
- Intracranial vascular malformation

Cardiovascular Defects

Some 15-35% of patients have defects.
- ASD, VSD, & ToF

ALAGILLE SYNDROME

Alagille syndrome is autosomal dominant and occurs in about 1:100,000 live births. Studies report mutations in *JAG1* or *NOTCH2* genes. The *JAG1* gene resides on chromosome 20p12, and the *NOTCH2* gene resides on chromosome 1p13-p11. These genes make proteins that are critical to fetal development. Genetic testing for *JAG1* and *NOTCH2* mutations is commercially available. [21, 22]

Noncardiovascular Features

Neurodevelopment
- Delayed

Head & face
- Broadened forehead & pointed chin
- Elongated nose with bulbous tip
- Corneal Axenfeld anomaly
- Retinitis pigmentosa & pupillary abnormalities
- Optic disc anomalies

Extremities & skeletal
- Butterfly hemivertebrae
- Rib anomalies
- Shortening of the radius, ulna, & phalanges

Hepatic
- Cholestatic jaundice
- Hepatosplenomegaly

Others
- Renal artery stenosis
- Lipoid nephrosis
- Glomerulosclerosis
- Xanthomas from hypercholesterolemia

Cardiovascular Defects

More than 75% have defects.
- Peripheral pulmonary artery stenosis
- ASD, VSD, PDA, CoA, & ToF
- Preexcitation (WPW)
- Arterial aneurysms of the CNS & aorta
- Moyamoya disease

CLINICAL VIGNETTES

5. You exam a newborn and find that he has abnormal facies that include hooded eyes, a small mouth, small chin, small ears, microcephaly, and cleft palate. A pediatric cardiologist tells you that the patient also has truncus arteriosus. You should order the following test:

a. Standard chromosomes to rule out trisomy 21
b. Standard chromosomes to check for XO, indicating Turner syndrome
c. Chromosomes with fluorescent in situ hybridization (FISH) to check for a chromosome 22q11 deletion
d. Standard chromosomes to rule out trisomy 18

6. The staff calls you to the newborn nursery to evaluate a baby with a heart murmur. You note the patient has anal atresia, and you are unable to pass a nasogastric tube. You also note the infant has a single umbilical artery. Before the cardiology or genetic consultants arrive, you suspect the patient has:

a. Down syndrome
b. VACTERL association
c. CHARGE syndrome
d. Marfan syndrome

3 Dysmorphic Features

REFERENCES

1 Jones KL. Smith's Recognizable Patterns of Human Malformations. Philadelphia, Elsevier Saunders, 2006

2 Marino BS, Bird GL, Wernovsky G. Diagnosis and management of the newborn with suspected congenital heart disease. Clinics in Perinatology 2001; 28: 91-136

3 Pierpont ME, Basson CT, Benson WD Jr, Gelb BD, Giglia TM, Goldmuntz E, McGee G, Sable CA, Srivastava D, Webb CL. Genetic basis for congenital heart defects: current knowledge. Circ 2007; 115: 3015-3038

4 McKusick VA. Mendelian Inheritance in Man: A Catalog of Human Genes and Genetic Disorders. Baltimore, Johns Hopkins University Press, 1998

5 Jones KL, Smith DW. Recognition of the fetal alcohol syndrome in early infancy. Lancet 1973; 302: 999-1001

6 Tartaglia M, Mehler EL, Goldberg R, Zampino G, Brunner HG, Kremer H, van der Burgt I, Crosby AH, Ion A, Jeffery S, Kalidas K, Patton MA, Kucherlapati RS, Gelb BD. Mutations in PTPN11, encoding the protein tyrosine phosphatase SHP-2, cause Noonan syndrome. Nat Genet 2001; 29: 465-468

7 Pandit B, Sarkozy A, Pennacchio LA, Carta C, Oishi K, Martinelli S, Pogna EA, Schackwitz W, Ustaszewska A, Landstrom A, Bos JM, Ommen SR, Esposito G, Lepri F, Faul C, Mundel P, López Siguero JP, Tenconi R, Selicorni A, Rossi C, Mazzanti L, Torrente I, Marino B, Digilio MC, Zampino G, Ackerman MJ, Dallapiccola B, Tartaglia M, Gelb BD. Gain-of-function RAF1 mutations cause Noonan and LEOPARD syndromes with hypertrophic cardiomyopathy. Nat Genet 2007; 39: 1007-1012

8 De la Chapelle A, Herva R, Koivisto M, Aula P. A deletion in chromosome 22 can cause DiGeorge syndrome. Hum Genet 1981; 57: 253-256

9 Quan L, Smith DW. The VATER association. Vertebral defects, anal atresia, T-E fistula with esophageal atresia, radial and renal dysplasia: a spectrum of associated defects. J Pediatr 1973; 82: 104-107

10 Shaw-Smith C. Genetic factors in esophageal atresia, tracheo-esophageal fistula and the VACTERL association: Roles for FOXF1 and the 16q24.1 FOX transcription factor gene cluster, and review of the literature. Eur J Med Genet 2010; 53: 6-13

11 Hayward C, Brock DJ. Fibrillin-1 mutations in Marfan syndrome and other type-1 fibrillinopathies. Hum Mutat. 1997; 10: 415-423

12 Dean JCS. Management of Marfan syndrome. Heart 2002; 88: 97-103

13 Timeline of Tuberous Sclerosis. http://en.wikipedia.org/wiki/Timeline_of_tuberous_sclerosis

14 Orlova KA, Crino PB. The tuberous sclerosis complex. Ann N Y Acad Sci 2010; 1184: 87-105

15 Pagon RA, Graham JM Jr, Zonana J, Yong SL. Coloboma, congenital heart disease, and choanal atresia with multiple anomalies: CHARGE association. J Pediatr 1981; 99: 223-237

16 Bajpai R, Chen DA, Rada-Iglesias A, Zhang J, Xiong Y, Helms J, Chang CP, Zhao Y, Swigut T, Wysocka J. CHD7 cooperates with PBAF to control multipotent neural crest formation. Nature 2010; 463: 958-962

17 Morris CA, Loker J, Ensing G, Stock AD. Supravalvular aortic stenosis cosegregates with a familial 6;7 translocation which disrupts the elastin gene. Am J Med Genet 1993; 46: 737-744

18 Fan C, Chen Q, Wang QK. Functional role of transcriptional factor TBX5 in pre-mRNA splicing and Holt-Oram syndrome via association with SC35. J Biol Chem 2009; 284: 25653-25663

19 Hall JG, Levin J, Kuhn JP, Ottenheimer EJ, van Berkum KA, McKusick VA. Thrombocytopenia with absent radius (TAR). Medicine (Baltimore) 1969; 48: 411-439

20 Klopocki E, Schulze H, Strauss G, Ott CE, Hall J, Trotier F, Fleischhauer S, Greenhalgh L, Newbury-Ecob RA, Neumann LM, Habenicht R, König R, Seemanova E, Megarbane A, Ropers HH, Ullmann R, Horn D, Mundlos S. Complex inheritance pattern resembling autosomal recessive inheritance involving a

microdeletion in thrombocytopenia-absent radius syndrome. Am J Hum Genet 2007; 80: 232-240

21 Li L, Krantz ID, Deng Y Genin A, Banta AB, Collins CC, Qi M, Trask BJ, Kuo WL, Cochran J, Costa T, Pierpont ME, Rand EB, Piccoli DA, Hood L, Spinner NB. Alagille syndrome is caused by mutations in human Jagged1, which encodes a ligand for Notch1. Nat Genet 1997; 16: 243-251

22 Lalani SR, Thakuria JV, Cox GF, Wang X, Bi W, Bray MS. 20p12.3 microdeletion predisposes to Wolff-Parkinson-White syndrome with variable neurocognitive deficits. J Med Genet 2009; 46: 168-175

3 Dysmorphic Features

4 Abnormal Heart Rates & Rhythms

Contents

Background	49
Diagnostic Devices	50
Fast Rates & Rhythms	52
Slow Rates & Rhythms	61
Irregular Rates & Rhythms	63
Clinical Vignettes	65

4 Abnormal Heart Rates & Rhythms

vincent thomas

BACKGROUND

A patient with an abnormal heart rate and rhythm can present in the outpatient clinic, emergency room, or hospital. Patient complaints may be vague and may include palpitations, chest pain, or syncope. Some patients have no complaints. However, patients may also present with symptoms and signs of congestive heart failure, myocarditis, or cardiovascular collapse. An accurate diagnosis may require 24-hour Holter monitoring, portable cardiac event monitors, exercise testing, a surgically implanted event monitor, or even an electrophysiology (EP) procedure. Testing and treatment depend on the clinical presentation. For infants and children, a pediatric cardiologist or pediatric electrophysiologist should direct arrhythmia management.

An EKG differentiates sinus rhythm from nonsinus rhythms. Sinus rhythm produces upright P-waves in lead I, II, and aVF; consistent PR intervals; and narrow-QRS complexes (figure on the right). Sinus tachycardia and sinus bradycardia are not abnormal heart rates and rhythms; rather, the are physiological adaptations. Sinus tachycardia and bradycardia are sinus rhythms with narrow-QRS complexes, normal P-waves, and consistent PR intervals.

Nonsinus rhythms fall into 3 clinical categories: fast, slow, and irregular. Nonsinus tachycardias and nonsinus bradycardias have abnormal P-QRS relationships and may have wide-QRS complexes. An irregular rhythm may be from sinus arrhythmia (variation in heart rate with respiration) or isolated premature atrial or ventricular contractions (PACs or PVCs). However, irregular rhythms may also arise from significant underlying cardiac disease. For more on EKG interpretation, see Chapter 21. For more on EP procedures, see Chapter 26. [1-4]

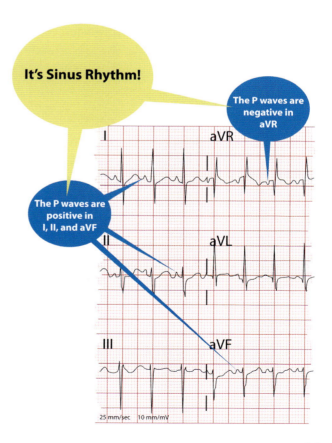

4 Abnormal Heart Rates & Rhythms

DIAGNOSTIC DEVICES

Abnormal heart rates and rhythms often occur intermittently. Diagnosis can be difficult from history and symptoms alone. Parents may bring their child to an urgent care facility or emergency room complaining of a fast heart rate, palpitations, or even syncope. There, the child's EKG is often normal. An EKG may be normal because an arrhythmia converts to normal sinus rhythm, because palpitations are often intermittent, or the because symptoms are not from an abnormal heart rate and rhythm.

Figure A on the facing page shows the placement of a Holter monitor. A Holter (capitalized for the inventor, Norman Holter) can be left on for 24 to 48 hours. Holter monitors work best for known arrhythmias that are persistent or at least occur daily. We also use Holter monitoring for patients with unknown rhythm disorders that complain of palpitations every day or have other daily symptoms. Holter monitors record every heart beat while worn. Later, a computer downloads the information. The analysis computer tabulates high and low heart rates, episodes of sustained tachycardia or bradycardia, and numbers and types of premature contractions. Patients keep timed-diaries of their symptoms, which we can correlate with the Holter's print out.

Figure B on the facing page displays the use of a portable cardiac event monitor. These devices do not connect to the patient with leads like a Holter monitor. Patients or parents can apply these devices to the child's chest during symptoms. Portable cardiac event monitors work best for unknown intermittent abnormal heart rates and rhythms, for intermittent palpitations, or for other intermittent symptoms. A "record" button can trigger the device, after which the device records an EKG for several seconds and stores the information. The Patient or parent then calls the office and downloads the information over the phone. The office receiver prints out an EKG tracing for interpretation. We can provide these devices to families for 30 to 60 days. Portable cardiac event monitors can be especially helpful when attempting to diagnose intermittent supraventricular tachycardia.

Figure C on the facing page demonstrates the placement of a surgically implantable event monitor (about the size of a flash drive). We use this device more rarely than either Holter or portable event monitors. Although for patients unable to wear a device, unable to trigger a device, or who are syncopal with an arrhythmia event, a surgically implanted event monitor can be diagnostic. The device's battery lasts for about 1 to 2 years, and it automatically records and stores arrhythmias. Also, the patient can trigger the device. Similar to a pacemaker, the device allows transcutaneous interrogation and downloading of stored information.

4 Abnormal Heart Rates & Rhythms

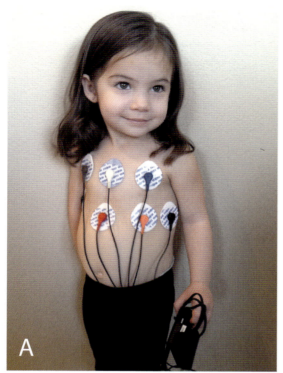

A

Holter Monitor

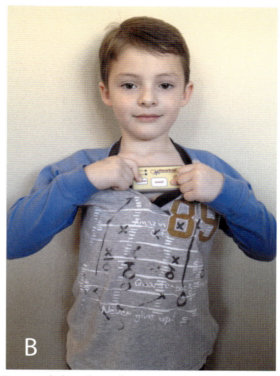

B

Portable Cardiac Event Monitor

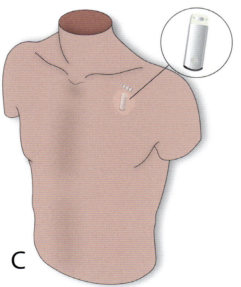

C

Implanted Event Monitor

FAST RATES & RHYTHMS

Sinus Tachycardia

- Pain
- Anxiety
- Hypovolemia
- Fever
- Anemia
- Increased catecholamines
- Prescription medications
- Illicit drugs
- Hyperthyroidism
- Congestive heart failure

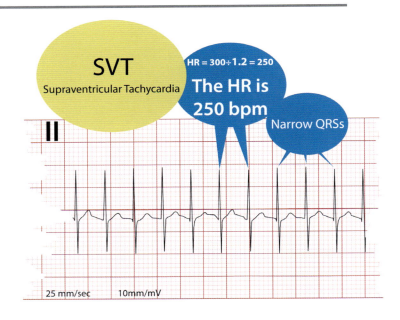

Supraventricular Tachycardia

As the tracing on the upper right displays, narrow-QRS Supraventricular tachycardia (SVT) is the most common nonsinus tachycardia. In infants and young children with SVT, the heart rate is > 220 bpm. The P-waves are often not evident, because the rapid rate "buries" them in the tracing. The heart rate usually shows little or no variation. SVT may occasionally have wide-QRS complexes, making wide-QRS SVT difficult to distinguish from ventricular tachycardia (VT). Wide-QRS SVT is often more hemodynamically stable than VT, but not always.

SVT common mechanisms

The primary SVT mechanism lies in abnormal congenital intracardiac electrical pathways that, with the normal conduction system, allow "reentrant circuits." Abnormal electrical pathways may exist between the atrium and the ventricles or within the atrioventricular node.

The figures on the facing page display atrioventricular reentrant circuits. Figure A illustrates the normal conduction system with an abnormal, congenital-bypass tract (or accessory pathway). When manifest, accessory pathways result in preexcitation or Wolff-Parkinson-White (WPW). WPW appears on an EKG as a short PR interval with QRS delta-waves (tracings below figure A) that can be positive (upstroke) or negative (downstroke). However, abnormal intracardiac pathways may also be present despite a normal EKG (concealed pathways). Concealed pathways require an electrophysiology (EP) procedure for diagnosis.

Bypass tracts can be a substrate for atrioventricular reentrant tachycardia (AVRT). AVRT is the most common SVT mechanism in infants and children. Atrioventricular nodal reentrant tachycardia (AVNRT) is more common than AVRT in adolescents and adults; the figures do not

4 Abnormal Heart Rates & Rhythms

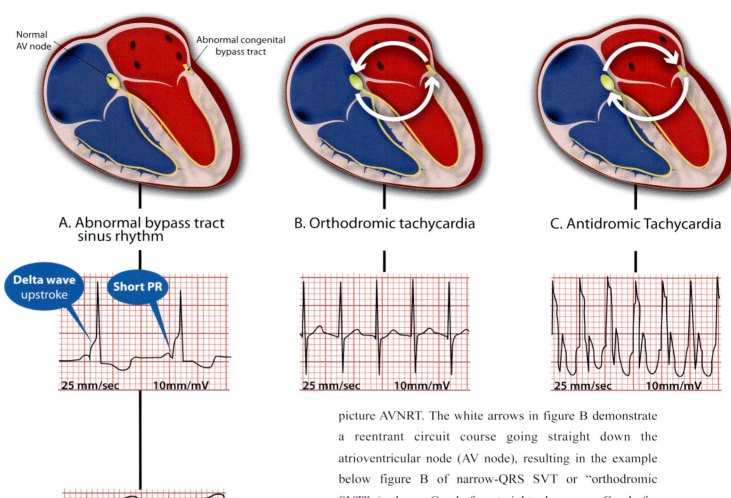

A. Abnormal bypass tract sinus rhythm

B. Orthodromic tachycardia

C. Antidromic Tachycardia

picture AVNRT. The white arrows in figure B demonstrate a reentrant circuit course going straight down the atrioventricular node (AV node), resulting in the example below figure B of narrow-QRS SVT or "orthodromic SVT" (ortho = Greek for straight, dromos = Greek for course). Figure C shows a reversed reentrant circuit course traveling in the opposite direction through the AV node, resulting in the example below figure C of wide-QRS SVT or "antidromic SVT" (antidromic = opposite course). Orthodromic circuits are more common than antidromic circuits.

Cardiac malformations including Ebstein anomaly, some cardiac tumors, and some glycogen storage diseases can have abnormal, intracardiac electrical pathways. Often, however, accessory pathways occur in structurally normal hearts.

SVT Clinical features

Patients with SVT may have vague past medical histories. With infants, parents may report paleness episodes and periods of irritability and lethargy. In older children and adolescents, patients may describe sudden onset and sudden cessation tachycardias (characteristic description for SVT), or they may note intermittent palpitations.

Upon initial presentation, obtain an echocardiogram (Echo) to rule out a structural malformation and to measure ventricular function, as patients with prolonged SVT frequently have ventricular dysfunction.

Infants often receive chronic medical therapy; although, rare infant cases require invasive ablation [5]. For older children and adolescents, we frequently recommend an EP procedure with pathway ablation.

SVT ℞ options

The clinical status directs treatment. Refer to Appendix C for medication dosing.

Acute conversion to sinus rhythm

- Vagal maneuvers for infants

For hemodynamically stable infants, use crushed ice mixed with water in a sealable plastic bag. Place the plastic bag on the infant's forehead and nose with moderate pressure for 10 to 15 seconds, then release. This maneuver simulates the "mammalian diving reflex," which occurs when mammals plunge into cold water. Vagal nerve stimulation causes the reflex bradycardia and SVT conversion. If the first application produces no effect, then repeat several times, allowing the infant to warm between applications.

- Vagal maneuvers for older children

For an older child or adolescent, encourage vagal maneuvers including valsalva or bearing down, blowing through an occluded straw, or even hanging upside down. However, ice to the face does not work well in older children. Carotid massage rarely works in children. Avoid eyeball pressure, as retinal detachments may result.

- IV adenosine

Adenosine works by blocking the AV node and interrupting the AV nodal path of the reentrant circuit. Use adenosine in patients who are hemodynamically stable and unresponsive to vagal maneuvers. Blood rapidly metabolizes adenosine; therefore, give adenosine by rapid IV push and quickly follow with a large flush volume, preferably through a central line. The expected response is tachycardia termination, often with a short asystolic period. As the rhythm returns to normal sinus, a slow junctional escape rhythm (narrow QRS without p-waves) may occur transiently along with temporary sinus tachycardia. Whenever possible, obtain a 12-lead EKG or rhythm strip during adenosine administration, as the tracing is useful for a pediatric cardiologist's review.

Adenosine can also be diagnostic for atrial flutter or atrial ectopic tachycardia. Following a dose, adenosine blocks the AV node, which disrupts ventricular conduction, allowing for better visualization of atrial activity on the cardiac monitor or EKG. The tracing below demonstrates this effect:

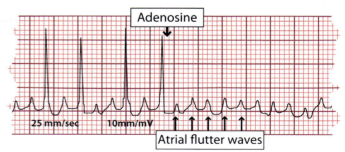

Response to Adenosine in a Patient with Atrial Flutter

Adenosine does not convert atrial flutter, atrial ectopic tachycardia, junctional ectopic tachycardia, or ventricular tachycardia to sinus rhythm. See the next section for more information about these abnormal rhythms.

- IV esmolol

Use esmolol in stable patients with normal ventricular function when several adenosine doses fail to convert SVT to normal sinus rhythm, or when SVT recurs quickly after conversion to normal sinus rhythm.

- IV amiodarone

As an alternative to esmolol, amiodarone may be effective in recalcitrant SVT [6]. However, amiodarone is longer lasting and has more side effects than esmolol. Also, administer IV amiodarone boluses slowly, as rapid infusions can cause cardiovascular collapse.

- IV digoxin

Cardiologists rarely use digoxin for SVT conversion. But if used and preexcitation is present on an EKG after conversion to sinus rhythm, then stop digoxin and start a beta-blocker like propranolol for chronic prevention.

- Electrical cardioversion in unstable patients

Cardioversion with 0.5 to 2.0 Joules/kg is appropriate for unstable patients or those with wide-QRS tachycardias, as wide-QRS SVT is difficult to distinguish from ventricular tachycardia. The cardioverter-defibrillator needs infant or pediatric paddles. Synchronize the equipment with the QRS. Unsynchronized defibrillation may cause ventricular fibrillation, requiring immediate repeat cardioversion. Patients require deep sedation for electrical cardioversion. Trained personnel should administer deep sedation.

➤Verapamil contraindicated

In the young, avoid verapamil and other calcium-channel blockers for SVT conversion, as calcium-channel blockers can cause cardiac arrest in such patients.

Chronic recurrence prevention

After conversion to normal sinus rhythm, obtain a 12-lead EKG to check for preexcitation. Preexcitation may underlie an increased risk of sudden death, especially if the patient is on digoxin.

Usually, we treat infants with medications. Often, we discontinue medications after about 6 to 12 months, if SVT does not recur during this time. Although SVT may not recur for months or years after discontinuing medications, patients can have episodes later in life.

Contrary to infants, older children with SVT (especially with WPW) often undergo an EP procedure and ablation. Nonetheless, observation is reasonable for some with a single SVT episode, occasional SVT, or even multiple short SVT episodes. However, most patients require treatment.

Treatment choices for all ages include:

- Oral beta-blockers like propranolol

With or without preexcitation.

- Oral digoxin

Without preexcitation.

- Other medications

According to a pediatric cardiology consultant.

- Electrophysiology procedure & ablation

According to an electrophysiologist. For more on EP procedures, see Chapter 26.

Other Nonsinus Tachycardias

Other nonsinus tachycardias include atrial flutter, atrial ectopic tachycardia, multifocal atrial tachycardia, junctional ectopic tachycardia, permanent junctional reciprocating tachycardia, or ventricular tachycardia. These are rarer than SVT and more often occur with underlying cardiac pathology from conditions such as myocarditis, some dilated cardiomyopathies, or post cardiac surgery. Atrial fibrillation is rare in children; thus, we do not address atrial fibrillation in this chapter.

Atrial flutter (AF)

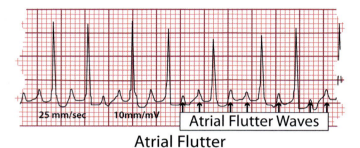

Atrial Flutter

In children, AF (tracing above) most often occurs in infants in the perinatal period. However, AF may also occur with congenital heart disease, especially with right or left atrial enlargement or previous atrial surgery. Obtain an Echo to rule out intracardiac clots, especially when the history is consistent with chronic AF.

AF acute ℞ options

- Electrical cardioversion

0.5 to 1.0 Joule/kg is the quickest means of cardioversion. Electrical cardioversion is appropriate even in stable patients. Always synchronize, as we previously described.

- IV digoxin

If digoxin precedes electrical cardioversion, then load with lidocaine before electrical cardioversion to protect against possible ventricular fibrillation with digoxin onboard.

- Transesophageal overdrive pacing

A pediatric cardiologist should perform this procedure (see Chapter 26).

AF chronic ℞ options

Infants with normal hearts rarely need chronic therapy, but those with congenital heart disease and AF may need acute and chronic treatment. A pediatric cardiologist or electrophysiologist should direct medical care. Options include:

- Digoxin for rate control
- Flecainide, sotalol, amiodarone for chronic suppression

Atrial ectopic tachycardia (AET)

Atrial ectopic tachycardia (AET) is the most common cause of chronic incessant tachycardia in children, and AET may present with ventricular dysfunction. Distinguishing AET from atrial flutter on EKG is difficult, and a diagnosis usually requires input from a pediatric cardiologist. Those < 3 years old may respond to medical therapy with dysrhythmia resolution. Those > 3 years old may need an invasive EP procedure with ablation. Beta-blockers may be effective when ventricular function is normal, and amiodarone may be preferable with ventricular dysfunction. If EP ablation is unsuccessful, then the patient may need surgical ablation of the AET focus. [7]

AET ℞ options with normal ventricular function

- IV esmolol
- IV amiodarone
- Oral beta-blockers like propranolol
- Others per pediatric cardiology consultant

AET ℞ options with decreased left ventricular function

- IV amiodarone
- Oral amiodarone

- Other medications per pediatric cardiology consultant
- EP procedure with ablation

Multifocal atrial tachycardia (MAT)

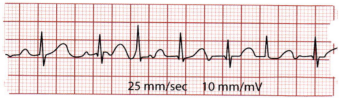

Multifocal Atrial Tachycardia

MAT (tracing above) is a rare dysrhythmia. MAT has multiple premature atrial contractions with diverse P-wave morphologies (> 3), irregular P-P intervals, isoelectric baseline between P-waves, and ventricular rates > 100 bpm (usually 150 to 250 bpm in children). Atrial rates may be as high as 400 bpm. MAT's etiology remains unknown, and it usually resolves spontaneously. [8]

MAT ℞ options

- Probably none when asymptomatic
- Occasionally digoxin to slow ventricular rate
- Occasionally amiodarone, flecainide, or sotalol

Junctional ectopic tachycardia (JET)

JET can occur after surgical repair. Usually, the characteristics of JET are atrioventricular disassociation with a narrow-QRS ventricular rate higher than the atrial rate (usually lower rate than SVT). The example tracing above on the right comes from postoperative, temporary pacing wires attached to an EKG machine. The tracing in black originates from a ventricular pacing lead and the tracing in blue comes from the atrial lead. The ventricular lead displays ventricular complexes; however, the atrial

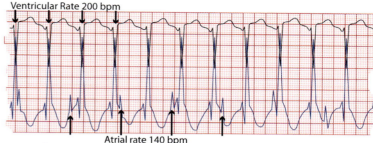

Postoperative Junctional Ectopic Tachycardia

lead shows atrial and ventricular complexes. The hallmark AV dissociation of JET is readily apparent, a finding usually not evident on a standard EKG tracing.

Congenital JET can also occur. Incessant congenital JET may cause left ventricular dysfunction. Postoperative and congenital JET may respond to amiodarone. If the patient with congenital JET is > 2 to 3 years old and the JET remains uncontrolled with medications, then proceed to an EP procedure with ablation. [9-12]

Postoperative JET ℞ options

- Normalize electrolytes, including calcium
- Correct acidosis
- Aim for high normal magnesium level
- Decrease doses of inotropes
- IV amiodarone
- Atrial pacing to rates above the JET rate, if temporary wires present
- Esophageal overdrive pacing
- IV dexmedetomidine (Precedex) for sedation
- Patient cooling on occasion

Congenital JET ℞ options

- IV amiodarone
- Oral amiodarone
- EP procedure with ablation

Permanent junctional reciprocating tachycardia (PJRT)

PJRT may present with incessant tachycardia and left ventricular dysfunction. Patients may respond to medical treatment. If PJRT does not respond to medical therapy, then proceed to an EP procedure with ablation. [13] PJRT usually has negative P-waves in leads II, III, and aVF but positive in aVL, as in the tracing below:

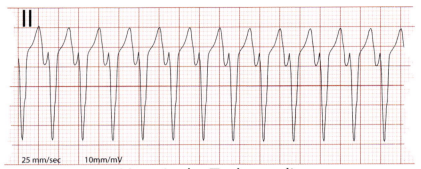

Ventricular Tachycardia

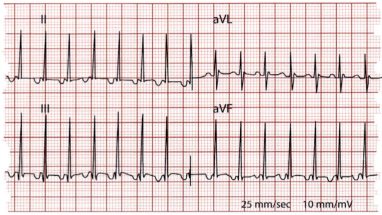

Permanent Junctional Reentrant Tachycardia

PJRT ℞ options

- Oral flecainide
- Oral sotalol
- IV or oral amiodarone
- EP procedure with ablation

Ventricular tachycardia (VT)

VT or accelerated idioventricular rhythm (AIVR) may be asymptomatic and require no therapy. Usually, however, VT needs immediate treatment like the example in the tracing above on the right.

VT causes

- **Inflammation**

All causes of myocarditis.

- **Structural or myocardial disease**

These can include hypertrophic or dilated cardiomyopathies, cardiac tumors, and arrhythmogenic right ventricular cardiomyopathy (ARVC). ARVC replaces myocardium with fibrous-fatty tissue. ARVC is autosomal dominant, has a male predominance, and most often presents at about 30 years old.

- **Ion channelopathies**

Ion channelopathies stem from mutations in genes that code for proteins found in cell-membrane channels that transport potassium, sodium, and calcium ions. Long QT syndrome (LQTS) is the most common channelopathy.

Phenotypically, LQTS is consistent with Romano-Ward (autosomal dominant without deafness) or Jervell and Lange-Nielsen (autosomal recessive with deafness). In the United States, 99% of LQTS fits the Romano-Ward pattern, or a long QTc without deafness.

As the table on the top of the facing page shows, LQTS types 1 to 3 account for about 70% of all forms of LQTS. The table also lists the chromosome for the gene mutation locations, the penetrance, the ion channel

4 Abnormal Heart Rates & Rhythms

Long QT Syndrome

Type	Chromosome	Penetrance	Current	Effect	% Among LQTS	EKG	Triggers Lethal Cardiac Event
LQTS1	3	62%	K	↓	30 - 35	Broad based T wave	Exercise (68%) Emotional stress (14%) Sleep, repose (9%) Others (19%)
LQTS2	7	75%	K	↓	25 - 30	Notched T wave	Exercise (29%) Emotional stress (49%) Sleep, repose (22%)
LQTS3	11	90%	Na	↑	5 - 10	Long ST segment Peaked T wave	Exercise (4%) Emotional stress (12%) Sleep, repose (64%) Others (20%)

involved, how the mutation affects the potassium (K) or sodium (Na) channel's ionic current, the percent occurrence, the EKG effects, and the clinical triggers.

LQTS may cause ventricular tachycardia/fibrillation know as *Torsades de pointes* (twisting around a point). A gradual change in the amplitude and twisting of the QRS complexes around the isoelectric line characterizes *Torsades de pointes* (tracing below).

Other ion channelopathies include catecholaminergic polymorphic VT (CPVT) and Brugada syndrome. Genetic abnormalities in patients and family members underlie these problems; however, confirmatory genetic testing is expensive. [14]

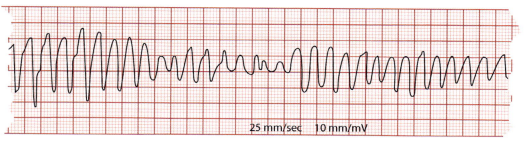

Torsades de Pointes

4 Abnormal Heart Rates & Rhythms

- **Drugs**

Especially methamphetamines, cocaine, digoxin toxicity, and medications that lengthen the QT interval, see http://www.sads.org/Living-with-SADS/Drugs-to-Avoid/Printable-Drug-List for a list of medications to avoid in LQTS.

- **Cardiac surgery**

Especially in postoperative tetralogy of Fallot or other surgical procedures with ventricular scarring.

- **Metabolic & electrolyte abnormalities**

Conditions can include hypoxia, acidosis, hypokalemia, and hyperkalemia. Hyperkalemia produces peaked T-waves and eventually a wide QRS. The figures below display a deteriorating QRS-T wave findings with serum potassium levels increasing from 6.5 to 9.0 mEq/dL.

Acute treatment of hyperkalemia	
Calcium	100 mg/kg IV slow push over 5 minutes
Dextrose & Insulin	glucose 0.5 g/kg + insulin 0.1 U/kg IV 30 minutes
Albuterol	0.05-0.15 mg/kg by inhalation
Furosemide	1-2 mg/kg/dose IV slow push
Na$^+$ Bicarbonate	1-2 mEq/kg/dose IV slow push over 10-30 minutes

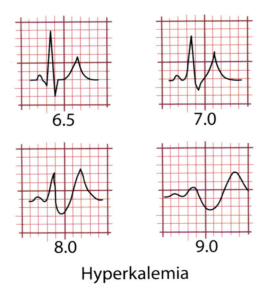

Hyperkalemia

➤The table above right outlines hyperkalemia treatment. May also give Kayexalate (sodium polystyrene sulfonate) at 1.0 g/kg orally or rectally; however, the potassium-lowering effect is not immediate, rather the effect occurs over time. Thus, Kayexalate has a limited role in the acute hyperkalemia treatment. Also, Kayexalate may cause bowel perforations in premature infants.

VT acute ℞ options

In unstable patients, be ready to perform CPR, administer resuscitation medications, and perform cardioversion when necessary.

- **Electrical cardioversion**

2.0 to 4.0 Joules/kg, repeat if no conversion to sinus rhythm.

- **Pharmacological ℞**

Medications include IV lidocaine or IV amiodarone.

VT chronic ℞ options

- Observation without medications for slow VT or AVIR
- Beta-blockers
- EP procedure with ablation if possible
- Implantable cardioverter defibrillator (ICD)

4 Abnormal Heart Rates & Rhythms

SLOW RATES & RHYTHMS

Sinus Bradycardia

Sinus bradycardia has many causes and most are benign. Nonetheless, some causes are pathological like LQTS. Even fetal bradycardia can herald a long QT [15]. Therefore, manually calculate the QTc in all sinus bradycardias (see Chapter 21). The tracing below is from a newborn with an extremely long QTc (0.70 sec or 700 msec and a sinus bradycardia with a heart rate of 99):

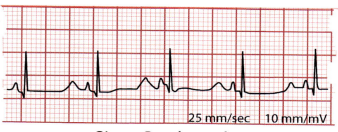
Sinus Bradycardia

Sinus bradycardia causes

- Increased vagal activity
- Hypothermia
- Hypothyroidism
- Apnea
- Hypoxia
- Asphyxia
- Increased intracranial pressure
- Medications such as beta-blockers
- Hyperkalemia
- LQTS (tracing above)

Nonsinus Bradycardias

Blocked premature atrial contractions

Nonpathological regularly blocked premature atrial contractions can present as a bradycardia at any age, even prenatally. The tracing below shows an example:

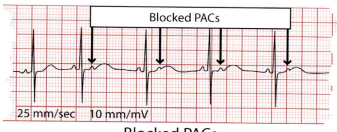
Blocked PACs

Atrioventricular block

The tracing below shows 3rd-degree AV block:

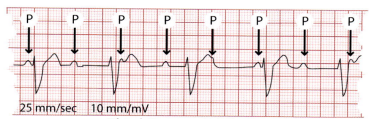
Third Degree AV Block

Congenital

Congenital heart block may accompany cardiovascular malformations, especially complex ones. Nonstructural related congenital complete heart block usually results from maternal systemic lupus erythematosus (SLE) autoantibodies. Maternal autoantibodies pass to the fetus

61

transplacentally where these antibodies damage the fetal cardiac conduction system. Regardless the etiology, congenital heart block is permanent.

Systemic connective tissue diseases, such as SLE and Sjögren syndrome, cause exposure of nuclear and cytoplasmic ribonucleic proteins (RNPs). These exposed RNPs stimulate maternal autoantibody production. The maternal autoantibodies cross the placenta and can damage the fetal conduction system. Researchers have not determined the exact function of RNPs, but their molecular structure is similar across species or "evolutionarily conserved."

Originally, investigators designated the Sjögren syndrome autoantibodies as anti-SSA (Sjögren syndrome antigen-A) and anti-SSB (Sjögren syndrome antigen-B), and the SLE autoantibodies as anti-Ro and anti-La (Ro and La were the first 2 letters of the first patients' names in whom researchers found antibodies). Further experiments determined anti-SSA was identical to anti-Ro and anti-SSB was identical to anti-La; consequently, the terms are now anti-SSA/Ro and anti-SSB/La. For more on these antibody tests, see Appendix D. [16-18]

Acquired

Heart block may result from heart surgery, progressive AV nodal disease, myocarditis, or drugs. Contrary to congenital heart block, acquired heart block may be temporary.

AV block ℞ options

- Consider prenatal maternal steroids & IVIG for 1st- & 2nd -degree AV block, but not effective for 3rd-degree block
- For infants and children consider isoproterenol, temporary, or permanent pacemaker
- Observation for those not meeting pacing indications; we list pacing indications in Chapter 26

4 Abnormal Heart Rates & Rhythms

IRREGULAR RATES & RHYTHMS

An irregular rhythm may be simple sinus arrhythmia or isolated premature atrial or ventricular contractions (PACs or PVCs, figures below).

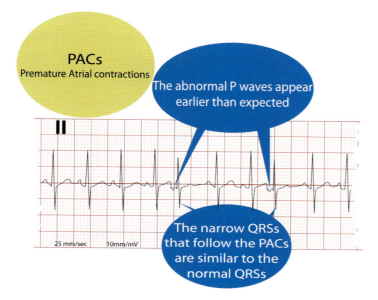

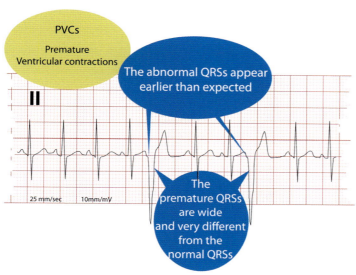

PACs and PVCs are usually benign if the patient is unaware of them; if ectopics are unifocal (all complexes appearing identical with identical relationship with previous normal QRSs); if ectopics disappear with increased heart rates like with exercise; and if the ectopics are not too frequent. Conversely, PACs and PVCs are worrisome if the ectopics are new onset, multifocal, occur in pairs or runs, occur with structural heart disease or myocarditis, do not suppress with increased heart rates, increase with exercise, or are frequent. We list ectopic frequency definitions in the table below:

Ectopic frequency noted from Holter	
Rare	<1/hour
Occasional	1-30/hour
Frequent	>30/hour

Benign Irregular Rhythms

Patients require no treatment for the following:
- Sinus arrhythmia
- Benign idiopathic PACs or PVCs at any age
- PACs in newborns with atrial septal aneurysms
➤ Although, 1 previous study reported fetal SVT with atrial septal aneurysms [19].

63

4 Abnormal Heart Rates & Rhythms

Pathological Irregular Rhythms

Pathological ectopics are also usually PACs or PVCs. Similar causes can produce atrial or ventricular ectopics. Excessive PVCs (≥ 20% of the total heart beats in a 24-hour Holter monitor recording) may cause ventricular dysfunction [20]. Occasionally, 2nd-degree heart block can also be the cause of an irregular rhythm from dropped beats.

Causes

- Digoxin toxicity
- Abnormal electrolytes
- Myocarditis
- Postoperative cardiac surgery
- Indwelling catheters
- Hyperthyroidism
- Brugada syndrome
- Arrhythmogenic RV cardiomyopathy (ARVC)
- Automatic foci
- Myocardial contusion
- Drugs such as caffeine or cocaine
- Other causes of catecholamine excess

℞ options

Similar to all arrhythmias, treating irregular rhythms may require alternative medications to those we list. Further, a pediatric cardiologist or pediatric electrophysiologist should direct care.

- **Treat underlying condition**

Treat myocarditis, remove indwelling catheter, correct electrolytes, or discontinue a potentially causative medication.

- **IV or oral beta-blockers like propranolol**

For pathological PACs or PVCs with normal LV function.

- **IV or oral amiodarone**

For pathological PACs or PVCs with impaired left ventricular function; although, ablation may be preferable.

- **IV lidocaine**

For acute hemodynamically significant PVCs.

- **Other antiarrhythmics**

As per pediatric electrophysiologist.

- **EP procedure with ablation**

For PVC induced cardiomyopathy.

CLINICAL VIGNETTES

7. The staff call you to see a baby in the newborn nursery with a low heart rate. The baby's mother has a past history of muscle and joint pains, but she is on no medications and has not seen a doctor lately. On exam, the baby is full term, pink and in no distress. The rhythm is regular with a heart rate of 57 bpm. The pulses are equal in the upper and lower extremities, and the liver is not palpable. The precordium is quiet, and there is no heart murmur. Before obtaining an EKG, the most likely diagnosis:

a. Normal heart with sinus bradycardia
b. Atrial ectopic tachycardia
c. Complex congenital heart disease with heart block
d. Congenital heart block likely from maternal autoantibodies.

8. A 2-month old female presents to the emergency room with a fast heart rate. She was full term and has had no pre- or postnatal problems. The mother describes episodes of paleness and irritability. On exam, she is in no marked distress, her respiratory rate is about 40 per minute. The heart rate is too fast to count, the pulses are thready, and the liver is just palpable below the right costal margin. The precordium is mildly hyperdynamic, and there is no murmur. The cardiac monitor shows a narrow-QRS tachycardia with a heart rate of 250 bpm without heart rate variation. The most appropriate initial intervention:

a. An IV calcium-channel blocker
b. Carotid massage
c. A sealed plastic bag with ice water to the face
d. Observation in the emergency room

REFERENCES

1 Hanisch D. Pediatric arrhythmias. J Pediatr Nurs 2001; 16: 351-362

2 Singh Harinder R, Garekar S, Epstein ML, L'Ecuyer T. Neonatal supraventricular tachycardia (SVT). Neo Reviews 2005; 6: e339-e350

3 Kothari DS, Skinner JR. Neonatal tachycardias: an update. Arch Dis Child Fetal Neonatal Ed 2006; 91: F136-F144

4 Massin MM, Benatar A, Rondia G. Epidemiology and outcome of tachyarrhythmias in tertiary pediatric cardiac centers. Cardiology 2008; 111: 191-196

5 Makhoul M, Von Bergen NH, Rabi F, Gingerich J, Evans WN, Law IH. Successful transcatheter cryoablation in infants with drug-resistant supraventricular tachycardia: a case series. J Interv Card Electrophysiol 2010; 29: 209-215

6 Celiker A, Ceviz N, Ozme S. Effectiveness and safety of intravenous amiodarone in drug-resistant tachyarrhythmias of children. Acta Paediatr Jpn 1998; 40: 567-572

7 Salerno J, Kertesz NJ, Friedman RA, Fenrich AL. Clinical course of atrial ectopic tachycardia is age-dependent: Results and treatment in children < 3 or ≥ 3 years of age. J AM Coll Cardiol 2004; 43: 438-444

8 Bradley DJ, Fischbach PS, Law IH, Serwer GA, Dick M 2nd. The clinical course of multifocal atrial tachycardia in infants and children. J Am Coll Cardiol 2001; 38: 401-408

9 Kovacikova L, Hakacova N, Dobos D, Skrak P, Zahorec M. Amiodarone as a first-line therapy for postoperative junctional ectopic tachycardia. Ann Thorac Surg 2009; 88: 616-622

10 Chrysostomou C, Beerman L, Shiderly D, Berry D, Morell VO, Munoz R. Dexmedetomidine: a novel drug for the treatment of atrial and junctional tachyarrhythmias during the perioperative period for congenital cardiac surgery: a preliminary study. Anesth Analg 2008; 107: 1514-1522

11 Law IH, Von Bergen NH, Gingerich JC, Saarel EV, Fischbach PS, Dick M 2nd. Transcatheter cryothermal ablation of junctional ectopic tachycardia in the normal heart. Heart Rhythm 2006; 8: 903-907

12 Collins KK, Van Hare GF, Kertesz NJ, Law IH, Bar-Cohen Y, Dubin AM, Etheridge SP, Berul CI, Avari JN, Tuzcu V, Sreeram N, Schaffer MS, Fournier A, Sanatani S, Snyder CS, Smith RT Jr, Arabia L, Hamilton R, Chun T, Liberman L, Kakavand B, Paul T, Tanel RE. Pediatric nonpost-operative junctional ectopic tachycardia medical management and interventional therapies. J Am Coll Cardiol 2009; 53: 690-697

13 Vaksmann G, D'Hoinne C, Lucet V, Guillaumont S, Lupoglazoff JM, Chantepie A, Denjoy I, Villain E, Marçon F. Permanent junctional reciprocating tachycardia in children: a multicentre study on clinical profile and outcome. Heart 2006; 92: 101-104

14 Schimpf R, Veltmann C, Wolpert C, Borggrefe M. Channelopathies: Brugada syndrome, long QT syndrome, short QT syndrome, and CPVT. Herz 2009; 34: 282-288

15 Collazos JC, Acherman RJ, Law IH, Wilkes P, Restrepo H, Evans WN. Sustained fetal bradycardia with 1:1 conduction and long QT syndrome. Prenat Diagn 2007; 27: 879-881

16 Acherman RJ, Evans WN, Luna CF, Castillo WJ, Rollins R, Kip K, Law IH, Collazos JC, Restrepo H. Fetal bradycardia. A practical approach. Fetal and Maternal Medicine Review 2007; 18: 225-255

17 Acherman RJ, Friedman DM, Buyon JP, Schwartz J, Castillo WJ, Rollins RC, Evans WN. Doppler fetal mechanical PR interval prolongation with positive maternal anti-RNP but negative SSA/Ro and SSB/La auto-antibodies. Prenat Diagn 2010; 30: 797-799

18 Pises N, Acherman RJ, Iriye BK, Rollins RC, Castillo W, Herceg E, Evans WN. Positive maternal anti-SSA/SSB antibody-related fetal right ventricular endocardial fibroelastosis without atrioventricular block, reversal of endocardial fibroelastosis. Prenat Diagn 2009; 29: 177-178

19 Respondek M, Wloch A, Kaczmarek P, Borowski D Wilczynski J, Helwich E. Diagnostic and perinatal management of fetal extrasystole. Pediatr Cardiol 1997; 18: 361-366

20 Takemoto M, Yoshimura H, Ohba Y, Matsumoto Y, Yamamoto H, Origuchi H. Radiofrequency catheter ablation of premature ventricular complexes from right ventricular outflow tract improves left ventricular dilation and clinical status in patients without structural heart disease. J Am Coll Cardiol 2005; 45: 1259-1265

4 Abnormal Heart Rates & Rhythms

5 Heart Failure

Contents	
Background	71
Causes	72
Evaluation	74
℞ Options	77
Clinical Vignettes	80

5 Heart Failure

kathleen cass

BACKGROUND

This chapter highlights subacute or chronic congestive heart failure rather than acute cardiovascular collapse. We discuss patients presenting in extremis in Chapter 8.

Congestive heart failure (CHF) results from the heart's inability to pump blood effectively. Usually, excess catecholamines, pulmonary venous congestion, and systemic venous congestion accompany CHF. Symptoms may include fatigability, failure-to-thrive, shortness of breath, or chronic abdominal pain from gastrointestinal-tract edema. Signs of CHF-related catecholamine excess may include tachycardia, diaphoresis, pallor, and cool extremities. Signs of pulmonary venous congestion may include tachypnea, wheezing, and râles. Signs of systemic venous congestion may include hepatomegaly, jugular venous distension, and peripheral edema. Other signs may include dysrhythmias, abnormal pulses, a hyperdynamic precordium, and heart murmurs.

CHF management's principal goal is to discover, if possible, an etiology amenable to definitive treatment. Treatable conditions may include a pericardial effusion with tamponade, a correctable cardiac defect, a treatable arrhythmia, metabolic abnormalities such as carnitine deficiency, or any other treatable cause.

Some CHF etiologies including rheumatic fever, muscular dystrophy, and drug abuse occur more often in older children and adolescents than in infants and young children. Nonetheless, consider all CHF causes despite the patient's age. If a clinicians group CHF etiologies too specifically by age, then they may not consider all potential causes. [1-6]

Mechanisms of CHF

- Tamponade physiology
- Volume overload
- Pressure overload
- Ventricular systolic dysfunction
- Ventricular diastolic dysfunction
- Arrhythmias

For simplicity, we list causes of CHF by principal mechanism; although, etiologies often affect the heart through multiple mechanisms. We also organize the treatment section by principal mechanism.

CHF CAUSES BY PRINCIPAL MECHANISM

Tamponade Physiology

A pericardial effusion causing cardiac tamponade can present subacutely, but patients usually require emergent treatment. Treating the pericardial effusion eliminates congestive heart failure without specific pharmacological agents (other than possibly a course of anti-inflammatory medications).

Etiologies include:
- Viral pericarditis, including HIV
- Bacterial pericarditis
- Kawasaki disease
- Rheumatic fever
- Systemic connective tissue disease
- Post-pericardiotomy syndrome

Volume Overload

- **Left-to-right shunts**

Ventricular septal defect (VSD), patent ductus arteriosus (PDA), and on rare occasion, a large atrial septal defect (ASD).

- **Valvular regurgitation**

Moderate to severe mitral, tricuspid, aortic, or pulmonary valve regurgitation.

- **High output states**

From anemia, hyperthyroidism, and arteriovenous malformations.

- **Iatrogenic**

Excessive IV fluid administration.

Pressure Overload

- **Defects with LV pressure overload**

Coarctation of the aorta (CoA) and aortic stenosis (AS).

- **Defects with RV pressure overload**

Severe pulmonic stenosis (PS), mitral stenosis, and cor triatriatum.

- **Systemic HTN with LV pressure overload**

Systemic hypertension (HTN) with ventricular dysfunction can result from post streptococcal acute glomerulonephritis (AGN), hyperthyroidism, neonatal indwelling umbilical artery lines (especially in premature infants), and other systemic HTN causes (see Chapter 14).

- **Pulmonary HTN with RV pressure overload**

Persistent pulmonary hypertension of the newborn (PPHN), primary pulmonary hypertension, or Eisenmenger syndrome in older children.

Ventricular Systolic Dysfunction

- **Viral myocarditis**

Adenovirus, CMV, Coxsackie A & B, EBV, echovirus hepatitis, herpes, HIV, influenza, mumps, parvovirus, or varicella.

- **Bacterial myocarditis**

Diphtheria, hemophilus influenzae, listeria, lyme disease, salmonella.

- **Other microbial myocarditis**

Aspergillus, ascaris, candida, cisticercosis, histoplasma, rickettsia, schistosoma, trypanosoma cruzi (Chagas disease), and visceral larva migrans.

- **Other myocarditis**

Kawasaki disease, rheumatic fever, or systemic connective tissue disease.

- **Structural coronary artery abnormalities**

Anomalous left coronary artery from the pulmonary artery (ALCAPA), coronary artery aneurysms, thrombosis or stenosis from Kawasaki disease.

- **Other structural defects**

CoA, AS, and complex malformations such as 1-functional ventricle or others.

- **Drugs & toxins**

Anthracyclines (anticancer medications), cocaine, arsenic, heavy metals, radiation, or alcohol.

- **Metabolic abnormalities**

Nutritional deficiencies, hypoxia, acidosis, hypothyroidism, hypoparathyroidism, or anemia.

- **Mitochondrial disorders**

Carnitine deficiency and fatty acid oxidation disorders.

- **Muscular dystrophies**

Duchenne and Becker.

- **Dilated cardiomyopathies**

Familial, postpartum, or idiopathic.

Ventricular Diastolic Dysfunction

- **Hypertrophic cardiomyopathies (HCM)**

Hereditary HCM, steroid induced, infants of diabetic mothers (IDM), Pompe disease, Noonan syndrome, or idiopathic.

- **Restrictive cardiomyopathy (RCM)**

RCM is rare and usually idiopathic in infants and young children. Other causes include hypereosinophilic syndrome, hemochromatosis, glycogen storage disease, post mediastinal radiation, amyloidosis, scleroderma, sickle cell anemia [7], and post-cardiac transplantation.

- **Constrictive pericarditis**

Constrictive pericarditis occurs occasionally following infectious or noninfectious pericarditis. Constrictive pericarditis causes impaired diastolic filling.

Arrhythmias

Arrhythmias can occur acutely or chronically and present either intermittently or incessantly. Arrhythmias may be a cause or consequence of congestive heart failure. Because heart failure and arrhythmias can occur together, determining which problem is primary may be difficult.

Arrhythmias from inflammation are usually ventricular ectopics, ventricular tachycardia, or heart block. Arrhythmias, not from inflammation, frequently have congenital mechanisms.

With heart rates > 220 bpm, supraventricular tachycardia is usually immediately evident, and conversion therapy often occurs quickly. However, tachyarrhythmias with heart rates in the high 100s can sometimes appear similar to sinus tachycardia, yet often present in CHF. Subtle EKG findings may help to differentiate between sinus tachycardia accompanying ventricular dysfunction and primary tachyarrhythmia-induced ventricular dysfunction. Heart block, however, is usually obvious on the EKG. For more on arrhythmias, see Chapter 4.

Arrhythmias that may cause CHF

- Supraventricular tachycardia (SVT)
- Atrial ectopic tachycardia (AET)
- Multifocal atrial tachycardia (MAT)
- Junctional ectopic tachycardia (JET)
- Permanent junctional reciprocating tachycardia (PJRT)
- Congenital or acquired heart block
- Frequent PVCs

5 Heart Failure

EVALUATION

History & Exam

Medical history questions should relate to possible causes because physical exam findings including heart murmurs, gallop rhythms, hepatomegaly, a hyperdynamic precordium, or other signs may be similar regardless the etiology. Check pulses to avoid missing a treatable coarctation of the aorta. The physical exam in cardiac tamponade has unique features including distant heart tones and "pulsus paradoxus" (the near disappearance of the radial pulse, and a significant fall in systolic blood pressure with inspiration).

Testing

Echocardiogram

Even though a chest X-ray (CXR) may precede an Echo, an Echo can be diagnostic or the study can guide additional testing. From the organigram on the top of the facing page, an Echo may demonstrate a clearly identifiable etiology for CHF including tamponade, a structural defect causing volume or pressure overload, a structural defect causing ventricular systolic dysfunction, or structural problem causing ventricular diastolic dysfunction.

However, from the organigram on the bottom of the pacing page, an Echo may demonstrate decreased ventricular function or pulmonary hypertension without elucidating an obvious cause. Such Echo findings require further workup. Cardiac catheterization or other imaging studies might reveal ALCAPA. Laboratory testing may help determine whether CHF stems from an acute myocarditis or chronic conditions like carnitine deficiency.

If all testing for decreased ventricular function is negative, then the patient has an idiopathic cardiomyopathy. For pulmonary hypertension, further investigation may find a pulmonary embolism or a systemic connective tissue disease. Negative testing may result in a diagnosis of primary pulmonary hypertension.

Electrocardiogram

Obtain an EKG quickly in every patient presenting with CHF. The EKG can identify an underlying arrhythmia or ST-T wave changes suggesting inflammation or myocardial ischemia. Failure to diagnose a CHF-causative arrhythmia may delay definitive treatment.

Chest X-ray

Every patient needs a CXR. Although a CXR may precede an Echo, CXR findings are far less specific. Always obtain an Echo before commencing CHF treatment, as cardiomegaly in a CXR may be from a pericardial effusion and not ventricular enlargement. For CXR evaluation, see Chapter 20.

CXR evaluation
- Heart size & position
- Pulmonary edema
- Pulmonary infiltrates
- Pleural effusions

Blood work

Blood work depends on the Echo and EKG findings. A B-natriuretic peptide (BNP) level may be clinically helpful in congenital and acquired disorders. The cardiac ventricles

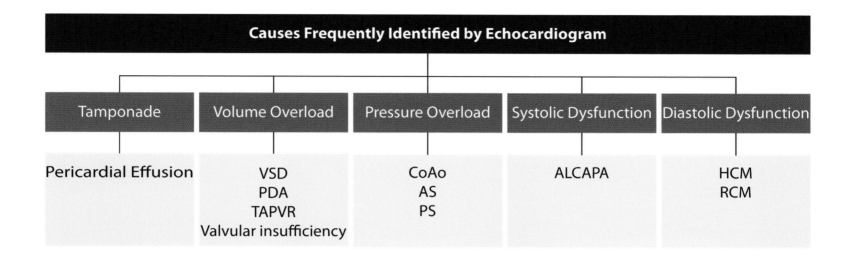

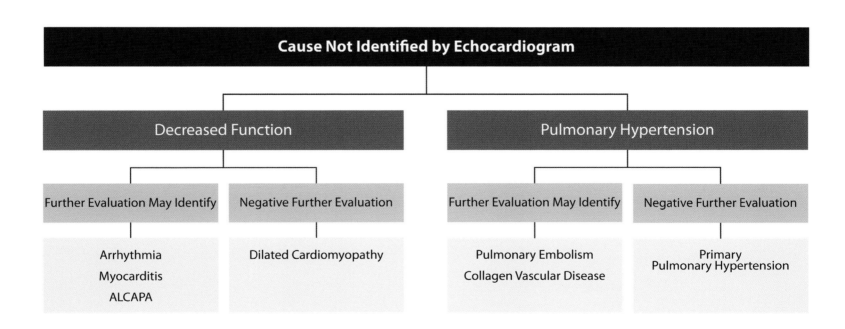

synthesize and secrete BNP. BNP levels increase with ventricular stress from abnormal volume or pressure loads [8, 9]. A patient with a structural problem does not need testing for acute phase reactants, viral titers, or streptococcal antibodies. Nonetheless, if ventricular dysfunction is not from a cardiovascular structural problem, then it is important to obtain additional blood work to evaluate for inflammatory markers, carnitine deficiency, or other metabolic abnormalities.

Tests
- Blood gases
- CBC
- Electrolytes
- BUN & creatinine
- Total protein & albumin
- Liver function tests
- Blood cultures
- Lyme disease titer (especially with heart block)
- Thyroid studies.
- Acute phase reactants (ESR & CRP)
- Streptococcal antibodies
- B-natriuretic peptide (BNP)
- Troponin I, CPK-MB, & CPK index
- Viral titers & cultures
- Urine amino & organic acids
- Serum carnitine & amino acids
- Consider genetic testing

Extended testing

Besides Echo, noninvasive testing may include magnetic resonance imaging (MRI) and computed tomography (CT). Invasive testing may include cardiac catheterization and an EP procedure. All these modalities usually come after an initial workup. Extended testing may discover treatable problems that other evaluation or testing does not disclose. For more on MRI and CT scanning, see Chapter 24. For more on cardiac catheterization and EP procedures, see Chapters 25 and 26.

- **MRI or CT scan**

To evaluate for pericardial thickening consistent with constrictive pericarditis, myocarditis changes, HCM, arrhythmogenic RV cardiomyopathy (ARVC), and to rule out ALCAPA.

- **Cardiac catheterization & angiography**

To rule out ALCAPA, as false positives and false negatives are possible with Echo. To determine pulmonary vascular resistance or the presence of restrictive physiology. Restrictive physiology may be consistent with constrictive pericarditis or restrictive cardiomyopathy.

- **Myocardial biopsy**

To diagnose myocarditis, hypereosinophilic syndrome, hemochromatosis, and other cardiomyopathy causes.

- **EP procedure**

To evaluate, diagnose, or treat an arrhythmia.

℞ OPTIONS

CHF management usually requires medications or procedures to improve the heart's performance. Additionally, treatment should not overlook comorbidities such as respiratory or systemic infections. In some patients, a single pharmacological agent or interventional procedure (like CoA balloon angioplasty) may be beneficial. In many patients, however, effective treatment may require multiple medications, catheter intervention, an EP procedure, or surgery. Begin medicines at minimal therapeutic doses and then titrate up depending on response and side effects. If CHF does not respond to maximal treatment efforts, then heart transplantation may become necessary, especially in deteriorating patients. See Appendix C for medication dosing information.

Tamponade Physiology

Deliver an IV fluid bolus before pericardiocentesis, as peripheral vasodilation usually occurs with preprocedure sedation. Vasodilation may cause a drop in cardiac output before the ameliorating effects of tamponade relief can occur. Although rare, a few reports exist of a paradoxical fall in cardiac output with rapid pericardial fluid removal. Usually, however, the cardiac output acutely rises with pericardial drainage.

Perform pericardiocentesis in an emergency room, intensive care unit, cardiac catheterization laboratory, or in the operating room with trained personnel and cardiac monitoring. Echocardiography guidance may help when performing the procedure outside the operating room.

Volume Overload

Cardiovascular malformations commonly cause CHF from ventricular-volume overload; thus, the definitive treatment is repair by surgery or interventional catheterization. However, circumstances such as infections or prematurity may delay repair. Even in patients old enough or well enough for repair, the medical treatment of CHF before either surgery or interventional catheterization reduces morbidity and mortality.

Acute medical ℞ options

- IV furosemide
- Dialysis for severe volume overload
- IV nesiritide [9]

Chronic medical ℞ options

- Oral furosemide
- Oral hydrochlorothiazide
- Oral angiotensin-converting enzyme (ACE) inhibitors like enalapril (may reduce left-to-right shunts)
- Maximize calories without fluid restriction
- Possibly restrict fluids if on TPN

Pressure Overload

Pressure overload from a coarctation of the aorta, valvular aortic stenosis, or valvular pulmonic stenosis is usually an indication for interventional cardiac catheterization or surgery. Systemic or pulmonary hypertension not arising from structural problems requires medical management.

Systemic HTN acute ℞ options

- IV nitroprusside
- IV nitroglycerine
- IV angiotensin-converting enzyme (ACE) inhibitors like enalapril

Systemic HTN chronic ℞ options

- Oral ACE inhibitors such as enalapril or captopril
- Oral angiotensin II-receptor blockers (ARBs)
- Oral hydralazine

Pulmonary HTN acute ℞ options

- Ventilation
- Inhaled nitric oxide

Pulmonary HTN chronic ℞ options

- Nasal cannula O_2
- Oral phosphodiesterase inhibitors like sildenafil
- Other pulmonary vasodilators per pediatric pulmonary or cardiology consultant

Ventricular Systolic Dysfunction

Treatment includes inotropes to increase ventricular contractility, afterload reducers to decrease the resistance the heart pumps against, diuretics, and possibly anti-inflammatory or anti-viral agents for myocarditis. Occasionally a CoA, AS, or ALCAPA causes decreased left ventricular contractility. These conditions require interventional cardiac catheterization or surgery. Nonetheless, patients with structural problems causing decreased ventricular contractility may experience less morbidity and mortality when such patients undergo stabilization with medical therapy before interventional cardiac catheterization or surgery.

Acute ℞ options

Inotropes

- IV milrinone
- IV dopamine
- IV dobutamine
- IV epinephrine
- IV calcium chloride

Afterload reduction

- IV milrinone

Diuretics

- IV furosemide

Anti-inflammatory & anti-viral agents

Currently, these agents are controversial in myocarditis.

- IV immunoglobulin (IVIG)

More accepted than steroids, but studies are unclear whether benefit exists.

- IV or oral steroids

Currently, controversial in acute viral replication phase.

- Antiviral agents

We rarely use antiviral agents unless tests identify a treatable virus.

- Novel anti-inflammatory agents

Some have used cytolytic therapy (OKT3 and ATG) in a few cases, but there is no consensus on employing these agents in myocarditis except for cardiac-transplant rejection myocarditis. [10]

ECMO or ventricular assist devices

Occasionally, patients need these devices for support, allowing time for improvement or providing a bridge to transplantation.

Chronic ℞ options

- Oral digoxin
- Oral diuretics
- Oral ACE inhibitors like enalapril
- Oral carvedilol [11, 12]
- Oral carnitine for carnitine deficiency
- Resynchronization therapy (a complex pacing method); see Chapter 26 for more information

Ventricular Diastolic Dysfunction

Restrictive cardiomyopathies lack effective medical therapy, and patients usually need heart transplantation. However, hypertrophic cardiomyopathies may occasionally improve with beta-blockers or calcium-channel blockers or both. Constrictive pericarditis may be amenable to pericardial stripping.

Acute ℞ options for HCM

- IV esmolol, especially for IDM cardiomyopathy

Chronic ℞ options for HCM

- Oral beta-blockers like propranolol
- Oral calcium-channel blockers like nifedipine
- Surgical myectomy

Arrhythmias

For more information, see Chapter 4.

Fast rhythms

℞ options for SVT

- Initial conversion
- Chronic medical management
- EP procedure with ablation

℞ options for ectopic tachycardias

Including AET, JET, and PJRT.

- Medications usually ineffective
- EP procedure with ablation

℞ options for ventricular tachycardia

- IV lidocaine
- Electrical cardioversion 2.0 to 4.0 Joules/kg

➤Repeat if no conversion to sinus rhythm. Use a defibrillator equipped with proper size paddles and synchronize with the QRS.

Slow rhythms

℞ options for heart block

- IV isoproterenol for an emergency
- Temporary or permanent pacemaker

Irregular rhythms

Frequent premature ventricular or atrial contractions may also need pharmacological suppression or even EP ablation.

5 Heart Failure

CLINICAL VIGNETTES

9. A 10-year old female presents with shortness of breath and abdominal pain. She was well until about 2 to 3 days before presentation when she developed fever and myalgias. On exam, her temperature is 38° C, respiratory rate of 30 per minute, heart rate of 130 bpm, and a blood pressure of 70/30 mmHg. Her pulses are equal but slightly diminished throughout, and her liver is 2 centimeters below the right costal margin. She has a mildly hyperdynamic precordium with a grade II holosystolic murmur at the apex. Initial laboratory work shows an elevated white blood cell count, an erythrocyte sedimentation rate (ESR) of 50 mm/hr (normal < 10 mm/hr), a troponin I of 5.0 ng/mL (normal < .05 ng/mL), and a B-natriuretic peptide of 850 pg/mL (normal < 100 pg/mL). Before further cardiac testing, her most likely diagnosis:

a. Acute rheumatic fever
b. Myocarditis
c. Idiopathic cardiomyopathy
d. Ventricular septal defect

10. A 3-year old male presents with lethargy. He was well until about 2 months before presentation when the parents noted him becoming tired quickly during play. On exam, he is afebrile, in no significant distress, the respiratory rate is 20 per minute, and the heart is 175 bpm with some heart rate variability. His pulses are equal throughout, and the liver is not palpable. The precordium is quiet, he has no audible murmur. His initial laboratory work shows a normal CBC, normal ESR, normal troponin I, and a BNP of 300 pg/mL. The EKG shows a narrow-QRS tachycardia with unusual P-waves. Before the pediatric cardiologist arrives, his most likely diagnosis:

a. An atrial ectopic tachycardia with cardiomyopathy
b. Pericarditis
c. Coarctation of the aorta
d. Endocarditis

References

1 Kay JD, Colan SD, Graham Jr TD. Congestive heart failure in pediatric patients. Am Heart J 2001; 142: 923-928

2 Hsu DT, Pearson GD. Heart failure in children: part I: history, etiology, and pathophysiology. Circ Heart Fail 2009; 2: 63-67

3 Hsu DT, Pearson GD. Heart failure in children: part II: diagnosis, treatment, and future directions. Circ Heart Fail 2009; 2: 490-498

4 Uhl TL. Viral myocarditis in children. Crit Care Nurse 2008; 28: 42-63

5 Haddad F, Berry G, Doyle RL, Martineau P, Leung TK, Racine N. Active bacterial myocarditis: a case report and review of the literature. J Heart Lung Transplant 2007; 26: 745-749

6 Gottesman GS, Hoffmann JW, Vogler C, Chen SC. Hypertrophic cardiomyopathy in the newborn infant. J Pediatr 1999; 134: 114-118

7 Batra AS, Acherman RJ, Wong WY, Wood JC, Chan LS, Ramicone E, Ebrahimi M, Wong PC. Cardiac abnormalities in children with sickle cell anemia. Am J Hematol 2002; 70: 306-312

8 Koulouri S, Acherman RJ, Wong PC, Chan LS, Lewis AB. Utility of B-type natriuretic peptide in differentiating congestive heart failure from lung disease in pediatric patients with respiratory distress. Pediatr Cardiol 2004; 25: 341-346

9 Favilli S, Frenos S, Lasagni D, Frenos F, Pollini I, Bernini G, Aricò M, Bini RM. The use of B-type natriuretic peptide in paediatric patients: a review of the literature. J Cardiovasc Med (Hagerstown) 2009; 10: 298-302

10 Simsic JM, Mahle WT, Cuadrado A, Kirshbom PM, Maher KO. Hemodynamic effects and safety of nesiritide in neonates with heart failure. J Intensive Care Med 2008; 23: 389-395

11 Ahdoot J, Galindo A, Alejos JC, George B, Burch C, Marelli D, Sadeghi A, Laks H. Use of OKT3 for acute myocarditis in infants and children. J Heart Lung Transplant. 2000; 19: 1118-1121

12 Shaddy RE, Boucek MM, Hsu DT, Boucek RJ, Canter CE Mahony L, Ross RD, Pahl E, Blume ED, Dodd DA, Rosenthal DN, Burr J, LaSalle B, Holubkov R, Lukas MA, Tani LY. Carvedilol for children and adolescents with heart failure: a randomized controlled trial. JAMA 2007; 298: 1171-1179

13 Nishiyama M, Park IS, Yoshikawa, Hatai Y, Ando M, Takahashi Y, Mori K, Murakami Y. Efficacy and safety of carvedilol for heart failure in children and patients with congenital heart disease. Heart Vessels 2009; 24: 187-192

5 Heart Failure

6 Patent Ductus Arteriosus & the Premature Infant

Contents

Background	85
Echo Guided Medical ℞	87
Surgery	88
Clinical Vignettes	90

6 PDA & the Premature Infant

william evans

BACKGROUND

In 1938, Robert Gross, at Boston Children's Hospital, performed the first successful patent ductus arteriosus (PDA) ligations in older infants and children. Twenty-five more years passed before the 1963 report from the Royal Children's Hospital in Melbourne by M.L. Powell. Powell first suggested a pathological association between premature infants and PDAs. In 1963, Helaire Decancq, at the University of Rochester in New York, first reported a PDA ligation in a premature infant. In 1966, Peter Auld at Cornell in New York and Delores Danilowicz and colleagues at Albert Einstein in New York first reported congestive heart failure in prematures with PDAs. Wanda Jegier and colleagues, from Montreal Children's Hospital, reported the first surgical-ligation series of PDAs in prematures with respiratory distress syndrome (RDS) in 1968. In 1969, at the University of California Los Angeles's Harbor General Hospital, Bijan Siassi and colleagues first suggested prolonged ventilation with a PDA may cause bronchopulmonary dysplasia. By the mid-1970s, numerous reports touted indomethacin's effectiveness for closing PDAs in premature infants. [1-8]

Even after more than 3 decades, controversy remains over the indications, modality, and timing of PDA treatment in premature infants with respiratory distress syndrome or other problems complicated by a PDA. In 2007, Ronald Clyman noted a solitary, small, controlled-treatment trial existed, a 1978 report of 15 patients by Robert Cotton. Cotton concluded that a persistent PDA increased respiratory support and pulmonary morbidity. [9,10]

More than 20 years ago, we retrospectively analyzed our approach using IV indomethacin for PDAs in 100 premature infants with RDS. We published our results in a letter-to-the editor format in 1987. Similar to others, we concluded, for premature infants < 1,000 grams, echocardiography-guided, indomethacin treatment within 24 hours of birth resulted in a > 90% closure rate. The closure rate in this group fell to about 50% if treatment were delayed to ≥ 48 hours old. In premature infants > 1,000 grams, we found a similar 85-95% closure rate persisting until about 5 to 6 days old. Beyond that age, the treatment closure rate fell to about 50%. We further discovered, by following this temporal treatment algorithm, our PDA reopening rate was < 5% in both groups, and our overall surgical ligation rate was also < 5%. [11]

Current treatment protocols include early or late indomethacin or ibuprofen, multiple dosing schedules, and surgical ligation. Treatment protocols vary among institutions and among providers within the same institutions. As there are no recent large, controlled studies for treating a patent ductus arteriosus in premature infants with RDS, therapeutic influences for physicians arise from the medical literature, individual or collective experience, and institutional bias. Additionally, recent studies reported a possible genetic risk for PDAs in preterm infants. Possible genetic factors introduce yet more variables [12].

PDA Potential Morbidity

- Worsens RDS
- Risk for pulmonary hemorrhage
- Congestive heart failure
- Bronchopulmonary dysplasia
- Necrotizing enterocolitis (NEC)
- Central nervous system bleed

MANAGEMENT

Diagnosis by Echo

In premature infants, a PDA's physical findings are unreliable. Echocardiography (Echo) is the diagnostic gold standard [13]. As the figure below demonstrates, Echo can determine a PDA's size and the direction of shunt, left-to-right or right-to-left. Echo can determine the shunt's hemodynamic effect including left atrial or left ventricular volume loading. Echo can also measure ventricular function, and rule out a potential complicating structural malformations such as coarctation or other ductal-dependent defects.

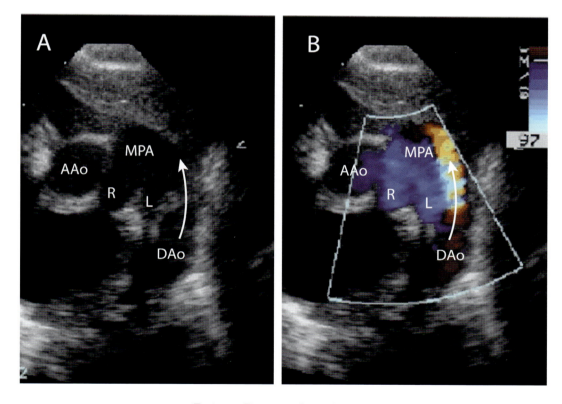

Patent Ductus Arteriosus

2-dimensional (A), and color Doppler evaluation (B). The arrows show the flow direction and the position of the ductus arteriosus connecting the descending aorta (DAo) with the main pulmonary artery (MPA). AAo, ascending aorta; L, left pulmonary artery; R, right pulmonary artery.

Echo-Guided ℞ Options

- < 1,000 grams with RDS

Obtain an Echo in the first 24 hours of age. If the study demonstrates a PDA with predominant left-to-right shunt, then strongly consider pharmacological treatment.

If the initial Echo shows a PDA shunt predominantly right-to-left, then the patient has pulmonary hypertension. As pulmonary hypertension therapy progresses, repeat the study within next 24 hours. If, after 24 hours, the shunt is chiefly left-to-right, then strongly consider treatment.

- > 1,000 grams with RDS

Obtain an Echo within the first 24 to 96 hours of age. If the study shows a PDA with a predominantly left-to-right shunt, then strongly consider pharmacological treatment.

If the initial Echo shows a PDA shunt chiefly right-to-left, then the patient has pulmonary hypertension. As pulmonary hypertension therapy progresses, perform serial Echos to determine whether the shunt becomes left-to-right, and then consider pharmacological treatment.

- Treated patients

Treated patients need followup Echos close in time to the last dose to confirm ductal closure or continued patency. If the PDA remains, then a 2nd treatment course may be necessary. If after 2 treatment courses, the ductus remains open and is a complicating clinical factor, then strongly consider surgical ligation. Ligation after 1 failed medical course, especially in patients < 28 weeks, is also appropriate [14].

- Exceptions

Clinical contraindications including CNS bleeds, NEC, thrombocytopenia, or other conditions may alter any or all the above.

Indomethacin or Ibuprofen ℞

Recent studies suggest indomethacin (Indocin) and ibuprofen (NeoProfen) both achieve similar PDA closure rates. However, studies show ibuprofen has less renal effects and may cause less necrotizing enterocolitis. [15, 16] We list dosing schedules for Indocin and NeoProfen in Appendix C.

Potential ℞ morbidity

Indomethacin

- Oliguria & possible renal failure
- Bleeding, including CNS bleed
- NEC
- Intestinal perforation in < 1.0 kg (apart from NEC [17])
- Hyponatremia & hyperkalemia

Ibuprofen

- Less oliguria & less renal failure than indomethacin
- Bleeding, including CNS bleed
- Studies suggest less NEC than indomethacin
- Hyperbilirubinemia

Surgical Support

Depending on the institution, a pediatric cardiac or pediatric general surgeon, who can perform PDA ligations, should be available. Usually, surgeons perform the procedure in an NICU to avoid possible morbidity associated with transport to an operating room. Obtain an Echo after surgery to confirm PDA closure and to ensure no obstruction to the left pulmonary artery or the aorta.

Surgical morbidities

- Residual PDA

- Obstruction of left pulmonary artery or aorta
- Transient ventricular dysfunction
- Infection
- Pneumothorax
- Chylothorax
- Phrenic nerve paralysis
- Vocal cord paralysis
- Risk of chronic lung disease and retinopathy
- Risk of neurodevelopment abnormalities [18]

CLINICAL VIGNETTES

11. You admit a 26-week gestation, 750 gram premature infant to the neonatal intensive care unit, and you place him on a ventilator for respiratory distress syndrome. At approximately 24 hours of age, an Echo shows a moderate-sized PDA with pure left-to-right shunt, a large left atrium, normal ventricular function, and no structural heart disease. The patient has a normal CBC, normal platelet count, and normal renal function. Appropriate management includes:

a. Prostaglandin to keep the ductus open
b. Indomethacin or ibuprofen for medical PDA closure
c. Antifungal agents for a candida infection
d. Digoxin for congestive heart failure

12. You admit a 32-week, 1,500 gram premature infant to the neonatal intensive care unit. and you place her on a ventilator for severe respiratory distress. At 24 hours of age, an Echo shows a large PDA with a right-to-left shunt, right ventricular enlargement, and significant tricuspid regurgitation. Appropriate management includes:

a. Indomethacin or ibuprofen to medically close the PDA
b. Digoxin for congestive heart failure
c. Treat pulmonary hypertension and repeat an Echo in 24 hours
d. Diuretics and a repeat Echo in 24 hours

References

1 Evans WN. The Blalock-Taussig shunt: the social history of an eponym. Cardiol Young 2009; 19: 119-128

2 Powell ML. Patent ductus arteriosus in premature infants. Med J Aust 1963; 2: 58-60

3 Decancq HG Jr. Repair of patent ductus arteriosus in a 1,417 gm infant. Am J Dis Child 1963; 106: 402-410

4 Auld PA. Delayed closure of the ductus arteriosus. J Pediatr 1966; 69: 61-66

5 Danilowicz D, Rudolph AM, Hoffman JI. Delayed closure of the ductus arteriosus in premature infants. Pediatrics 1966; 37: 74-78

6 Jegier W, Karn G, Stern L. Operative treatment of patent ductus arteriosus complicating respiratory distress syndrome of the premature. Can Med Assoc J 1968; 98:105

7 Siassi B, Emmanouilides GC, Cleveland RJ, Hirose F. Patent ductus arteriosus complicating prolonged assisted ventilation in respiratory distress syndrome. J Pediatr 1969; 74: 11-19

8 Heyman MA, Rudolph AM, Silverman NH. Closure of the ductus arteriosus in premature infants by inhibition of prostaglandin synthesis. NEJM 1976; 295: 530-533

9 Clyman RI, Chorne N. Patent ductus arteriosus: evidence for and against treatment. J Pediatr 2007; 150: 216-219

10 Cotton RB, Stahlman MT, Bender HW, Graham TP, Catterton WZ, Kovar I. Randomized trial of early closure of symptomatic patent ductus arteriosus in small preterm infants. J Pediatr 1978; 93: 647-651

11 Evans WN, Cass KA, Feldman BH. Indomethacin therapy for patent ductus arteriosus. Am J Dis Child 1987; 141: 1042

12 Dagle JM, Lepp NT, Cooper ME, Schaa KL, Kelsey KJ, Orr KL, Caprau D, Zimmerman CR, Steffen KM, Johnson KJ, Marazita ML, Murray JC. Determination of genetic predisposition to patent ductus arteriosus in preterm infants. Pediatrics 2009; 123: 1116-1123

13 Skelton R, Evans N, Smythe J. A blinded comparison of clinical and echocardiographic evaluation of the preterm infant for patent ductus arteriosus. J Paediatr Child Health 1994; 30: 406-411

14 Hafeez U, Watkinson M. When is a second course of indomethacin effective in ventilated neonates with patent ductus arteriosus? http://www.neonatal-nursing.co.uk/pdf/inf_016_acs.pdf

15 Van Overmeire B, Smets K, Lecoutere D, Van de Broek H, Weyler J, Degroote K, Langhendries JP. A comparison of ibuprofen and indomethacin for closure of patent ductus arteriosus. N Engl J Med 2000; 343: 674-681

16 Ohlsson A, Walia R, Shah SS. Ibuprofen for the treatment of patent ductus arteriosus in preterm and/or low birth weight infants. Cochrane Database Syst Rev. 2008; 1: CD003481

17 Novack CM, Waffam F, Sills JH, Pousti TJ, Warden MJ, Cunningham MD. Focal intestinal perforation in the extremely-low-birth-weight infant. J Perinatol 1994; 14: 450-456

18 Kabra NS, Schmidt B, Roberts RS, Doyle LW, Papile L, Fanaroff A. Neurosensory impairment after surgical closure of patent ductus arteriosus in extremely low birth weight infants: results from the Trial of Indomethacin Prophylaxis in Preterms. J Pediatr 2007; 150: 229-234

6 PDA & the Premature Infant

7 Oxygen Desaturation

Contents

Background	95
Newborns	96
Newborn Workup	98
Newborn management	101
Older infant & Child	103
Clinical Vignettes	106

7 Oxygen Desaturation

carlos luna

BACKGROUND

As a presenting problem, a low pulse-oximeter reading is more common than visible cyanosis. In blood, oxygen binds chiefly to hemoglobin. A pulse-oximeter measures the percentage of hemoglobin saturated with oxygen, but the common nomenclature is "oxygen saturation." Oxygen saturation at sea level is ≥ 95%. Clinical cyanosis is often lacking with mild oxygen desaturation (> 85% but < 94% in room air); nonetheless, some patients with "cyanotic" congenital heart disease can present with oxygen saturations in this range. Most patients with oxygen desaturation present as newborns, but occasionally an older infant or child presents with oxygen desaturation.

Etiologies

- Persistent pulmonary hypertension of the newborn (PPHN)
- Primary respiratory problems
- Cardiovascular malformations
- Acrocyanosis
- Methemoglobinemia

Right-to-Left Shunts

The term "right-to-left shunt" may cause confusion. The term originated with cardiovascular defects. Normally, deoxygenated blood is on the right side of heart and saturated blood on the left side. When desaturated blood mixes with saturated blood through an atrial or a ventricular septal defect, the blood moves from the right side of the heart to the left side of the heart, a "right-to-left shunt" (left figure below). However, in dextrocardia or other conditions, deoxygenated blood is often on the left side of the heart and the oxygenated blood is on the right side. The term "right-to-left shunt" persists when desaturated blood mixes with saturated blood (right figure below). Therefore, a "right-to-left shunt" is the pathological condition of desaturated blood mixing with saturated blood regardless of the anatomical direction of blood flow, or even when the "right-to-left" shunt occurs outside the heart. A similar but opposite explanation exists for left-to-right shunts. [1-8]

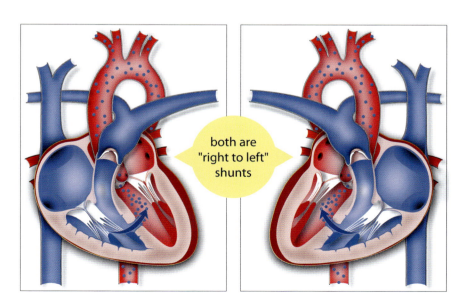

both are "right to left" shunts

CAUSES IN NEWBORNS

PPHN

Persistent pulmonary hypertension of the newborn usually presents immediately at birth. PPHN is a failure in the normal, newborn drop of pulmonary arterial pressure and pulmonary vascular resistance. For more on normal neonatal-physiological changes, see Chapter 18. "Persistent fetal circulation (PFC)" is a misnomer, as the fetal circulation does not persist in its entirety postnatally.

PPHN is either primary (unidentifiable cause), or secondary to a another problem. Primary and secondary PPHN have decreased pulmonary blood flow and a right-to-left ductus arteriosus shunt. Furthermore, both conditions usually have a foramen ovale right-to-left shunt. Intrapulmonary right-to-left shunts also frequently complicate secondary PPHN.

- Primary

Primary PPHN results from unclear mechanisms; however, the condition likely arises through abnormal in utero fetal pulmonary-arteriolar development. Maldeveloped, fetal pulmonary arterioles fail to relax at birth, preventing the normal, neonatal drop in pulmonary vascular resistance and pressure. Since primary PPHN occurs without obvious lung or airway disease, a clear chest X-ray is typical.

- Secondary

Perinatal asphyxia, meconium aspiration syndrome, pneumonia, sepsis, hyaline membrane disease, pneumothorax, pleural effusions, chest masses, pulmonary hypoplasia, and diaphragmatic hernia. Plus, airway pathology we list under "Primary respiratory problems." An abnormal chest X-ray typifies secondary PPHN.

Primary Respiratory Problems

Respiratory problems can cause intrapulmonary right-to-left shunts because diseased lung segments prevent normal oxygenation of desaturated pulmonary-arterial blood. Instead, desaturated blood from the lung's diseased parts passes directly to the pulmonary veins where the desaturated blood mixes with oxygenated blood from normal lung segments. These conditions may or may not occur with pulmonary hypertension.

- Airway pathology

Choanal atresia, macroglossia, micrognathia, nasopharyngeal mass, laryngo- and bronchomalacia, laryngeal web, vocal cord paralysis, mucous plug, or vascular ring.

- Lung pathology

All the conditions we note under secondary PPHN.

- Gastrointestinal

Gastroesophageal reflux and bronchoaspiration.

- Central nervous system

Apnea, hypoxic induced encephalopathy, or neuromuscular mediated hypoventilation.

Cardiovascular Problems

For more on the following cardiovascular malformations, see Chapter 19.

The 5 "Ts"

- **T**etralogy of Fallot (ToF)
- **T**ransposition of the great arteries (TGA)
- **T**otal anomalous pulmonary venous return (TAPVR)

- **T**ricuspid atresia
- **T**runcus arteriosus

Other defects

- Double outlet right ventricle (DORV)
- Pulmonary atresia with intact ventricular septum
- Ebstein anomaly of the tricuspid valve
- 1-functional ventricles
- Congenital pulmonary arteriovenous malformations

Special circumstances

- **AVSD with pulmonary hypertension**

Right-to-left intracardiac shunts are possible in patients with complete atrioventricular septal defects (AVSD).

- **Critical valvular pulmonic stenosis**

Pulmonary blood flow may become so restricted with severe obstruction that the obstruction forces blood to cross the right atrium into the left atrium or to cross a VSD into the left ventricle, thereby creating a right-to-left shunt.

- **The hypoplastic left heart syndrome**

The hypoplastic left heart syndrome (HLHS), with the ductus arteriosus open in the first hours after birth, can present with subtle oxygen desaturation because a severely underdeveloped left ventricle forces the saturated pulmonary venous blood to the right atrium. From the right atrium, the pulmonary venous blood mixes with all the desaturated systemic venous blood, and the right ventricle pumps the mixture of saturated and desaturated blood to the lungs and to the body via the ductus arteriosus. The ductus arteriosus provides all the systemic blood flow and maintains normal cardiac output. Desaturated blood coming from the ductus is the right-to-left shunt causing oxygen desaturation. However, extremis results when the ductus closes.

Acrocyanosis

Observable cyanosis can also be peripheral (acrocyanosis). Peripheral cyanosis can occur in newborns or older patients. Acrocyanosis usually does not arise from a pathological process. An anatomic right-to-left shunt does not underlie acrocyanosis; consequently, contrary to central cyanosis, mucous membranes remain pink. Acrocyanosis usually stems from a physiological response to cold stress, chiefly affecting the hands and feet and the area around the mouth (especially in light complexioned infants). Increased oxygen extraction in areas with sluggish blood flow causes acrocyanosis. Pulse-oximeter recordings are normal in a warmed hand or foot. Occasionally acrocyanosis can also result from polycythemia with hyperviscosity or low cardiac output.

Methemoglobinemia

Methemoglobinemia is a rare cause of low pulse-oximeter readings or visible cyanosis. An anatomic right-to-left shunt is not present with methemoglobinemia. Methemoglobinemia can occur in newborns or older patients. Methemoglobinemia has congenital and acquired causes. These conditions prevent oxygen from binding to hemoglobin. Besides central cyanosis, patients may also have shortness of breath, mental status changes, headache, fatigue, dysrhythmias, seizures, and coma. As methemoglobinemia does not affect dissolved oxygen, arterial blood gas (ABG) PaO_2 is normal.

Congenital

- NADH-methemoglobin reductase deficiency
- Abnormal hemoglobins

Acquired

- Drugs, including benzocaine, lidocaine, and sulfa
- Toxins, including nitrates (occasionally in well water)

NEWBORN WORKUP

The first observation or question should be: Is the desaturated patient comfortable or tachypneic with respiratory distress? Generally, comfortable oxygen desaturation means a congenital cardiovascular defect, and oxygen desaturation with distress indicates PPHN or a primary respiratory problem. Nevertheless, newborns can have PPHN complicated by both a cardiac problem and meconium aspiration or other combinations. Furthermore, cardiac problems with pulmonary edema or obstructed pulmonary venous return can present with oxygen desaturation and respiratory distress.

History & Exam

Place the newborn in a neutral thermal environment and check the airway patency and general condition. The evaluation's intensity and management should mirror the clinical severity. With a stable patient or one in minimal distress, give oxygen via hood, mask, or nasal cannula, and monitor oxygen saturations and blood gases before and after starting oxygen (also called an oxygen challenge test). A neonate with severe hypoxia, respiratory distress, or hemodynamic instability needs intubation and umbilical lines. These actions may be unnecessary, and may even be harmful, in a neonate without distress. Simultaneous to initial evaluation and management, ask relevant medical history questions and note pertinent positive or negative physical exam findings.

Prenatal history

- Advanced maternal age
- Pregnancy induced hypertension (PIH)
- Preeclampsia
- Maternal diabetes & elevated maternal BMI
- Maternal reactive airway disease
- Maternal fever & group B streptococcus status
- Maternal medications
- Maternal or other family history of heart defects
- Oligo- & polyhydramnios
- Fetal distress

Delivery history

- Maternal anesthesia
- C-section
- Placental abruption
- Uterine rupture
- Maternal hemorrhage
- Premature rupture of membranes
- Prenatal distress & difficult delivery
- Cord prolapse or nuchal cord

Postnatal history

- Delivery room resuscitation
- Low Apgar scores
- Meconium aspiration

Exam

- Small or large for gestational age
- Post dates
- Presence of dysmorphic features
- Presence or absence of retractions
- Stridor or airway noise
- Scaphoid abdomen in diaphragmatic hernia
- Abnormal heart rate & rhythm

- Abnormal 4-extremity pulses & blood pressures
- Hyperdynamic precordium or quiet precordium
- Presence or absence of murmurs
- Decreased breath sounds in hyaline membrane disease
- Unilateral breath sounds
- Wheezing in meconium aspiration or pulmonary edema
- Presence or absence of hepatomegaly

Oxygen Response

A patient's response to oxygen underlies the initial evaluation and management. Oxygen response helps distinguish primary cardiovascular defects from PPHN or respiratory pathology. If the initial arterial blood gas demonstrates a high PCO_2 and a low PaO_2, and supplemental oxygen and ventilation improve both, then the condition is likely a respiratory problem or PPHN. Further, pre- and post-ductal pulse-oximeter measurements can be helpful. If the preductal (upper extremity) oxygen saturation is > 5% higher than the post-ductal (lower extremity) oxygen saturation, then usually PPHN is present. The difference in oxygen saturation values arises from the right-to-left shunt across the ductus arteriosus, as a right-to-left ductus shunt delivers blood with low oxygen saturation to the descending aorta and lower extremities. However, cardiac malformations may complicate these findings, as some defects can also produce differential oxygen saturations values.

Without PPHN or a primary respiratory problem, blood gases in cardiovascular causes of oxygen desaturation show a low PaO_2 with a normal or low PCO_2. In cardiovascular causes, oxygen supplementation, even with an FiO_2 of 100%, may show no significant increase in PaO_2; although, the pulse-oximeter readings may rise to > 90%.

Tests

Principal ones include laboratory tests, chest X-ray (CXR), and an echocardiogram (Echo). An EKG is not helpful unless for arrhythmia evaluation or to check for myocardial stress related ST-T wave changes. An EKG rarely rules congenital heart disease in or out.

Laboratory tests

Common

- Blood gases
- Glucose
- Electrolytes
- Blood cultures

B-natriuretic peptide (BNP)

The cardiac ventricles synthesize and secrete BNP. BNP levels increase with ventricular volume or pressure overload.

Chest X-ray

Have the CXR film brought to the bedside for direct visualization, or go personally to radiology and review the film rather than waiting for a report.

Important observations

- Endotracheal tube position
- Heart size
- Heart position (left, right, or midline)
- Stomach bubble & liver positions
- Pulmonary vascularity
- Aeration of lung fields
- Presence or absence of parenchymal disease
- Masses or other space occupying conditions
- Effusions
- Rib or vertebral anomalies

Echo

An Echo can differentiate a cardiovascular malformation from PPHN or other respiratory problems. An Echo can further provide a structural and functional cardiovascular diagnosis.

Additionally, we can diagnose right-to-left shunts (intracardiac or across a PDA) using color-flow Doppler or with contrast Echo. For contrast Echo, we inject a small volume of agitated normal saline in a peripheral or central vein. The microbubbles formed during normal saline agitation appear as a fine "white mist" on the Echo image. With a right-to-left shunt, we can image the "white mist" as it passes from right atrium to left atrium through an atrial communication or from right ventricle to left ventricle through a VSD.

Continuous-wave (CW) Doppler Echo can provide quantitative measurements of right ventricular systolic pressure by measuring the velocity of the tricuspid regurgitation jet. If the absence of pulmonic stenosis, the RV systolic pressure equates to the pulmonary artery systolic pressure.

Another method to estimate pulmonary pressure employs CW Doppler for measuring the pressure difference across a PDA. With a high pulmonary artery (PA) pressure, the pressure difference is minimal between the pulmonary artery and the aorta through the ductus. Therefore, the CW Doppler flow velocity through the PDA is minimal when the PA pressure is equal or nearly equal to the aortic pressure. The CW Doppler velocity through the PDA is high when the PA pressure is low compared to the aortic pressure.

Doppler Echo can guide PPHN treatment via reevaluation of pulmonary arterial pressures primarily by CW Doppler interrogation of the tricuspid regurgitation jet peak velocity. For more on Echo, see Chapter 22.

NEWBORN MANAGEMENT

PPHN

Treating PPHN may include oxygen, ventilation, additional pulmonary artery vasodilators, and management of underlying problems. Underlying problems can include a combination of conditions such as an infection and a diaphragmatic hernia. A few patients, not improving with aggressive ventilation and optimal medical management, may need extracorporeal membrane oxygenation (ECMO). ECMO equipment uses a artificial-membrane oxygenator to function as the patient's lungs. Specialized centers perform ECMO.

Interventions

- Oxygen at high FiO_2s
- High-frequency ventilation
- Minimal handling
- Sedate or paralyze
- Optimize systemic blood pressure
- High normal blood PH, avoid acidosis
- Optimize hemoglobin & hematocrit
- Antibiotics
- Correct hypoglycemia
- Inhaled nitric oxide
- IV magnesium sulfate (if nitric oxide unavailable)
- Oral sildenafil & IV sildenafil [9-11]
- Follow progress with Echo
- May need ECMO

Primary Respiratory Problems

Respiratory problems include myriad conditions. The primary disease process influences the management.

Interventions

- Surfactant for hyaline membrane disease
- Antibiotics for pneumonias
- Chest tubes for a pneumothorax or effusions
- Oxygen & ventilation
- Surgery for diaphragmatic hernia or other lung masses
- Tracheostomy for proximal airway problems
- May need ECMO for severe problems

Cardiovascular Problems

An Echo can define the anatomy of most cardiovascular malformations. CT and MRI are important tools that can help refine a complex anatomical diagnosis. Still, some patients may need cardiac catheterization with or without an interventional procedure. Most patients require palliative or corrective therapeutic procedures. Before cardiac catheterization or surgery, infants with serious heart disease often need initial treatment with prostaglandin E1 (PGE1). A pharmacologically-maintained patent ductus arteriosus allows steady pulmonary blood flow with severe pulmonary artery obstruction and systemic flow to the body in aortic obstruction. See the chapters on Cardiac Catheter Intervention and Cardiovascular Surgery for further explanation.

Diagnostic & ℞ options

Prostaglandin E1

Prostaglandin side effects are common and include the following:

- Apnea

- CNS depression & occasional seizures
- Hypotension
- Flushing
- Fever
- Bleeding, as PGE1 inhibits platelet aggregation

Diagnostic & interventional cardiac catheterization

- Angiography

Angiography can detail complex intra and extracardiac anatomy, and the images assist surgical planning.

- Balloon atrial septostomy

Transposition of the great arteries usually requires a balloon atrial septostomy (BAS). BAS improves mixing at atrial level, allowing the heart to pump additional saturated blood to the body, reducing cyanosis.

- Balloon valvuloplasty

Valvuloplasty of a critically stenotic pulmonary valve increases pulmonary blood flow and reduces the right-to-left shunt at atrial level, improving oxygen saturation.

3D imaging with CT or MRI

- May help define extracardiac anatomy

Surgical palliation for restricted pulmonary blood flow

- Systemic artery-to-pulmonary artery shunt
- Interventional cath for PDA or RV outflow tract stents

Surgical palliation for unrestricted pulmonary blood flow

- Pulmonary artery band
- Pulmonary artery transection & systemic-to-pulmonary artery shunt

Surgical correction

- Arterial switch operation (ASO) for TGA
- Repair TAPVR
- Repair of truncus arteriosus

Surgical palliation with the Norwood or Sano procedure

- Hypoplastic left heart syndrome & its variants

Hybrid procedure

In newborns, the hybrid procedure includes initial surgical palliation, usually without cardiopulmonary bypass (CPB), and the placement of intracardiovascular devices in the cardiac catheterization laboratory. More recently, surgeons and cardiologists can accomplish their respective procedures in a hybrid operating room-catheterization laboratory. In small infants, hybrid procedures avoid the potential negative effects of CPB, as complex surgical repairs require CPB. [12] For more on hybrid procedures, see Chapters 25 and 27. Defects treatable with the hybrid procedure include the following:

- Hypoplastic left heart syndrome
- Complex aortic arch problems

Methemoglobinemia

- IV methylene blue
- Oral methylene blue for congenital forms

OLDER INFANTS & CHILDREN

An older infant or child presenting with oxygen desaturation is less common than a newborn presentation. Respiratory causes are far more common than cardiovascular causes, as newborn cyanotic congenital heart disease rarely escapes detection.

A B-natriuretic peptide (BNP) level can help differentiate a primary respiratory problem from congestive heart failure [13]. However, pulmonary hypertension also elevates BNP levels.

Primary Respiratory Problems

- **Pneumonias**

Pneumonias often have desaturation from intrapulmonary right-to-left shunts.

- **Respiratory syncitial virus (RSV)**

RSV pneumonia causes significant morbidity and mortality, especially in infants and young children with congenital heart disease. During the fall and winter when RSV is common, a series of monthly-parenteral doses of palivizumab (Synagis) may prevent RSV pneumonia in patients ≤ 2 years. Synagis is a humanized monoclonal antibody (IgG), which acts against the RSV particle.

- **Reactive airway disease (asthma)**

Asthma with oxygen desaturation is a dangerous clinical finding, usually preceding respiratory failure. Such patients require intensive care observation and treatment.

Cardiovascular Problems

A few conditions can escape early detection. The 3 most common malformations that cause desaturation or cyanosis that can present in later infancy or childhood include tetralogy of Fallot, unobstructed total anomalous pulmonary venous return, and pulmonary arteriovenous malformations.

Rare conditions include primary pulmonary hypertension (PPH) and Eisenmenger syndrome. PPH requires complex evaluation and management. If a large VSD or other cardiovascular abnormalities escape detection, then the patient may eventually develop Eisenmenger syndrome that includes pulmonary hypertension and desaturation. Please refer to comprehensive textbooks for descriptions of PPH and Eisenmenger syndrome.

Tetralogy of Fallot

Occasionally, a newborn with tetralogy of Fallot (ToF) escapes detection at birth. The initial newborn exam may consist of an easily missed soft murmur and no cyanosis. The murmur may be soft as the pulmonic stenosis may be initially mild. Pulmonic stenosis in ToF often progressively worsens. Thus, the first presentation may be a hypercyanotic episode or "Tet spell."

Events that increase heart rate and contractility may trigger a Tet spell. Increased heart rate, contractility, and peripheral vasodilation—especially in combination—cause a further decrease in pulmonary blood flow. Conditions causing this cascade include fever, irritability, crying, dehydration, or even a warm bath or shower.

A vicious circle may develop where the initial events decrease pulmonary blood flow and increase the right-to-left shunt through the VSD, followed by increasing cyanosis. Increasing cyanosis stimulates the respiratory

7 Oxygen Desaturation

drive causing hyperpnea. Hyperpnea increases systemic venous return, increasing the blood in the right ventricle. The extra right-ventricular blood shunts right-to-left through the VSD, further decreasing arterial PaO_2. Severe cyanosis may cause seizures, apnea, and occasionally death. A patient presenting with a Tet spell can appear in extremis, leading some to initiate inotropic therapy. Inotropes worsen a Tet spell. A patient having a Tet spell requires targeted treatment.

Tet spell ℞ options

General

- **Comfort**

Calming the infant reduces intrathoracic pressure, allowing enhanced pulmonary blood flow, which decrease the right-to-left shunt through the VSD. Calming also decreases circulating catecholamines. Excess catecholamines accentuate muscle contraction of the RV outflow tract, which limits pulmonary flow.

- **Knee chest position**

This maneuver increases the systemic vascular resistance. Increased systemic vascular resistance increases left ventricular pressure and drives additional blood across the VSD to the lungs, increasing pulmonary blood flow and oxygen saturation.

- **IV fluids**

Patients experiencing a Tet spell may be ill or febrile, leading to dehydration.

- **Oxygen**

Oxygen is of questionable benefit. If the mask or hood causes the patient distress, then stop giving oxygen.

- **Avoid inotropes**

Dopamine, dobutamine, epinephrine, or milrinone all increase the contraction of the RV outflow tract, further decreasing pulmonary blood flow and accentuating the right-to-left shunt through the VSD. Milrinone also decreases systemic vascular resistance, which increases the right-to-left shunt. Therefore, avoid milrinone for both reasons.

Specific

- **Subcutaneous or intramuscular morphine**

For deeper sedation, but watch for respiratory depression.

- **IV esmolol**

Beta-blockers help relax a hypercontractile right ventricular outflow tract, allowing additional desaturated blood to enter the lungs. This process increases the arterial oxygen saturation. Although short-term beta-blockers have a role, avoid long-term beta-blockers as palliation before surgery; rather, any patient experiencing a Tet spell should have emergent or semi-urgent surgery.

- **IV sodium bicarbonate**

Correct acidosis, as acidosis also decreases pulmonary blood flow.

- **IV phenylephrine**

Increases the systemic vascular resistance by causing vasoconstriction, driving desaturated blood into the lungs and increasing the oxygen saturation.

- **General anesthesia**

Occasionally, a Tet spell requires relief via general anesthesia. However, an expert in pediatric anesthesiology should administer the medications.

- **Emergency surgery**

Patient may require emergent repair or a systemic-to-pulmonary artery shunt.

Unobstructed Total Anomalous Pulmonary Venous Return

Total anomalous pulmonary venous return (TAPVR) usually presents with oxygen desaturation or cyanosis shortly after birth. Nonetheless, symptoms may occur late if the patient has unobstructed anomalous pulmonary veins. Oxygen desaturation may be insignificant enough to cause visible cyanosis. If symptoms are absent and oxygen desaturation fails detection at birth, then an infant with TAPVR may go home from the newborn nursery. Infants invariably present later with respiratory distress from pulmonary overcirculation or with pneumonia, especially RSV. Reports of late presentations in infancy and even in young children exist. Echocardiography is usually diagnostic, but a CT scan may also help plan surgical treatment.

Pulmonary arteriovenous malformations

Pulmonary arteriovenous malformations (PAVMs) are communications between pulmonary arteries and pulmonary veins that bypass the pulmonary alveoli. Most PAVMs are congenital and are more common in females. Some occur with hereditary hemorrhagic telangiectasia. Other conditions with PAVMs include liver disease, trauma, and chronic pulmonary inflammatory problems. Most PAVMs occur in the lower lung lobes and most are unilateral. Some PAVMs are microscopic but most have vessels a few millimeters to several centimeters in diameter.

The clinical presentation may include cough, dyspnea, hemoptysis, clubbing, and progressive cyanosis. PAVMs increase the risk for paradoxical embolization, stroke, and brain abscess. Imaging includes contrast echocardiography, chest X-ray, CT or MRI scans, and pulmonary angiography.

Small PAVMs may need no treatment, but significant cases may benefit from cardiac catheterization and embolization or surgical resection of affected lung segments.

7 Oxygen Desaturation

CLINICAL VIGNETTES

13. The staff calls you to see a 12-hour old full-term male infant with an oxygen saturation of 70%, not improving with supplemental oxygen by nasal cannula. On exam, the infant is in no distress, features suggest possible chromosome 22q11 deletion (see Chapter 3). The pulses are equal throughout, and the liver is not palpable. The precordium is slightly hyperdynamic and there is a grade III systolic ejection murmur. The chest X-ray shows a normal-sized heart and hyperlucent lung fields. Before cardiac testing, the most likely diagnosis:

a. Small VSD
b. Persistent pulmonary hypertension of the newborn
c. Transposition of the great arteries without VSD
d. Tetralogy of Fallot with significant PS

14. The staff calls you to the delivery room to evaluate an infant in distress. On exam, the respiratory rate is > 100, the oxygen saturation in the right upper extremity is 90% and 75% in the lower extremity, the abdomen appears scaphoid. The heart rate is 195 bpm, and you hear heart tones best on the right, and there is no murmur. The chest X-ray shows the heart in the right chest and the stomach bubble in the left chest. The most likely diagnosis:

a. Left-sided diaphragmatic hernia with secondary PPHN
b. Transposition of the great arteries
c. Primary PPHN
d. Methemoglobinemia

References

1 Steinhorn RH. Evaluation and management of the cyanotic neonate. Clin Pediatr Emerg Med 2008; 9: 169-175

2 Marino BS, Bird GL, Wernovsky G. Diagnosis and management of the newborn with suspected congenital heart disease. Clinics in Perinatology 2001; 28: 91-136

3 Rohan AJ, Golombek SG. Hypoxia in the term newborn: part one-cardiopulmonary physiology and assessment. MCN Am J Matern Child Nurs. 2009; 34: 106-112

4 Konduri GG, Kim UO. Advances in the diagnosis and management of persistent pulmonary hypertension of the newborn. Pediatr Clin North Am 2009; 56: 579-600

5 Hernández-Díaz S, Van Marter LJ, Werler MM, Louik C, Mitchell AA. Risk factors for persistent pulmonary hypertension of the newborn. Pediatrics 2007; 120: e272-e282

6 Tibballs J, Chow CW. Incidence of alveolar capillary dysplasia in severe idiopathic persistent pulmonary hypertension of the newborn. J Paediatr Child Health 2002; 38: 397-400

7 Van Heijst A, Haasdijk R, Groenman F, van der Staak F, Hulsbergen-van de Kaa C, de Krijger R, Tibboel D. Morphometric analysis of the lung vasculature after extracorporeal membrane oxygenation treatment for pulmonary hypertension in newborns. Virchows Arch. 2004; 445: 36-44

8 Rehman HU. Methemoglobinemia. West J Med 2001; 175: 193-196

9 Baquero H, Soliz A, Neira F, Venegas ME, Sola A. Oral sildenafil in infants with persistent pulmonary hypertension of the newborn: a pilot randomized blinded study. Pediatrics 2006; 117: 1077-1083

10 Krishnan U. Management of pulmonary arterial hypertension in the neonatal unit. Cardiol Rev 2010; 18:73-75

11 Steinhorn RH, Kinsella JP, Pierce C, Butrous G, Dilleen M, Oakes M, Wessel DL. Intravenous sildenafil in the treatment of neonates with persistent pulmonary hypertension. J Pediatr 2009; 155: 841-847 e1

12 Honjo O, Caldarone CA. Hybrid palliation for neonates with hypoplastic left heart syndrome: current strategies and outcomes. Korean Circ J 2010; 40: 103-111

13 Koulouri S, Acherman RJ, Wong PC, Chan LS, Lewis AB. Utility of B-type natriuretic peptide in differentiating congestive heart failure from lung disease in pediatric patients with respiratory distress. Pediatr Cardiol 2004; 25: 341-346

7 Oxygen Desaturation

8 Extremis

Contents

Background	**111**
Delivery room	**112**
Later Presentation	**114**
℞ options	**116**
Clinical Vignettes	**118**

8 Extremis

william evans

BACKGROUND

A patient presenting *"in extremis"* (Latin for "at the point of death") needs resuscitation and a quick, etiology-category assessment, even when a clinician cannot rapidly make a definite diagnosis. Fundamentally, severe abnormalities in cardiac output or gas exchange cause extremis. Newborns and young infants more often present in extremis than older infants and children. Using a checklist of etiology categories, quickly consider each one. If, for example, a clinician presumes sepsis without considering any other cause, then an infant with hypoplastic left heart syndrome can die without the benefit of prostaglandin. [1-4]

Etiology Categories
- Cardiovascular
- Hydrops (newborn specific)
- Respiratory
- Gastrointestinal
- Sepsis
- Anemia & hypovolemia
- Trauma
- Drugs or toxins
- Endocrine & inborn errors of metabolism (IEM)
- Anaphylaxis

Every patient presenting in extremis needs an immediate cardiac rhythm assessment via a cardiac monitor and a 12-lead EKG, a chest X-ray, an abdominal X-ray, and an echocardiogram (Echo). Immediate blood work should include CBC, arterial blood gases, blood cultures, urine analysis, and a comprehensive metabolic panel. If trauma is the differential diagnosis, then patients should quickly undergo additional radiography studies like a head CT scan. Also, obtain toxicology studies when you suspect poisoning or drug ingestion. Anaphylaxis requires immediate recognition and administration of epinephrine.

DELIVERY ROOM PRESENTATION

A newborn can present in extremis in the delivery room. If a mother has had no prenatal care or poor prenatal care, then significant fetal abnormalities may escape detection until delivery. Beyond standard delivery room resuscitation, a neonate with a cardiovascular condition may need immediate transfer to a cardiac catheterization laboratory or operating room. Newborns presenting in extremis have dismal outcomes.

Cardiovascular Problems
Malformations

- Ebstein anomaly of the tricuspid valve

Severe tricuspid regurgitation in utero can cause severe hydrops and "wall-to-wall" heart size on chest X-ray.

- HLHS with an intact atrial septum

An intact atrial septum, in hypoplastic left heart syndrome (HLHS), obstructs all the pulmonary venous blood within the left atrium. The intact atrial septum completely blocks pulmonary venous blood, causing severe respiratory distress and extremely low oxygen saturations.

- TGA with intact atrial & ventricular septa

Transposition of the great arteries (TGA) with intact septa prevents intracardiac mixing of saturated and desaturated blood, causing extremely low oxygen saturations.

- Severe ToF with an absent PDA

Tetralogy of Fallot (ToF) with severe obstruction to essentially all pulmonary blood flow results in severe oxygen desaturation.

- TAPVR with pulmonary venous obstruction

Total anomalous pulmonary venous return (TAPVR) with severe obstruction blocks all pulmonary venous blood returning to the heart, causing severe respiratory distress and extremely low oxygen saturations.

Arrhythmias

- Heart block

Fetal heart rates less < 50s may cause severe in utero heart failure.

- SVT or atrial flutter

Rapid fetal heart rates from supraventricular tachycardia or atrial flutter may also cause severe in utero heart failure.

Inflammation

- Myocarditis

In utero myocarditis, whether viral, bacterial, or from other causes, may cause severe in utero heart failure.

- Pericardial effusion

Pericardial effusions can occur with in utero heart failure, immune hydrops, nonimmue hydrops, or from other inflammatory reactions.

Asphyxia

- Myocardial depression

Myocardial depression can occur from perinatal asphyxia either chronically or acutely.

Idiopathic cardiomyopathy

- In utero cardiomyopathy

An idiopathic cardiomyopathy may present in the delivery room with severe CHF and hydrops.

Hydrops

- **Immune hydrops**

90% of immune hydrops results from Rh disease, 1% from ABO incompatibility, and 9% from other incompatibilities.

- **Nonimmune hydrops**

Nonimmune hydrops can result from the cardiovascular problems we list above, and from chromosomal syndromes, chest masses, tumors, infections, gastrointestinal abnormalities, genitourinary malformations, twin-twin transfusion, thyroid disorders, some inborn errors of metabolism, or be idiopathic.

Respiratory

- **Diaphragmatic hernia or chest mass**

A diaphragmatic hernia or chest mass may severely compromise lung function and present with severe respiratory distress and extremely low oxygen saturations.

- **Airway obstruction**

Airway obstruction from multiple causes presents with severe respiratory distress and extremely low oxygen saturations.

- **Meconium aspiration syndrome**

Meconium aspiration can cause severe respiratory distress with extremely low oxygen saturations.

Gastrointestinal

Abdominal wall defects can present unexpectedly in the delivery room, but newborns seldom present in extremis.

- Gastroschisis
- Omphalocele

Sepsis

Premature rupture of membranes significantly increases the risk of fetal sepsis and cardiovascular collapse.

- Group B streptococcus
- Candida
- Herpes
- Others

Anemia & Hypovolemia

- Hydrops per above
- Placenta previa
- Placental abruption
- Uterine rupture
- Umbilical cord rupture
- Severe twin-twin transfusion

Trauma

- Spleen & liver rupture from birth trauma
- Fetal injury from maternal trauma

Drugs or Toxins

- Maternal anesthetic agents
- Maternal illicit drug use

Endocrine & IEM

Endocrine

Maternal Graves disease may cause fetal thyrotoxicosis via transplacental maternal thyrotropin receptor-stimulating antibodies (TSHR-Ab) that increase fetal thyroxine levels, causing severe hydrops.

Inborn errors of metabolism (IEM)

IEM usually do not present in the delivery room, except for some glycogen and lysosomal storage diseases.

Anaphylaxis

- Rare in neonates

LATER PRESENTATION

Cardiovascular

If a cardiovascular malformation is ductus arteriosus dependent, then presentation can occur within hours or a few days after birth (depending on when the ductus closes). Nonductal-dependent conditions have variable presentations. Newborns can present quickly with arrhythmias that affect cardiac function. An inflammatory process may develop rapidly, and a patient may present suddenly with severe myocardial dysfunction. Similar presentations may occur in patients with pericardial effusion and tamponade.

Malformations

For more on each malformation, see Chapter 19.

Ductal-dependent systemic circulation
- Hypoplastic left heart syndrome
- Coarctation with large a VSD
- Interrupted aortic arch
- Severe aortic stenosis

Ductal-dependent pulmonary circulation
- Severe tetralogy of Fallot
- Pulmonary atresia with or without VSD
- Tricuspid atresia

Early severe heart failure
- Truncus arteriosus with truncal valve regurgitation
- Ebstein anomaly

Hypercyanotic episode
- Tetralogy of Fallot "Tet spell," see Chapter 7

Arrhythmias
- Supraventricular tachycardia
- Ventricular tachycardia
- Heart block

Inflammation
- Myocarditis
- Pericardial effusion with tamponade

Respiratory
- Severe PPHN
- Severe pneumonia
- Severe airway obstruction or lung mass
- Pneumothorax
- Severe bronchiolitis

Gastrointestinal
- Volvulus
- Intussusception
- Toxic megacolon
- Necrotizing entercolitis

Sepsis

Sepsis may cause cardiovascular collapse. Sepsis may also be associated with meningoencephalitis, which may increase intracranial pressure or cause status epilepticus.

Bacterial
Gram negative
- E. coli
- Meningococcus

- Klebsiella
- Enterobacter
- Pseudomonas
- Proteus

Gram positive
- Group B streptococcus
- Staphylococcus
- Listeria
- Enterococcus
- Group A streptococcus
- Meningoccemia

Viral
- Herpes

Anemia & Hypovolemia
- Severe diarrhea or vomiting or both
- Blood loss
- Other severe anemias

Trauma
- Accidental trauma
- Nonaccidental trauma

Drugs or Toxins
- Accidental overdose
- Nonaccidental overdose
- Botulism

Endocrine & IEM

Postnatal screens can detect significant inborn errors of metabolism. For diverse reasons, however, some infants escape screening.

Endocrine
- Neonatal thyrotoxicosis
- Congenital adrenal hyperplasia (CAH)

IEM

Postnatally, an IEM can present quickly within 24 hours or after several days. Conditions include urea cycle disorders, aminoacidemias, organic acidemias, disorders of carbohydrate metabolism, and fatty acid oxidation abnormalities.

Findings
- Dysmorphic features
- Encephalopathy from elevated serum ammonia
- Metabolic acidosis
- Hypoglycemia
- Liver enzyme abnormalities
- Abnormal body or urine odor

Anaphylaxis
- Medications
- Food & environmental allergy
- Insect sting or bite

℞ OPTIONS

Cardiovascular

Malformations
- PGE1 to maintain a PDA or open a closed ductus
- Pericardiocentesis for tamponade
- Inotropes, but avoid in "Tet" spells & HCM
- May need emergent surgery or cath intervention

Arrhythmias
- **Fast**

Electrical cardioversion may be the quickest method of converting a symptomatic supraventricular tachycardia or ventricular tachycardia. For more on arrhythmias, see Chapter 4.

- **Slow**

Symptomatic heart block requires isuprel and or an emergent temporary or permanent pacemaker.

Inflammation
- Inotropes
- Pericardiocentesis for tamponade
- IV gammaglobulin

Hydrops
- Pericardiocentesis or thoracentesis
- Diuretics
- Transfusion
- Occasionally hemofiltration [5]

Respiratory
- Airway management & ventilation
- Nitric oxide
- Evacuate pneumothorax or pleural effusion
- Surgery for chest mass

Gastrointestinal
- Surgery

Sepsis
- Antibiotics
- Antivirals

Anemia & Hypovolemia
- Volume expanders
- Transfusion

Trauma
- Surgery may be necessary for abdominal trauma

Drugs or Toxins

Call poison control or consult appropriate texts on childhood poisonings. Administer supportive care and identify counteracting agents if available.

Common
- Aspirin
- Iron
- Household cleaning supplies
- Unguarded drugs either illicit or prescription

Endocrine & IEM

Endocrine

Thyrotoxicosis

- First, IV (esmolol) or oral beta-blockers (propranolol)
- Oral propylthiouracil (PTU)
- Oral potassium iodide (SSKI)
- Oral Lugol solution
- Oral methimazole
- Oral prednisone

Congenital adrenal hyperplasia
- IV hydrocortisone
- Hyperkalemia treatment, see Chapter 4

IEM
- IV sodium bicarbonate
- IV sodium benzoate + sodium phenylacetate for hyperammonemia
- IV glucose to prevent ketosis
- Oral carnitine
- Hemodialysis

Anaphylaxis
- Epinephrine SC, IM, or IV

CLINICAL VIGNETTES

15. The staff calls you to the delivery room for a female infant profoundly cyanotic with oxygen saturation of 30%. The mother received no prenatal care. On exam, there is significant hydrops. Pulses are equal throughout. Her precordium is hyperdynamic and there is a grade III holosystolic murmur at the left lower sternal border. A chest X-ray shows marked cardiomegaly with a wall-to-wall heart. The lung fields appear hyperlucent. Before cardiac testing, her most likely diagnosis:

a. An inborn error of metabolism
b. Severe tetralogy of Fallot
c. Severe Ebstein anomaly with tricuspid regurgitation
d. A diaphragmatic hernia with severe PPHN

16. A 3-day old male infant, a newborn nursery discharged the previous day, presents to the emergency room in shock. His upper extremity pulses are present but weak, and the lower extremity pulses are nonpalpable. The liver is 5 cm below the right costal margin. The precordium is hyperdynamic. There is a loud second sound and a low frequency grade I to II holosystolic murmur heard over the entire precordium. Before additional testing, his most likely diagnosis:

a. An idiopathic cardiomyopathy
b. A severe coarctation of the aorta and large VSD
c. A small VSD with sepsis
d. Birth trauma with a ruptured liver and spleen

REFERENCES

1 Burton, BK. Inborn errors of metabolism in infancy: a guide to diagnosis. Pediatrics 1998; 102: E69

2 Colletti JE, Homme JL, Woodridge DP. Unsuspected neonatal killers in emergency medicine. Emerg Med Clin North Am 2004; 22: 929-960

3 Brousseau T, Sharieff GQ. Newborn emergencies: the first 30 days of life. Pediatr Clin North Am 2006; 53: 69-84

4 Yee L. Cardiac emergencies in the first year of life. Emerg Med Clin North Am 2007; 25: 981-1008

5 Castillo F, Nieto J, Salcedo S, Peguero G, Castello F. Treatment of hydrops fetalis with hemofiltration. Pediatr Nephrology 2000; 15: 14-16

8 Extremis

9 Aborted or Sudden Cardiac Death

Contents

Background	**123**
Causes SCD	**124**
Primary Prevention	**126**
Aborted SCD	**127**
Fatal SCD	**128**
Clinical Vignettes	**129**

9 Aborted or Sudden Cardiac Death

joseph ludwick

BACKGROUND

Sudden cardiac death (SCD) is natural death from a cardiovascular cause within 1 hour of acute symptoms. Most patients are younger than 40 years old. In patients > 21 years old, SCD is primarily from coronary artery disease. In patients < 21 years old, SCD is often from ventricular fibrillation or rapid ventricular tachycardia arising from diverse cardiovascular pathology. Although the incidence of SCD is low, SCD is devastating because it usually occurs in otherwise healthy appearing individuals.

Contrary to SCD, an underlying cardiovascular abnormality rarely causes infant aborted life threatening events or ALTEs. In 2004, McGovern published a population study that reported a < 1% incidence of cardiovascular etiologies for infant ALTEs. Gastroesophageal reflux, seizures, or unknown events cause most infant ALTEs. However, an ALTE workup should include an EKG to rule out long QT syndrome, Wolff-Parkinson-White (WPW) syndrome, or other rhythm or electrical disorders. Echocardiography can rule out pericardial effusions, structural abnormalities, cardiomyopathies, or ventricular dysfunction. [1-8]

Demographics
SCD in individuals < 21 years old in the United States.
- 500 to 1,000 cases per year
- 10% of deaths in those < 21 years old
- Most deaths occur during sports
- About 1 to 5 per 100,000 young athletes per year
- 90% of sports related SCD events occur in males
- Primarily during high school & college sports
➤ The most common are basketball, football, or track and field. About ⅓ of SCD events occur during a competitive sporting event, and the remaining ⅔ occur during practice.

SCD CAUSES

The table below provides estimates of SCD related conditions found at autopsy; however, the ultimate cause of death from the listed structural problems is most often a fatal arrhythmia.

	SCD causes at autopsy	
Rank	Cause	%
1	Hypertrophic cardiomyopathy	35-40
2	No clear cause (although most are likely ion channelopaties)	10-35
3	Idiopathic left ventricular hypertrophy	10-15
4	Coronary artery anomalies	10-15
5	Coronary artery disease	5-10
6	Aortic rupture	5-10

Arrhythmias

Cardiomyopathy induced

- Hypertrophic cardiomyopathy (HCM)
- Idiopathic left ventricular hypertrophy
- Dilated cardiomyopathy (DCM)
- Arrhythmogenic RV cardiomyopathy (ARVC)
- Noncompaction cardiomyopathy

Ion Channelopathies

Ion channelopathies are disorders characterized by mutations in genes coding for proteins that underlie cell-membrane transport systems for sodium, potassium, and calcium. Also, see Chapter 4.

- Long QT syndrome (LQTS)
- Short QT syndrome (currently ill-defined)
- Catecholaminergic polymorphic ventricular tachycardia (CPVT)
- Brugada syndrome

Wolff-Parkinson-White (WPW)

- Conduction bypass tracts (see Chapters 4 & 21)
- Atrial fibrillation or flutter may lead to ventricular tachycardia (VT) or fibrillation (VF)

Atrioventricular block

- Congenital
- Acquired

Myocardial ischemia induced

- Coronary artery abnormalities
- Coronary artery spasm
- Coronary artery thrombosis from Kawasaki disease
- Early atherosclerosis
- Significant aortic or pulmonic stenosis

Drug induced

- Cocaine
- Ephedrine
- Medications that prolong the QT interval, list at http://www.sads.org/Living-with-SADS/Drugs-to-Avoid/Printable-Drug-List

Trauma induced or *Commotio cordis*

- Fatal cardiac arrhythmia from trauma like a fast moving baseball to the chest

Inflammation induced

- Myocarditis

Other arrhythmia causes

- Pheochromocytoma
- Electrolyte abnormality
- Idiopathic VT or VF
- Primary pulmonary hypertension

Structural Cardiovascular Causes

Aortic dissection with rupture

- Marfan syndrome with aortic root dilation
- Bicuspid aortic valve with aortic root dilation
- Coarctation with aortic root dilation

CLINICAL SCENARIOS

The clinician's role includes detecting individuals at risk for SCD; managing patients surviving an aborted SCD event; and diagnosing and counseling families of patients dying suddenly.

Primary Prevention

Patients with underlying genetic causes of SCD, such as mutations for HCM or LQTS, may have normal phenotypes or normal echocardiograms and EKGs. Also, a small percentage of children, without an identifiable genotype for LQTS or HCM, have EKGs with above normal QTc values or ventricular hypertrophy on Echo. Other EKG findings such as WPW or Brugada syndrome may be intermittent. The challenge is to accurately identify risks for SCD.

Refer patients with a positive medical history, significant family history, abnormal physical examination, or an abnormal EKG to pediatric cardiology for further evaluation. Further testing may include an echocardiogram, Holter monitor, treadmill testing, or other procedures.

Patient & family medical history

- Evaluation for high risk patients and families
- Use the form in Appendix B for screening

Exam

- Physical features suggesting Marfan syndrome
- Hypertension
- Pulse discrepancy
- Irregular heart rate or rhythm
- Heart murmurs or extra heart sounds

Tests

Electrocardiogram

- Prolonged QTc ≥ 450 msec (see Chapter 21)
- T-wave inversion
- Abnormal T-wave repolarization
- Preexcitation
- Left ventricular hypertrophy
- Obtain EKGs on family members also
- Blowup of lead V1 below, contrasting Brugada syndrome findings with typical right bundle branch block (RBBB)

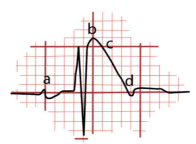

Brugada Syndrome
EKG characteristics
a. Broad P wave with PQ prolongation
b. J point elevation
c. Coved type ST segment elevation
d. Inverted T wave

Complete RBBB
EKG characteristic
- rSR' in V1

Echocardiogram

- Cardiovascular malformations
- Abnormal systolic or diastolic function
- Ventricular hypertrophy
- Dilated right ventricle in ARVC
- Noncompacted myocardium
- Abnormal coronary artery

Treadmill

- **Evaluation of symptoms**

A treadmill test may elucidate the causes of syncope, near syncope, chest pain, palpitations, or shortness of breath during exertion.

- **Evaluation of abnormal findings on EKG**

A treadmill test may provide additional information when an EKG shows abnormal T-waves, prolonged QTc, or ventricular arrhythmias.

Prevention

- **Prevention of Commotio cordis**

Protective-chest vests for participation in sports such as baseball or hockey.

- **Restriction from activity**

Patients deemed high risk from medical history, physical exam, and test results.

Aborted SCD

As sudden cardiac arrest in young people occurs most often during sporting events, either at practice or at competitive events. Resuscitation efforts can be successful in these settings. Following resuscitation, paramedics transport patients to appropriate emergency facilities. The following outlines the approach to such patients and their family.

History

- Triggers, including exertion, strong emotions, loud noises
- Exercise induced syncope
- Medications or drugs both prescription & illicit

Exam

- Hypertension or hypotension
- Abnormal heart rates & rhythms
- Heart murmurs or extra heart sounds

Tests

Basic Laboratory tests

- Electrolytes
- Thyroid function tests
- Serum & urine toxicology screen
- Urine catecholamines
- Freeze extra serum for future analysis

Electrocardiogram

- Check paramedic recordings
- Note myocardial-ischemia changes
- Long QTc, WPW
- Brugada syndrome (figure on previous page)
- Any arrhythmia

Holter, portable event monitor, implantable event monitor

- **Holter monitor**

Holter monitoring provides longer EKG tracings with daily activities.

- **Event monitor**

Best for intermittent palpitations. The patient self-applies the device and can trigger the monitor at home, school, or at a sporting event.

- **Implantable event monitor**

Surgeons place these devices under the skin. The devices allow automatically tracking of heart rate and rhythm. Implantable devices also allow transcutaneous interrogation and download of information, similar to a pacemaker.

Echocardiogram

Following aborted SCD, obtain an Echo to evaluate the following conditions:

- Transient decreased ventricular function
- Ventricular hypertrophy

- Cardiomyopathy
- Abnormal coronary artery
- Other cardiovascular malformations

Additional tests

Additional testing may unmask etiologies including LQTS, CPVT, ARVC, Brugada syndrome, or myocarditis.
- MRI
- Signal-averaged EKG (a specialized cardiology test)
- Exercise testing
- Drug challenges
- Electrophysiology procedure
- Cardiac catheterization & myocardial biopsy

Preventing recurrences

Resuscitated patients, after a ventricular arrhythmia without clear precipitating factors, are at high risk for recurrence. Such patients require restriction from intense physical activity and competitive sports.

- **Patients with a normal workup**

Normal testing complicates recommendations. However, such patients require followup, as some may show later abnormalities on EKGs, Holter monitoring, Echo, MRI, or other tests.

- **Patients with abnormal phenotypes**

If testing shows Long QTc, Brugada syndrome, CPVT, HCM, ARVC, then clinicians should consider genetic testing of patients and family members.

Cause guided ℞ options

- Beta-blockers for HCM, long QTc, CPVT
- Beta-blocker with possible left sympathectomy for LQTS
- Other medications for arrhythmias
- Implantable cardioverter defibrillators (ICDs)

➤An ICD is the safest and most effective therapy, and we may recommend an ICD in cases of resuscitated SCD and asymptomatic high-risk individuals with HCM, LQTS, or Brugada syndrome, especially with positive family histories. Patients requiring an ICD for LQTS should remain on beta-blockers.

Fatal SCD

Postmortem examination may reveal a previously undiagnosed cardiomyopathy, severe valvular stenosis, or a coronary artery abnormality. With a normal appearing heart, an arrhythmia is the most likely diagnosis. For cardiomyopathies, 1st-degree relatives need a cardiac evaluation and an echocardiogram. Young relatives of those dying from SCD should undergo echocardiography at regular intervals until adulthood. In suspected primary arrhythmic death, 1st-degree relatives need evaluation with resting and exercise EKGs to detect cases of LQTS, short QTc, Brugada syndrome, CPVT, and ARVC. Some authors suggest also evaluating 2nd-degree relatives [9]. Some genetically affected individuals have false negative or normal EKGs. Consider molecular autopsy to obtain myocardial tissue for genetic analysis to specifically look for channelopathy gene mutations. An identified mutation may lead to targeted screening of relatives.

CLINICAL VIGNETTES

17. A 17-year old football player collapses with a cardiac arrest during a game and dies. The autopsy shows a significantly thick interventricular septum consistent with a hypertrophic cardiomyopathy. The parents seek your advice about their 2 other children. Your recommendations should be:

a. Obtain EKGs and Echos on them and the parents
b. Restrict the siblings from all activity
c. Reassure the parents that the siblings are fine
d. Recommend beta-blockers for the siblings

18. A 10-year old collapses with a cardiac arrest after her teacher yells at her for a wrong answer. The teacher knows CPR and resuscitates her, and paramedics transport her to the local hospital. On exam, she has normal pulses, normally active precordium, and no murmur. An EKG shows a QTc of 500 msec. She has no siblings, but her mother has a sister with 2 children, and her father is adopted with no known siblings. Which of the following recommendation is the most correct:

a. Thank the teacher for CPR, but fire him for verbal abuse
b. Reassure the parents that she had a simple faint
c. Place the child on beta-blockers without further workup
d. Obtain EKGs on her 1° and 2° relatives, place her on beta-blockers, refer her for an ICD, and consider genetic testing for her and her family members

REFERENCES

1 Maron BJ. Sudden death in young athletes. N Engl J Med 2003; 349: 1064-1075

2 Berger S, Kugler JD, Thomas JA, Friedberg DZ. Sudden cardiac death in children and adolescents: introduction and overview. Pediatr Clin North Am 2004; 51: 1201-1209

3 Myerburg RJ, Castellanos A. Cardiac arrest and sudden cardiac death. In: Braunwald E, Zipes DP, Libby P (eds). Heart Disease: A Textbook of Cardiovascular Medicine. Philadelphia, WB Saunders, 2007, p 933-974

4 Maron BJ, Chaitman BR, Ackerman MJ, Bayés de Luna A, Corrado D, Crosson JE, Deal J, Driscoll DJ, Estes NA 3rd, Araújo CG, Liang DH, Mitten MJ, Myerburg RJ, Pelliccia A, Thompson PD, Towbin JA, Van Camp SP. Recommendations for physical activity and recreational sports participation for young patients with genetic cardiovascular diseases. Circulation 2004; 109: 2807-2816

5 Drezner J, Berger S, Campbell R. Current controversies in the cardiovascular screening of athletes. Curr Sports Med Rep 2010; 9: 86-92

6 McGovern MC, Smith MB. Causes of apparent life threatening events in infants: a systematic review. Arch Dis Child 2004; 89: 1043-1048

7 Krahn AD, Healey JS, Chauhan V, Birnie DH, Simpson CS, Champagne J, Gardner M, Sanatani S, Exner DV, Klein GJ, Yee R, Skanes AC, Gula LJ, Gollob MH. Systematic assessment of patients with unexplained cardiac arrest. Circulation. 2009; 120: 278-285

8 Tester DJ, Ackerman MJ. Postmortem long QT syndrome genetic testing for sudden unexplained death in the young. J Am Coll Cardiol 2007; 49: 240-246

9 Tan HL, Hofman N, van Langen IM, van der Wal AC, Wilde AA. Sudden unexplained death. Heritability and diagnostic yield of cardiological and genetic examination in surviving relatives. Circulation. 2005; 112: 207-213

10 Late Post-Procedure Problems

Contents

Background	133
Murmurs & Arrhythmias	134
Oxygen Desaturation	134
Post-Procedure Fever	135
Other Problems	136
Clinical Vignettes	137

10 Late Post-Procedure Problems

robert rollins

BACKGROUND

Most children undergoing surgical or catheter-interventional procedures experience no short-term (< 1 week), late post-procedure (1 to 6 weeks), or long-term problems (> 6 weeks). Long-term, post-procedure issues encompass regular pediatric cardiology followup, and we do not discuss them here. Short-term problems occur in the pediatric or cardiac intensive care units, and we do not cover them here either.

Late post-procedure problems often present to noncardiologists and noncardiac intensivists. Such problems may present during post-procedure recovery in intermediate care units, secondary-level neonatal intensive care units, pediatric units, in emergency rooms after discharge, or in a primary care office. Some late post-procedure problems are minor while others are emergencies. [1-4]

PROBLEMS

Heart Murmurs

Murmurs are common after surgery or catheter intervention from either trivial and significant residual malformations.

Some expected murmurs

- Loud systolic murmurs

A loud systolic murmur may persist in patients following ventricular septal defect (VSD) repair with a small residual VSD patch leak and other expected residual high flow turbulent lesions.

- Loud systolic & diastolic murmurs

Patients with asymptomatic complex congenital heart disease may have loud murmurs despite surgical or catheter-interventional procedures.

- Soft systolic & diastolic murmurs

Such murmurs are common after pulmonary or aortic valve balloon valvuloplasty, and following tetralogy of Fallot repair. Frequently, patients with D-transposition of the great arteries have a soft systolic murmur following the arterial switch operation.

Some unexpected murmurs

- Any murmur in symptomatic patients
- Loud murmurs after valvuloplasty or valvotomy

Abnormal Heart Rate & Rhythm

Late postoperative arrhythmias are possible after surgery or catheter intervention. Most post-procedure arrhythmias are benign, but patients with postoperative tetralogy of Fallot are at increased risk for pathological rhythm disorders. Also, any syncopal event needs prompt evaluation.

Fast rhythms

- Sinus tachycardia

Sinus tachycardia may occur with late postoperative fever, from post-pericardiotomy syndrome, infection, unexpected desaturation, or unexpected heart failure.

- Nonsinus tachycardias

Supraventricular tachycardia (SVT), atrial or junctional tachycardias, ventricular tachycardia (VT), or other tachyarrhythmias can all occur post procedures.

Slow rhythms

- Sinus node dysfunction from surgical cannulas
- Junctional bradycardias (narrow QRS without p-waves)
- Atrioventricular block may present late

Irregular rhythms

- Ectopics of any kind

Desaturation

Any child with complex cardiovascular malformations, following a surgery or catheter intervention procedure, may continue desaturated. However, fully-repaired cyanotic congenital heart disease should not have persistent oxygen desaturation.

Conditions with expected desaturation

- Tetralogy of Fallot

Desaturation persists following a palliative procedure such as a shunt or a stent in the ductus arteriosus.

- Palliated 1-functional ventricles

Patients remain desaturated after systemic-to-pulmonary artery shunts, Glenn procedures, pulmonary artery bands, or a pulmonary artery band and a systemic-to-pulmonary artery shunt. A fenestrated modified Fontan procedure has an opening between the Fontan conduit and the atrial chambers, resulting in desaturation.

- Other complex congenital heart disease

Any cardiovascular malformation with a persistent right-to-left shunt.

Conditions with unexpected desaturation

- Following a repair

After a successful complete repair for tetralogy of Fallot, transposition of the great arteries, or total anomalous pulmonary venous return, no significant desaturation should be present.

- Sudden fall in oxygen saturation

A sudden drop in saturation following palliation with a systemic-to-pulmonary artery shunt may be from shunt stenosis or thrombosis.

- Others

Post-pericardiotomy syndrome with tamponade or post-procedure pneumonia can present as medical emergencies.

Fever & Irritability
Post-pericardiotomy syndrome

- Etiology

The cause is unclear, but possibly an autoimmune etiology.

- Open heart

The condition most commonly follows surgeries that require opening the pericardium.

- Nonopen heart

Pacemaker placement where leads screw into the heart through the pericardium can also cause post-pericardiotomy syndrome.

- Symptoms & signs

Findings may develop a few days after surgery to as long as 6 weeks afterwards. Symptoms and signs include fever, irritability, tachycardia, chest pain (worsening with inspiration), and shortness of breath.

- Laboratory findings

Elevated acute phase reactants (ESR or CRP). Increased troponin I or CPK-MB may occur. A chest X-ray may show cardiomegaly and pleural effusions.

- Pericardial effusions & pericardiocentesis

Pericardial effusions usually occur in post-pericardiotomy syndrome. Obtain an Echo, as the absence of a pericardial friction rub does not rule out a pericardial effusion. Cardiac tamponade is a medical emergency. Tamponade requires emergency pericardiocentesis. Further, pericardiocentesis may be the preferable mode of therapy for treating moderate to large pericardial effusions without tamponade.

- NSAIDs or steroids

Anti-inflammatory treatment is appropriate for small to moderate-sized pericardial effusions without tamponade.

- Recurrence

After the initial episode of post-pericardiotomy syndrome, pericardial effusions occasionally recur over months or years

Sepsis
- Procedures can introduce bacteria
- Endocarditis possible with a positive blood culture

Wound infections
Incisions & tube sites

Benign problems include the extrusion of biodegradable

10 Late Post-Procedure Problems

sutures and noninfected open chest tube sites that later heal. Occasionally healed chest tube sites may have postoperative hernias. The following conditions need evaluation:
- Any incisional redness, swelling, or drainage
- A skin infection may portend a deep abscess

Monitoring line sites
- Infections can occur at monitoring line sites in the neck, groin, or extremities

Device Dislodgment

Interventional cardiac catheterization frequently includes placing devices for eliminating a PDA, ASD, VSD, or stents in the pulmonary arteries or aorta. A post-procedure chest X-ray may be the first indication of a dislodged device. Device dislodgment usually occurs shortly after placement, and late dislodgment is rare. All the following can embolize or migrate:
- PDA coils or vascular plugs
- ASD occluder devices
- VSD occluder devices
- Pulmonary artery stents
- Coarctation of the aorta stents
- Occasionally pacemaker leads may dislodge

Miscellaneous Concerns

Postoperative behavior changes

Neurocognitive impairments can occur in children following open-heart surgery, but such disorders are rare after most procedures. The following may occur:
- Attention deficit
- Concentration or short-term memory problems
- Fine motor function problems
- Regressive behavior & fearfulness

Post-procedure seizures
- Rare
- Consult neurology
- Need MRI or CT scans to rule out stroke

Post-procedure activity restrictions
- None for preschool children
- 4 to 6 weeks for postoperative school-age children
- Variable for catheterization procedures

SBE prophylaxis
- See the Appendix A.

Immunizations
- Usually no limits, unless post-heart transplant

CLINICAL VIGNETTES

19. A 5-year old female who underwent surgery 3 weeks ago for an ASD presents with fever, chest pain, and shortness of breath. She missed the first post-operative office visit. On exam, her temperature is 38.5° C, she is anxious and prefers sitting up. She is in moderate distress with a respiratory rate of 35 per minute, and a heart rate of 135 bpm. Her blood pressure is difficult to obtain. Her pulses are equal but intermittently palpable. Her precordium is quiet, and the heart tones are distant. A chest-X ray shows cardiomegaly and a small pleural effusion. What do you predict an echocardiogram will show?

a. A significant residual ASD
b. Endocarditis
c. Dilated cardiomyopathy
d. A large pericardial effusion

20. A 6-month male with a known complex cardiac anomaly presents to your office, and the mother reports he had a Glenn procedure. On exam, he is afebrile, comfortable, with normal vital signs and an oxygen saturation of 80%. He has normal pulses, and his liver is not palpable. He has a hyperdynamic precordium but no murmur. The mother appears unconcerned. What should you do?

a. Call 911
b. Relax, a saturation of 80% is expected after a Glenn
c. Recommend cardiology consultation ASAP
d. Call child-protective services

REFERENCES

1 Scarfone RJ, Donoghue AJ, Alessandrini EA. Cardiac tamponade complicating postpericardiotomy syndrome. Pediatr Emerg Care 2003 Aug; 19: 268-271

2 Cheung EWY, Ho SA, Tang KKY, Chau AKT, Chiu, CSW, Cheung, YF. Pericardial effusion after open heart surgery for congenital heart disease. Heart 2003; 89: 780-783

3 Miatton M, De Wolf D, François K, Thiery E, Vingerhoets G. Neurocognitive consequences of surgically corrected congenital heart defects: A review. Neuropsychol Rev 2006; 16: 65-85

4 Creighton DE, Robertson CM, Sauve RS, Moddemann DM, Alton GY, Nettel-Aguirre A, Ross DB, Rebeyka IM. Neurocognitive, functional, and health outcomes at 5 years of age for children after complex cardiac surgery at 6 weeks of age or younger. Pediatrics 2007; 120: e478-e486

11 Prolonged Fever

Contents

Background	141
Kawasaki Disease	142
Myocarditis / Pericarditis	145
Endocarditis	147
Rheumatic Fever	150
Clinical Vignettes	152

11 Prolonged Fever

william evans

BACKGROUND

In order of occurrence, the 4 most common conditions presenting with prolonged fever and possible cardiovascular abnormalities are Kawasaki disease, myopericarditis, endocarditis, and rheumatic fever. However, in the developing world, rheumatic fever is the most common. All these problems share some symptoms, signs, and laboratory findings. In addition, the varied cardiovascular pathology resulting from these 4 conditions may cause similar symptoms and signs such as congestive heart failure and heart murmurs. A careful review of the medical history, pertinent positive and negative physical findings, and selected laboratory tests can usually differentiate these conditions from each other and from other prolonged febrile illnesses that do not have specific associated cardiac abnormalities such as juvenile rheumatoid arthritis, Stevens-Johnson syndrome, measles, or drug reactions. Dosing information for disease specific medications is in Appendix C.

KAWASAKI DISEASE

Typical Presentation

Japanese physician Tomisaku Kawasaki initially described KD in 1967. Kawasaki suggested the name "mucocutaneous lymph node syndrome or MLNS." Not surprisingly, physicians quickly began using "Kawasaki disease." Patients are usually < 5 years old, with a peak incidence between 18 to 24 months old. Most patients are male with a ratio of 1.5:1. The etiology remains unknown; however, its features suggest an infection. Autoimmune mechanisms may also be possible. Manifestations result from a generalized vasculitis. KD has some genetic predisposition, as KD occurs more often in Asians than other ethnic groups. KD predominately occurs in late winter and early spring. Reports of transmission are infrequent, and KD rarely recurs. KD is likely present when the patient has 5 of 6 cardinal features (table below left). Although not a cardinal feature, patients are usually quite irritable. To minimize the chance of cardiac complications, treat with gammaglobulin within 10 days of the onset of fever. [1]

Atypical Presentation

Atypical KD is common. An atypical presentation can include patients younger or older than is typical. Also, atypical presentations have fewer than 5 cardinal signs, but usually ≥ 2. Infants with fever of unknown origin constitute a particularly difficult group. Infants, especially males, develop coronary aneurysms more often than those beyond 2 years old. A delay in diagnosis increases the risk for cardiovascular abnormalities, especially coronary artery aneurysms. Thus, always include KD in the differential diagnosis for infants with fevers of unknown origin, as prompt gammaglobulin treatment can significantly reduce the incidence of coronary artery aneurysms, especially giant aneurysms. Also, children > 5 years old may present sicker, leading them to often require more aggressive treatment such as > 1 IVIG dose, steroids, or other medications.

#	Kawasaki Cardinal Features
1	Fever ≥ 5 days
2	Bilateral nonpurulent conjunctivitis
3	Oral mucosa redness and swelling with cracked bleeding lips
4	Palmar & plantar swelling and erythema, late peeling of fingers & toes
5	Polymorphous erythematous rash
6	Cervical adenopathy

Noncardinal Symptoms & Signs
- Irritability
- Abdominal pain
- Diarrhea
- Hepatitis
- Cholecystitis

- Hydrops of the gallbladder
- Aseptic meningitis
- Pleural effusions
- Uveitis

Laboratory Values

- Elevated ESR & CRP
- Elevated white blood count & anemia
- Thrombocytosis or thrombocytopenia
- Urine analysis showing white blood cells
- Elevated liver enzymes
- Hypoalbuminemia
- Cerebral spinal fluid pleocytosis

Echocardiography Findings

Echocardiography (Echo) can image KD's cardiovascular effects. Cardiovascular effects may include endocardial, myocardial, and pericardial pathology. Even though KD may affect other systemic arteries, its most significant effect is coronary artery pathology.

Coronary artery pathology

- Perivascular Echo brightness
- Coronary artery dilatation
- Coronary artery aneurysms (figure above right)
- Coronary artery constrictions

➤Mild coronary artery abnormalities usually regress. As many as 25% of untreated KD patients may develop coronary artery pathology, and up to 5% of treated KD patients may still develop coronary artery changes.

Other possible Echo findings

- Pericardial effusion
- Myocardial dysfunction
- Mitral & aortic valvular regurgitation

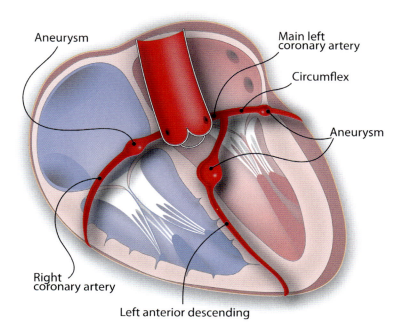

℞ Options

For medication dosing information, see Appendix C.

- **Intravenous gammaglobulin (IVIG)**

Slow infusion over 12 hrs. Pretreat with diphenhydramine (Benadryl) before starting the IVIG infusion to decrease possible side effects.

- **High dose aspirin for acute phase**

Use high-dose aspirin until the patient is afebrile, usually about 3 to 4 days total. Aspirin levels may help when questions arise about effectiveness, compliance, or toxicity. Therapeutic aspirin levels range from 10-20 mg/dL.

- **Steroids**

Currently, no steroids for initial therapy [2].

- **Low dose aspirin for chronic phase**

Use low-dose aspirin until approximately 6 weeks after the acute onset of KD, and stop aspirin if an Echo then shows no coronary artery abnormalities. Continue aspirin, when the Echo demonstrates persistent coronary artery changes (for giant aneurysm see warfarin below).

- **Dipyridamole (Persantine)**

May use persantine alone for persistent coronary artery abnormalities, but not as sole therapy for giant coronary artery aneurysms.

- **Warfarin**

Use warfarin, rather than aspirin or dipyridamole, for giant aneurysms ($\geq$ 8 mm in diameter by Echo). Keep INR between 2.0-3.0.

Recurrent Fever or Recalcitrant Kawasaki Disease

- **IVIG**

If fever persists or recurs within 24 to 48 hours of the 1st IVIG dose, then administer a 2nd dose.

- **Infliximab (Remicade)**

If a recurrent fever appears after a 2nd IVIG dose, then consider infliximab. Before using infliximab, pretreat with acetaminophen and diphenhydramine. [3, 4]

- **Steroids**

Rather than infliximab for recalcitrant KD, some recommend pulsed-methylprednisolone dosing over 3 days.

Followup

Followup frequency, including echocardiography, should mirror the clinical course. With a normal initial echocardiogram, we usually perform a followup Echo at 2 weeks and then at 6 weeks after onset of fever. If, however, the initial echocardiogram is abnormal, then we perform followup studies more frequently. A consulting pediatric cardiologist should direct long-term cardiology followup. Primary care physicians should consult the current edition of the American Academy of Pediatrics *Red Book* for guidelines regarding immunizations after IVIG treatment [5].

MYOCARDITIS / PERICARDITIS

Pathologically, myocarditis and pericarditis can occur independently. Clinically, however, the 2 conditions can overlap or be indistinguishable, as the history, physical exam, and test findings can be similar. Myocarditis and pericarditis arise from viruses, bacteria, other microbes, autoimmune or unexplained vasculitis, toxins, and physical agents. As clinically differentiating these 2 conditions may be impossible, we prefer the term "myopericarditis." Myopericarditis can occur at any age. For more information, see Chapter 5. [6, 7]

Etiologies

Some older sources claim Coxsackie virus is the most common cause of myocarditis in children, but recent reports dispute this claim. No etiology is clearly more common than another. We list causes alphabetically under each etiological category.

- Viral

Adenovirus, CMV, Coxsackie A & B, echovirus, Epstein-Barr, hepatitis, herpes, HIV, influenza, mumps, parvovirus, varicella.

- Bacterial

Diphtheria, hemophilus influenzae, Lyme disease, listeria, salmonella, and any bacterial endotoxin.

- Other microbes

Aspergillus, ascaris, candida, cisticercosis, histoplasma, rickettsia, schistosoma, trypanosoma cruzi (Chagas disease), and visceral larva migrans.

- Autoimmune & unexplained vasculitis

Kawasaki disease, rheumatic fever, and systemic connective tissue diseases.

- Toxins

Amphotericin B, anthracyclines (anticancer medications), arsenic, ethanol, heavy metals, snake venom, sulfonamides, and tetracycline.

- Other

Electrocution, hyperpyrexia, and radiation.

Evaluation

History

- Fever
- Persistent chest pain
- Left shoulder pain
- Patients feel better upright & leaning forward
- Occasionally cough
- Rash
- Diarrhea & vomiting
- A preceding viral illness

Exam

- Tachypnea
- Tachycardia
- Arrhythmia
- Hypotension or pulsus paradoxus
- Pericardial friction rub
- Distant heart sounds
- Gallop rhythm
- Mitral & aortic regurgitation murmurs
- Hepatosplenomegaly
- Extremities cool & clammy

Diagnostic tests

Chest X-ray

- Cardiomegaly
- Pulmonary venous congestion
- Pleural effusions

Electrocardiogram

- Sinus tachycardia
- Generalized ST-wave elevation (pericarditis)
- Flat or inverted T-waves
- Any arrhythmia, but mostly ventricular

Echocardiogram

- Pericardial effusion & tamponade findings
- Decreased ventricular function
- Mitral or aortic valve regurgitation

Laboratory

Primary tests

- CBC
- Acute phase reactants (ESR & CRP)
- Troponin I, CPK-MB, CPK index
- B-natriuretic peptide
- Blood cultures
- Viral titers & cultures
- Lyme disease titer (especially with heart block)

Secondary tests

- Blood gases
- Electrolytes
- BUN & creatinine
- Total protein & albumin
- Liver function tests
- Thyroid studies
- Streptococcal antibodies

Cardiac catheterization & myocardial biopsy

- Controversial
- Weigh risks & possible benefits

℞ Options

- See Chapter 5

ENDOCARDITIS

Endocarditis can occur at any age; however, presentation in children and adolescents is more common than in infants. Endocarditis can be acute (more virulent organisms) or subacute (less virulent organisms). Endocarditis occurs more often in those with cardiovascular malformations than those with normal hearts. Cardiovascular conditions may be significant or trivial and be pre- or postoperative. Many associated cardiovascular malformations are mild, such as a bicuspid aortic valve without stenosis, mitral valve prolapse, and a small PDA. As the auscultatory findings in these conditions are subtle, clinicians commonly overlook them. Therefore, a negative past medical history is not surprising in cases of endocarditis with a bicuspid aortic valve. Endocarditis may occur in structurally normal hearts, especially in the presence of indwelling intracardiac catheters. Most endocarditis is bacterial, but other organisms can also cause endocarditis. Infections can also occur as an endarteritis in the pulmonary artery, ductus arteriosus, and aorta, especially with a coarctation. Clinical presentation can vary widely. Pathogenesis begins with a bacteremia, followed by adhesion of bacteria to cardiac or arterial structures, and subsequent organism proliferation along with fibrin and platelet deposition. [8-10]

Evaluation

General symptoms & signs

- Persistent fever
- Chills
- Anorexia
- Malaise
- Arthralgias
- Gastrointestinal distress
- Chest pain
- Splenomegaly
- New or changing heart murmur
- Arrhythmias
- Congestive heart failure

Specific signs

- Emboli

Petechiae, splinter hemorrhage, strokes, and Janeway lesions (flat, painless, ecchymotic lesions on the palms and soles).

- Immune-complex depositions

Osler nodes (painful, palpable, erythematous lesions chiefly involving finger and toe pads), Roth spots (lesions on the retina), and glomerulonephritis.

Tests

Usual blood culture results

Endocarditis Blood Culture Results	
%	Organism
±35	Strep viridans
±30	Staph aureus
±30	Others
±5	Negative

Echo findings

Transthoracic Echo may be diagnostic. However, if the Echo windows are poor, transesophageal Echo may be needed.

- Oscillating intracardiac masses like a mitral valve vegetation in the figure below:

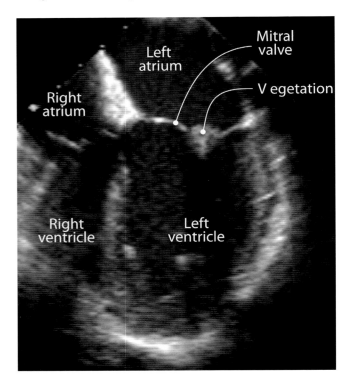

- New or acutely worsening valvular regurgitation
- Intracardiac abscess
- Dehiscence of prosthetic surgical material
- Dehiscence of a prosthetic valve

Diagnosis by Duke Criteria

In 1994, David Durack and his colleagues from Duke University established the Duke criteria for diagnosing endocarditis. Similar to the Jones criteria for rheumatic fever, followup reports have modified the Duke criteria over the last several years. We list a summary of the Duke criteria. Please consult a comprehensive textbook for an extensive description.

Major criteria

- **Positive blood culture**

At least 2 positive blood cultures with a typical organism.

- **Positive Echo**

Includes a vegetation, an abscess, an infected artificial valve or prosthetic material, or new or acutely worsening valvular regurgitation.

Minor criteria

- Predisposing heart condition
- Fever > 38° C
- Emboli, mycotic aneurysm, or Janeway lesions
- Glomerulonephritis (hematuria), Osler nodes, or Roth spots
- Positive blood cultures with atypical organism

Diagnosis

- **Definite endocarditis**

2 major criteria; or 1 major criterion and 3 minor criteria; or 5 minor criteria.

- **Possible endocarditis**

1 major criterion and 1 minor criterion, or 3 minor criteria.

- **No endocarditis**

Criteria above not met; or alternative diagnosis; or resolution of symptoms and signs suggesting endocarditis with ≤ 4 days of antibiotics; or negative pathology at surgery with ≤ 4 days of antibiotics.

℞ Options

Antibiotics

A pediatric infectious disease specialist should direct treatment. Antimicrobial therapy is IV. Placing a peripherally inserted central catheter (PICC line), for home IV therapy, avoids long-term hospitalization. Start empiric treatment before the results of cultures and sensitivities. Once culture and sensitivities are back, then modify the antibiotic regimen appropriately. Treatment usually lasts for 4 to 8 weeks, depending on the organism and presence of artificial intracardiac material. After discontinuing antibiotics, obtain new blood cultures to ensure sterility. If blood cultures are again positive, then resume treatment and consider surgical intervention.

Empiric antibiotic treatment:

- **Without prosthetic valves**

  Ampicillin (or vancomycin if penicillin allergic) + ciprofloxacin + gentamicin.

- **With prosthetic valves in patients ≤ 1 year old**

  Vancomycin + gentamicin + cefepime + rifampin.

- **With prosthetic valves in patients > 1 year old**

  Ampicillin (or vancomycin if penicillin allergic) + ciprofloxacin + gentamicin + rifampin.

Relative surgical indications

- Ongoing bacteremia despite antibiotics
- Embolism, especially to the brain
- Severe valvular dysfunction with CHF
- Intracardiac abscesses
- Persistent infection of prosthetic valves
- Persistent infection of prosthetic material
- Relapsing infection after stopping antibiotics
- Difficult to treat organisms

ACUTE RHEUMATIC FEVER

Acute rheumatic fever (ARF) is the most common worldwide cause of pediatric heart disease, but ARF is now rare in the developed world. Rheumatic fever is a delayed (1 to 6 weeks) autoimmune disorder, following a group A β-hemolytic streptococcal (GABHS) pharyngitis or upper respiratory infection. Rheumatic fever predominately occurs in fall, winter, or early spring. Skin infections from GABHS cause post-streptococcal glomerulonephritis, not ARF. Although rare in some locales, clinicians should include ARF in a differential diagnosis for prolonged fever. ARF usually occurs between the ages of 5 and 15. Rheumatic fever is rare in patients under 3 years old. The incidence in boys and girls is about equal except for Sydenham chorea, which is more common in girls. [11-14]

Jones Criteria

Followup reports have modified the Jones criteria over the last 6 decades, but the term persists.

Major criteria

- **Migratory polyarthritis**

Migratory polyarthritis involving the knees, ankles, elbows, and wrists that does not progress to chronic disease.

- **Carditis**

Valvular regurgitation may be inaudible; therefore, echocardiography is the gold standard for detecting carditis. Carditis may include endocarditis, myocarditis, and pericarditis. Mitral and aortic valve disease and pericardial effusions are especially common in ARF. Chronic rheumatic fever may progress to fibrosis and calcification usually of the mitral valve or aortic valve or both.

- **Sydenham chorea**

May manifest as clumsiness, deterioration of handwriting, emotional lability, grimacing, or fast-clonic involuntary movements. Sydenham chorea usually occurs late and may persist for months. Also, Sydenham chorea may be the solitary manifestation of ARF. Some may refer to Sydenham chorea as Saint Vitus dance, at term that dates back to the middle ages.

- **Erythema marginatum**

Transient, serpiginous lesions of 1 to 2 inches in size with pale centers and red, irregular margin, predominately on the trunk and limbs. Erythema marginatum is not itchy, and it worsens with application of warmth.

- **Subcutaneous nodules**

Painless, pea-sized, palpable nodules mainly over extensor surfaces of joints, spine, scapulae, and scalp.

Minor criteria

- Fever
- Arthralgia
- Elevated CRP or ESR
- Prolonged PR interval on EKG

Tests

- Throat culture positive for GABH streptococci
- Elevated CRP
- Elevated ESR (but may be normal in CHF)
- Anemia & elevated white blood count
- ASO titer > 250 Todd units
- Other positive streptococcal antibody tests
- Head CT or MRI with chorea to rule out other pathology

Diagnosis

Rheumatic fever is a clinical diagnosis without a unique confirmatory laboratory test. Three different combinations of major and minor criteria lead to an ARF diagnosis.

- 1st set of clinical criteria

2 major criteria, plus evidence of streptococcal infection from a positive throat culture or a positive antibody test.

- 2nd set of clinical criteria

1 major criterion and 2 minor criteria, plus evidence of streptococcal infection.

- 3rd set of clinical criteria

Isolated Sydenham chorea, ideally with positive evidence of strep. Sydenham chorea may occur months after the initial strep infection, and antibody tests may then be negative.

℞ Options

- Penicillin or equivalent to eradicate streptococci
- Aspirin at anti-inflammatory doses
- Possibly naproxen (no randomized studies)
- Restrict activities during acute phase
- No protracted bed rest after improvement in carditis
- Oral steroids for significant carditis
- Oral steroids are more effective than IV
- Anticongestive medications for CHF
- Diazepam or haloperidol for chorea

Preventing Recurrences

Rheumatic fever can recur; consequently, long-term antibiotic prophylaxis is important. Prophylaxis includes daily oral penicillin, monthly penicillin injections, or alternative antibiotics for penicillin sensitive individuals. Consult the current edition of the American Academy of Pediatrics *Red Book* for comprehensive recommendations [6]. A summary for rheumatic fever antibiotic prophylaxis duration follows:

- ARF without carditis

5 years or until 21 years old, whichever is longer.

- ARF with carditis & recovery

10 years or until 21 years old, whichever is longer

- ARF with carditis and chronic changes

10 years since last episode and until 40 years old, sometimes lifelong prophylaxis

11 Prolonged Fever

CLINICAL VIGNETTES

21. A 12-year old male presents with a 3 week history of fever and lethargy. The mother relates that a previous physician told her that he had a "valve problem." He has has not seen a doctor for 5 years. On exam, his temperature is 38° C and his vital signs are otherwise normal. He has petechiae and flat, painless, ecchymotic lesions on the palms and soles. His pulses are bounding, and his spleen is palpable. His precordium is hyperdynamic, he has a grade III systolic ejection murmur, and a grade II early diastolic murmur. Before additional testing, his most likely diagnosis:

a. Endocarditis
b. Myopericarditis
c. Kawasaki disease
d. Acute rheumatic fever

22. A 9-year old Asian male presents with fever and irritability for 6 days. He has had no other recent illnesses. A previous physician placed him on antibiotics for an ear infection, but he has remained febrile. His eyes have been red without discharge. On exam, his temperature is 39° C, his blood pressure is 70/30 mmHg, and his heart rate is 145 beats per minute. He has no rash, he has injected sclera, and his mucous membrane are normal. He has shotty lymphadenopathy, his pulses are thready, and the liver is felt just below the right costal margin. His precordium is normally active, and there is no murmur. Initial blood tests show an ESR of 100, a CBC with a WBC of 20,000, and a platelet count of 95,000. Before additional testing, his most likely diagnosis:

a. Acute rheumatic fever with congestive heart failure
b. Myopericarditis with congestive heart failure
c. Atypical Kawasaki disease with myocarditis
d. Endocarditis with congestive heart failure

REFERENCES

1 Newburger JW, Takahashi M, Gerber MA, Gewitz MH, Tani LY, Burns JC, Shulman ST, Bolger AF, Ferrieri P, Baltimore RS, Wilson WR, Baddour LM, Levison ME, Pallasch TJ, Falace DA, Taubert KA. Diagnosis, treatment, and long-term management of Kawasaki disease: a statement for health professionals from the Committee on Rheumatic Fever, Endocarditis, and Kawasaki Disease, Council on Cardiovascular Disease in the Young, American Heart Association. Pediatrics. 2004; 114: 1708-1733

2 Newburger JW, Sleeper LA, McCrindle BW, Minich LL, Gersony W, Vetter VL, Atz AM, Li JS, Takahashi M, Baker AL, Colan SD, Mitchell PD, Klein GL, Sundel RP. Randomized trial of pulsed corticosteroid therapy for primary treatment of Kawasaki disease. N Engl J Med 2007; 356: 663-675

3 Burns JC, Mason WH, Hauger SB, Janai H, Bastian JF, Wohrley JD, Balfour I, Shen CA, Michel ED, Shulman ST, Melish ME. Infliximab treatment for refractory Kawasaki syndrome. J Pediatr 2005; 146: 662-667

4 Son MB, Gauvreau K, Ma L, Baker AL, Sundel RP, Fulton DR, Newburger JW. Treatment of Kawasaki disease: analysis of 27 US pediatric hospitals from 2001 to 2006. Pediatrics 2009; 124: 1-8

5 American Academy of Pediatrics. Red Book 2006: Report of the Committee on Infectious Diseases. Washington, D.C., American Academy of Pediatrics, 2006

6 Dancea AB. Myocarditis in infants and children: a review for the paediatrician. Paediatr Child Health 2001; 6: 543-545

7 Fong IW. New perspectives of infections in cardiovascular disease. Current Cardiology Reviews 2009; 5: 87-104

8 Durack DT, Lukes AS, Bright DK. New criteria for diagnosis of infective endocarditis: utilization of specific echocardiographic findings. Am J Med 1994; 96: 200-209

9 Ferrieri P, Gewitz MH, Gerber MA, Newburger JW, Dajani AS, Shulman ST, Wilson W, Bolger AF, Bayer A, Levison ME, Pallasch TJ, Gage TW, Taubert KA. Unique features of infective endocarditis in childhood. Committee on Rheumatic Fever, Endocarditis, and Kawasaki Disease, Council on Cardiovascular Disease in the Young, American Heart Association. Pediatrics 2002; 109: 931-943

10 Baddour LM, Wilson WR, Bayer AS, et al. Infective endocarditis: diagnosis, antimicrobial therapy, and management of complications: a statement for healthcare professionals from the Committee on Rheumatic Fever, Endocarditis, and Kawasaki Disease. Circulation 2005; 111: e394-434

11 Steer AC, Carapetis JR. Prevention and treatment of rheumatic heart disease in the developing world. Nat Rev Cardiol 2009; 6: 689-698

12 Veasy LG. Rheumatic fever. Lancet Infect Dis 2004; 4: 661

13 Veasy LG, Tani LY, Minich L. The logic for extending the use of echocardiography beyond childhood to detect subclinical rheumatic heart disease. Cardiol Young 2009; 19: 30-33

14 Cilliers AM. Rheumatic fever and its management. BMJ 2006; 333: 1153-1156

11 Prolonged Fever

12 Chest Pain

Contents

Background	**157**
Noncardiac Causes	**158**
Cardiovascular Causes	**159**
Evaluation & ℞ Options	**160**
Clinical Vignettes	**162**

12 Chest Pain

william evans

BACKGROUND

Chest pain (CP) is common in children and adolescents. Although CP arises from many noncardiovascular causes, it leads to patient and family stress over concern that the heart is the cause. Further, because of CP's typical location, parents and children often describe it as "heart pain." Most patients describe their CP as midsternal to subcostal, sudden, sharp or stabbing, brief, and without pattern. Patients may report random CP occurring for months or even years. Usually, no other symptoms or signs accompany CP. Often adolescents describe pain radiating down their left arm, possibly from the popular knowledge that "heart attacks" often have associated left arm pain.

The most common causes for CP, even with known heart disease, are anxiety, gastroesophageal reflux, musculoskeletal, or simply unknown. Constant CP with additional symptoms or signs is uncommon, but such pain may have underlying pathology. Because some etiologies of CP have significant cardiovascular pathology, primary care providers may appropriately request pediatric cardiology consultation for patients causing them concern. [1, 2]

NONCARDIOVASCULAR CAUSES OF CHEST PAIN

Approximately 95% of CP in children is noncardiovascular, and up to 40% is idiopathic.

- Musculoskeletal

Costochondritis, trauma, muscle spasm, or sickle-cell crisis.

- Respiratory

Reactive airway disease, bronchitis, pneumonia, chronic cough, pneumothorax or pneumomediastinum from trauma, or pleurisy.

- Gastrointestinal

Gatroesophageal reflux and esophageal irritation or esophagitis especially from chronic oral antibiotics (tetracycline) for acne. Also ulcers or splenic infarcts.

- Psychosomatic

Stress induced anxiety, or panic disorder.

- Other

Varicella zoster (shingles), and most importantly idiopathic.

CARDIOVASCULAR CAUSES

Cardiovascular causes are rare, but some are potentially fatal.

- **Myopericarditis**

Post-pericardiotomy syndrome, viral or bacterial infection, Kawasaki disease, systemic connective tissue disease, or hypereosinophilic syndrome [3].

- **Arrhythmias**

Especially ectopics and intermittent SVT that a patient may describe as chest pain.

- **Myocardial ischemia with normal coronaries**

Ventricular hypertrophy from severe semilunar valve stenosis, hypertrophic cardiomyopathy, cardiac trauma, hypertensive crisis, allergic myocardial infarction (Kounis syndrome), diabetic ketoacidosis [4], or significant aortic regurgitation.

- **Myocardial ischemia with abnormal coronaries**

From postoperative changes, especially after arterial switch operation for TGA. Also from anomalous left coronary artery from the pulmonary artery (ALCAPA), coronary artery spasm (especially cocaine and amphetamine use), coronary artery occlusion (complications of Kawasaki disease), and other congenital coronary artery abnormalities.

- **Aortic dissection**

Marfan and Turner syndromes may present with aortic dissection.

- **Pulmonary embolism**

Resulting from lower extremity trauma, occult neoplasm, birth control pills, or hypercoagulable disorders.

- **Pulmonary hypertension**

Especially from primary pulmonary hypertension and may escape diagnosis for years.

- **Mitral valve prolapse**

Mitral valve prolapse is a questionable cause of chest pain.

12 Chest Pain

EVALUATION & ℞ OPTIONS

History

History is the most important, as history can frequently pinpoint a cause. A chronic history of nonpatterned, recurrent chest pain is almost never cardiac. Acute onset significant chest pain, without chest wall tenderness, is more likely cardiac; nevertheless, most presentations fitting this category are also noncardiac. Acute onset chest pain may result in an emergency room evaluation, leading usually to diagnostic tests that include CXR, EKG, troponin I levels, BNP, and usually echocardiography.

- **Family history**

Sudden death, arrhythmias, and cardiomyopathies.

- **Psychological stresses**

School, activities, friends, home, and child abuse.

- **General health**

Fever, fatigue, nausea, dizziness, syncope, and drugs.

- **Review of systems**

Cough, wheezing suggesting reactive airway disease, palpitations, nausea and vomiting, diarrhea and constipation, tetracycline use for acne, or rash suggesting varicella zoster.

- **History of trauma**

Sports, dance, carrying heavy objects, roughhousing, and nonaccidental.

- **Chest pain description**

Type, intensity, location, frequency, duration, pattern or none, with meals, changes with position, changes with inspiration, aggravating and relieving factors.

Exam

- Fever
- Hypertension
- Pulsus paradoxus suggests pericardial effusion
- Dysmorphic features suggest cardiovascular defect
- Pectus, scoliosis, or gynecomastia
- Chest wall pain on palpation suggests costochondritis
- Rales, rhonchi, or wheezes
- Pulses
- Murmurs
- Clicks, gallops, or rubs
- Loud S_2 suggests pulmonary hypertension
- Hepatosplenomegaly & peripheral edema

Initial Tests

Individualize testing consistent with the history and exam. Initial testing may include the following:

- Chest X-ray
- EKG
- Troponin I
- B-natriuretic peptide (BNP)
- D-dimer levels
- Acute phase reactants such as ESR or CRP
- Pulmonary function testing
- Upper GI

Additional Cardiac Tests

A consulting pediatric cardiologist should direct the cardiac testing and management. Tests may include:

- Echocardiogram

- Cardiac event monitor
- Holter monitor
- Treadmill
- Occasionally cardiac CT scan
- Occasionally cardiac catheterization
- Occasionally electrophysiology procedure

℞ Options

Noncardiac ℞ options

- Reassurance
- Rest
- Anti-inflammatories
- Antacids
- Reactive airway disease medications

Cardiac ℞ options

- Directed towards cause

12 Chest Pain

CLINICAL VIGNETTES

23. A 6-year old African-American female presents with sudden onset chest pain. She had an upper respiratory infection a week or so ago. On exam she is in moderate to severe distress and says she feels better sitting up. Her temperature is 38.5° C, and her respiratory rate is 35 per minute with a heart rate of 130 beats per minute. Her chest is not tender to palpation. Her pulses are equal throughout and there is no respiratory variation in pulse intensity. Her precordium is not hyperdynamic, there are no murmurs, but a rub is present. Her laboratory tests show a troponin I of 50 ng/mL and a normal BNP value. Her EKG shows elevated ST-T waves. Her most likely diagnosis:

a. Chest patin from gastroesophageal reflux
b. Pericarditis
c. Pulmonary embolism
d. Sickle cell crisis

24. A 12-year old male presents with chest pain for about a week. He has not been physically active and denies any chest wall injury. The pain is constant and does not vary with meals or any other activity. He reports ibuprofen has helped. On exam, he is afebrile, vital signs are normal. He has significant pain upon chest palpation. His pulses are equal throughout, and his liver is not palpable. He has a normally active precordium with no murmurs and no rub. His most likely diagnosis:

a. Costochondritis
b. Pericarditis
c. Pulmonary embolism
d. Severe aortic stenosis

REFERENCES

1 Reddy SRV, Singh HR. Chest pain in children and adolescents. Pediatr Rev 2010; 31: e1-e9

2 Cava JR, Sayger PL. Chest pain in children and adolescents. Pediatr Clin N Am 2004: 51: 1553-1568

3 Alomran H, AlGhamdi F, AlKhattabi F. Chest pain in a 12-year-old boy: when is it a harbinger of poor outcome? Int J Emerg Med 2009; 2: 179-185

4 Batra AS, Acherman RJ, Wong P, Silka MJ. Acute myocardial infarction in a 12-year-old as a complication of hyperosmolar diabetic ketoacidosis. Pediatr Crit Care Med 2002; 3: 194-196

12 Chest Pain

13 Syncope

Contents

Background	**167**
Evaluation	**168**
Testing	**169**
℞ Options	**171**
Clinical Vignettes	**172**

13 Syncope

katrinka kip

BACKGROUND

This chapter covers nonmalignant syncope. We address malignant syncope with aborted sudden cardiac death in Chapter 9.

Syncope is a transient loss of consciousness. Presyncope is a collection of symptoms occurring with or without a subsequent loss of consciousness. Presyncopal symptoms may include, among others, dizziness, disorientation, flushing, tingling, loss of vision, and nausea. About 80% of syncope is "neurocardiogenic" or "vasovagal syncope."

At least 15% of adolescents experience syncope at least once, and the incidence is higher in girls than boys. Nevertheless, patients of any age can faint. Evidence suggests that patients who had breath-holding spells in infancy may be prone to syncopal events later. In some families, a genetic predisposition for vasovagal syncope exists with multiple family members relating histories of episodic fainting, especially mothers of daughters.

Neurocardiogenic syncope (NCS) occurs with a drop in blood pressure, with or without bradycardia, resulting in decreased cerebral perfusion. Initially, patients may have prodromes of feeling faint, often noting dizziness, nausea, or vision "going black." Frequently patients are standing, sometimes rising to a stand, or in the act of sitting. Once fainting to a supine position, normal blood pressure and heart rate return.

Abnormal responses of vascular baroreceptors cause a drop in blood pressure and pulse. It is unclear why some are prone to abnormal autonomic responses and others are not. In patients with abnormal baroreceptor responses, stimuli including blood drawing, pain, micturition (urination), and hair grooming may also cause syncope. Further, venous pooling can accentuate abnormal autonomic responses.

History underlies the diagnosis of vasovagal syncope, as the physical examination and laboratory testing are usually normal. The primary goal for syncope evaluation is to exclude a malignant cause. NCS's primary treatment is nonpharmacological, as patients rarely need medications. [1-9]

13 Syncope

EVALUATION

History

- **Position before syncope**

NCS occurs most often while standing, walking, or getting up from lying or sitting down.

- **Time**

Morning is common, as dehydration can occur during sleep.

- **Location**

In or after a shower or bath that accentuates vasodilation.

- **Activities**

Hair grooming [8], blood drawing, pain, cough, or urination. Dance, sports, cheerleading, may cause chronic dehydration. However, an association with exercise is worrisome because of potentially lethal arrhythmias or structural heart defects such as hypertrophic cardiomyopathy or a coronary artery abnormality. For more on malignant syncope, see Chapter 9.

- **Stress**

Psychological stress from social conflict, school, or apprehension from other activities or situations. Physical stress from upper respiratory infections and gastroenteritis.

- **Prodrome**

Nausea, seeing "black spots," dizziness, or palpitations.

- **History of wheezing**

Occasionally, syncope results from exercise-induced asthma and hypoxia.

- **Presyncopal hyperventilation**

Suggests anxiety disorder.

- **Loss of bladder or bowel control**

Suggests seizures or possible malignant causes.

- **Frequent episodes**

If multiple episodes occur in a day and in any position including lying flat, then there may be psychiatric cause.

- **Migraines**

Migraine headaches can occur with syncope.

- **Drugs**

Prescription or illicit.

- **Family members**

Family history of NCS is common. However, if multiple family members have syncope, seizure disorders, or history of sudden death, then the chance of malignant syncope increases.

Exam

The physical exam is usually normal, although there may be orthostatic changes consisting of a decrease in blood pressure or an increase in heart rate with standing.

- **Orthostatic blood pressure & heart rate changes**

The recording of heart rate and blood pressure (BP) changes with change in position can be helpful. An immediate fall in BP with standing, following several minutes of recumbency, may suggest significant dehydration. Another possible response to standing upright, from a recumbent position, is a significant increase in heart rate without a significant fall in BP, consistent with postural orthostatic tachycardia syndrome (POTS). Some individuals have minimal initial vital sign changes, but in a few minutes they develop hypotension and syncope. Clinicians use various protocols to elicit these responses.

- **Chest**

Wheezing suggests reactive airway disease.

- **Heart**

Cardiac findings with a loud S_2 suggest pulmonary hypertension. Pathological murmurs suggest structural heart disease such as aortic stenosis or hypertrophic cardiomyopathy.

- **Pulses**

Check femoral and brachial pulses to rule out coarctation of the aorta.

- **Abdomen**

Hepatosplenomegaly may suggest a systemic illness or congestive heart failure.

Laboratory Testing

Primary care providers should order an EKG, urine analysis, and CBC. Pediatric cardiologists may perform additional tests commensurate with the history and exam.

Noncardiologists

- **Urine analysis**

Especially for urine specific gravity or other abnormalities. High specific gravity suggests dehydration.

- **CBC**

For anemia or polycythemia.

- **EKG**

An EKG can rule out arrhythmias; preexcitation; long QTS; right ventricular hypertrophy suggesting pulmonary hypertension or structural heart disease; left ventricular hypertrophy possibly from systemic hypertension; structural heart disease; hypertrophic cardiomyopathy; and ST-T wave changes suggesting myopericarditis.

Cardiologists

Standard testing

- **EKG**

To rule out all the findings above.

- **Echocardiography**

An Echo can rule out structural heart disease, ventricular dysfunction, pulmonary hypertension, or pericardial effusion.

- **Holter monitor**

In patients fainting several times per day, a Holter monitor allows direct correlation between symptoms and cardiac rhythm including sinus tachycardia preceding syncope in POTS syndrome, bradycardias with heart block, or other related arrhythmias. A Holter monitor may also help discern psychogenic factors; for example, when a patient reports palpitation, but the Holter simultaneously records normal sinus rhythm.

- **Exercise stress test**

To look for potential arrhythmias and for blunted blood pressure responses.

Extended testing

- **Implantable event monitor**

A small device surgically implanted under the skin continuously monitors the patient's rhythm and records arrhythmia triggered events, useful especially in young patients incapable of providing an adequate history.

- **Tilt table or head-up tilt (HUT)**

A tilt table test includes EKG and vital sign recordings while supine and at an 80° upright tilt. A tilt table test is a detailed and protracted means of evaluating heart and blood pressure changes that accompany change in position. We can perform the procedure with or without provoking agents such as isoproterenol or nitroglycerin. A positive test for NCS exists when symptoms coexist with a blood pressure drop or heart rate changes. A patient may have POTS when the heart rate increases significantly (> 30 bpm) with little or no drop in blood pressure. Some centers do cerebral blood flow studies, and a change in cerebral blood flow with symptoms and signs is consistent with a positive test. Without any pulse or blood pressure changes or decrease in cerebral perfusion, the test is negative for NCS. Rarely does the patient have a syncopal event with none of the above. In these cases, suspect a conversion reaction. [10]

℞ OPTIONS

The cause of syncope influences treatment. We rarely use medications. If Holter monitoring or an implantable event monitor reveals a significant bradycardia with syncope, then a pacemaker may be necessary. Also, a Holter or event monitor may record a tachyarrhythmia such as supraventricular tachycardia or ventricular tachycardia, which need further evaluation and treatment.

Nonpharmacological

- **Hydration recommendations**

Encourage fluid until the urine is colorless. Add salt to food to promote fluid retention. Use water or electrolyte sports drinks. Other fluids including juice, milk, and sodas do not count. Patients should avoid caffeinated drinks, as caffeine is a stimulant and a diuretic; diuretic agents compound dehydration and accentuates POTS.

- **Positional recommendations**

Patients should sit or lie down during a prodrome or with the onset of presyncopal symptoms. Patients should not lock their knees while standing; rather, they should move to augment venous return. Isometric exercise, like tightening extremity muscles, prevents venous pooling. The lack of venous pooling during movement is one reason NCS does not occur during exercise but may occur after exercise, when venous pooling suddenly increases. Cool down periods after exercise can prevent this sudden change in venous return.

Pharmacological

Medications are rarely necessary. However, when clinically indicated, probably the most successful agents are midodrine and fludrocortisone. Nonetheless, reserve these medications for recalcitrant NCS in patients that have undergone extensive workups.

- **Midodrine (ProAmatine)**

An alpha-agonist, which increases blood pressure.

- **Fludrocortisone (Florinef)**

Augments fluid and salt retention.

- **Beta-blockers like Inderal**

For patients with documented initial tachycardia before syncope, suppression of the tachycardia response may prevent subsequent bradycardia and hypotension.

- **Selective serotonin reuptake inhibitor or SSRI like Zoloft**

Some studies suggest the serotonin system's role in syncope mechanisms. [11]

- **Disopyramide (Norpace)**

Norpace is primarily an antiarrhythmic, but secondary anticholinergic, negative inotropic, and alpha-agonist effects may help prevent syncope.

13 Syncope

CLINICAL VIGNETTES

25. A 14-year old male presents with a single episode of syncope. He has been participating in cross-country for about 2 weeks, and he describes feeling dizzy with change of position. His episode of syncope occurred at school at about 10 AM, and he admits to not eating breakfast or drinking anything before he left for school. The syncopal episode duration was about 30 seconds. He went to the school nurses office and she sent him home. On exam, his vital signs are normal except for a 20 bpm increase in heart rate and a 10 to 20 mm Hg fall in systolic blood pressure with standing for 1 minute. His pulses and cardiac exam are normal. His most likely diagnosis:

a. A seizure disorder
b. An anomalous coronary artery
c. Neurocardiogenic syncope from chronic dehydration
d. Hypertrophic cardiomyopathy

26. A 7-year old female presents with a history of several episodes of syncope. She has been good health in the past. The mother had syncope when she was a teenager. The child's syncopal episodes have all occurred in the morning when she is getting ready for school. Each syncopal event has occurred with the mother brushing her daughter's hair. Each episode has lasted a few seconds, but the mother describes that she occasionally displays twitching. Her exam is normal, including lack of heart rate or blood pressure changes with standing for 1 minute. Her most likely diagnosis:

a. Long QT syndrome
b. Hair-grooming syncope
c. A psychiatric disorder
d. Breath holding spells

REFERENCES

1 Dermksian G, Lamb LE. Syncope in a population of healthy young adults incidence, mechanisms, and significance. J Am Med Assoc 1958; 168: 1200-1207

2 Ruckman RN. Cardiac causes of syncope. Pediatr Rev 1987; 9 : 101-108

3 Strasberg B, Sagie A, Rechavia E, Sclarovsky S, Agmon J. The noninvasive evaluation of syncope of suspected cardiovascular origin. Am Heart J 1989; 117: 160-163

4 Scott WA. Evaluating the child with syncope. Pediatr Ann 1991; 20: 350-359

5 Driscoll DJ, Jacobsen SJ, Porter CBJ, Wollan PC. Syncope in children and adolescents. J Am Coll Cardiol 1997; 29: 1039-1045

6 Kanter RJ. Syncope and sudden death. In: Garson A, Bricker JU McNamara DG (eds): The Science and Practice of Pediatric Cardiology. Baltimore, Lippincott Williams & Wilkins, 1998, p 2169-2199

7 Boehm KE, Morris EJ, Kip KT, Karas B, Grubb BP. Diagnosis and management of neurally mediated syncope and related conditions in adolescents. J Adolesc Health 2001; 28: 2-9

8 Evans WN, Acherman R, Kip K, Restrepo H. Hair-grooming syncope in children. Clin Pediatr (Phila) 2009; 48:834-836

9 Karas B, Grubb BP, Boehm K, Kip K. The postural orthostatic tachycardia syndrome: a potentially treatable cause of chronic fatigue, exercise intolerance, and cognitive impairment in adolescents. Pacing Clin Electrophysiol 2000; 23: 344-351

10 Samoil D, Grubb BP, Kip K, Kosinski DJ. Head-upright tilt table testing in children with unexplained syncope. Pediatrics 1993; 92: 426-430

11 Grubb BP, Samoil D, Kosinski D, Kip K, Brewster P. Use of sertraline hydrochloride in the treatment of refractory neurocardiogenic syncope in children and adolescents. J Am Coll Cardiol 1994; 24: 490-494

13 Syncope

14 Hypertension

Contents

Background	**177**
Definitions	**178**
Etiologies	**180**
Infants & Young Children	**181**
Older Child & Adolescent	**183**
Clinical Vignettes	**184**

14 Hypertension

william evans

BACKGROUND

For centuries, medicine has employed the terms "essential" or "idiopathic" for diseases with unknown etiologies. According to the *Oxford English Dictionary*, we now call nearly all unknown disease etiologies "idiopathic." The notable exception is "essential" hypertension. Rather than "essential hypertension," we prefer using the term "idiopathic hypertension," similar to other diseases with unknown causes.

In pediatrics, systemic hypertension (HTN) usually confronts a clinician in 1 of 2 scenarios: (1) Infants or young children with a renal, endocrine, neoplastic, or cardiovascular cause; or (2) Older children or adolescents with obesity, a family history of HTN, or idiopathic HTN.

Discernible HTN causes found in infants and young children can also occur in older children and adolescents. Nonetheless, discernible causes are rare in the older group. Infants and young children can present acutely with seizures, congestive heart failure, or even cardiovascular collapse. Infants and young children may also present less dramatically with feeding difficulties, lethargy, irritability, and mottling. Older children and adolescents often present via a routine exam or a sports clearance physical.

Short of recording values from an indwelling arterial line in a calm patient, blood pressure is the most difficult vital sign to measure. Standard tables of noninvasive blood pressure contain precise values; however, inaccuracy often plagues blood pressure (BP) recording. Inaccuracies can occur with any BP method, whether one uses an automated system, a cuff with palpation of the radial pulse, a cuff with manual Doppler radial-artery interrogation; or a cuff with standard antecubital fossa auscultation. The same limitations exist for measuring lower extremity blood pressure.

Factors Affecting BP Values

- Examiner

Inexperienced examiners may use the wrong size cuff, may position the arm above or below the heart level (both cause inaccuracies), or may be unfamiliar with operating automated devices or unskilled in the auscultatory method.

- Device calibration

Automated devices require routine calibration. Check manual and automated systems for leaks in the tubing, and ensure all connections are tight and in working order.

- Anxiety

Anxiety for older children and adolescents or "white-coat hypertension" temporarily elevates the BP. In infants and young children irritability, crying, or movement, including the discomfort of cuff inflation, can all introduce error.

- Cuff

The BP cuff's air bladder should encircle the arm, and the

14 Hypertension

cuff should cover at least ⅔ of the upper arm, as we display in the figure below:

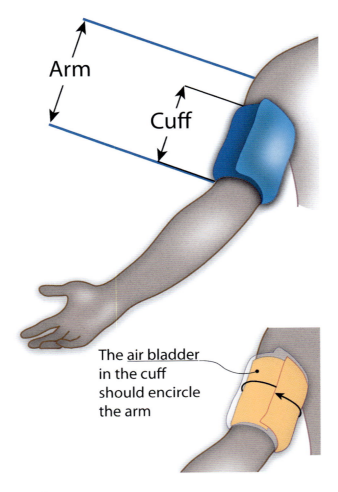

Definitions

Korotkoff (Korotkov) sounds noninvasively signify systolic and diastolic blood pressure. Auscultation and the oscillometric method (automated blood pressure machines) detect Korotkoff sounds. Clinicians universally accept systolic pressure as a continuous 1st Korotkoff sound (the minimum cuff pressure allowing blood to flow continuously). However, controversy exists whether the diastolic pressure occurs with the 4th, 5th, or other Korotkoff sounds. Also, detecting the radial pulse's appearance by a Doppler device or by palpation determines systolic pressure; neither method, however, allows determination of the diastolic pressure. Nevertheless, diastolic hypertension rarely exists without systolic hypertension, especially in children. Thus, measuring the systolic pressure is the simplest way to determine whether blood pressure is normal or high.

Blood pressure increases with age and size. Figures A and B on the facing page display graphs of systolic BP values for increasing gestational ages and newborn weights. Values on table C (on the facing page) stem from a study that meticulously recorded systolic BPs from 1 day to 30 days old. Values on table D (on the facing page) tabulate upper limits of normal systolic BP values for age categories from 1 to 18 years old. Table D also includes systolic blood pressure values for borderline, moderate, and severe HTN. We compiled the date for table D from both pediatric and adult references.

Unless clear evidence for significant HTN exists, base a HTN diagnosis on several measurements over time, in a relaxed state as possible. Ambulatory blood pressure systems are valuable for evaluating HTN, but ambulatory systems are rare in primary care. Whenever possible, instruct parents to obtain home blood pressure measurements. Such measurements are more likely to reflect relaxed values than those obtained in a clinician's office.

Systemic HTN can cause left ventricular hypertrophy, coronary artery disease, congestive heart failure, renal disease, retinopathy, and premature death. Therefore, investigate and treat true and persistent systemic HTN. [1-13]

14 Hypertension

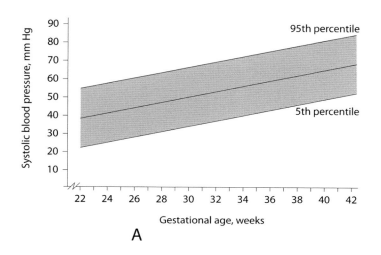

A. Systolic blood pressure vs. Gestational age

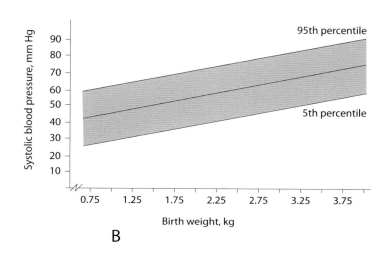

B. Systolic blood pressure vs. Birth weight

Systolic blood pressure vs. Postnatal age	
Postnatal age	Systolic blood pressure
1-2 days	69.7 ± 7.3
3 days	71.4 ± 8.6
4 days	75.7 ± 8.1
5-7 days	76.1 ± 9.7
8-14 days	77.5 ± 9.9
15-21 days	79.3 ± 8.3
1 month	84.9 ± 10.2

C

Systolic blood pressure 1 to 18 years				
Age	Upper Normal	Borderline Hypertension	Moderate Hypertension	Severe Hypertension
1-12 months	90	100	115	≥120
1-5 years	100	110	125	≥135
6-10 years	110	120	135	≥150
11-15 years	115	125	140	≥155
15-18 years	120	130	150	≥160

D

14 Hypertension

ETIOLOGIES

Cardiovascular
- Coarctation of the aorta (CoA)
- Hypertension may persist even after CoA repair

Renal
- **Vascular**

Renal artery stenosis (RAS) and renal vein thrombosis. Renal vascular abnormalities in Noonan, Turner, Williams, neurofibromatosis, and tuberous sclerosis.

- **Cystic disease**

Polycystic kidney disease either as autosomal dominant (approximately 1:500) or recessive (< 1:10,000). Multicystic-dysplastic kidney disease occurs in 1:4,000 and results in nonfunctional kidneys. Potter syndrome results when multicystic-dysplastic kidneys are bilateral.

- **Collecting system**

Ureteropelvic junction (UPJ) obstruction. UPJ obstruction activates the renin-angiotensin system. Posterior urethral valves.

- **Umbilical arterial & venous catheters**

HTN form umbilical artery catheters (UACs) likely originates from renal microthrombi. Premature infants with UAC related HTN can present with LV dysfunction and congestive heart failure. Umbilical venous catheters (UVC) can cause renal vein thrombosis. Hypertension resulting from UACs is usually worse than HTN from UVCs.

- **Others**

Hemolytic uremic syndrome, post-streptococcus acute glomerulonephritis (post-strep AGN), acute tubular necrosis (ATN), chronic pyelonephritis, and congenital nephrotic syndrome.

Endocrine & Metabolic
- Congenital adrenal hyperplasia (CAH)
- Hyperaldosteronism
- Hyperthyroidism
- Adrenal hemorrhage
- Hypercalcemia

Neoplasms
- Mass compression of renal vessels & ureters
- Vasoactive substances from a pheochromocytoma
- Neuroblastoma
- Mesoblastic nephropathy
- Wilms tumor

Other Causes
- Medications such as theophylline
- Steroids (anabolic, gluco-, & mineralocorticoids)
- Caffeine
- Illicit drugs like cocaine & anabolic steroids
- Prolonged total parenteral nutrition (TPN)
- Closure of abdominal wall defects
- Maternal medication in newborns
- Neonatal drug withdrawal
- Birth asphyxia
- Bronchopulmonary dysplasia
- Seizures & increased intracranial pressure
- Pain
- Obesity
- Familial hypertension
- Idiopathic

INFANTS & YOUNG CHILDREN

History

In neonates, important historical information may include prenatal exposures to illicit drugs, maternal prescription medications, umbilical artery and venous catheter use, history of chronic lung disease, and excessive fluid administration. In older infants and young children, the medical history may also include many of the same neonatal factors, occurrence of headaches, excessive caffeinated drinks, and a positive family history. Alternatively, the medical history may be negative.

Exam

- Small for gestational age
- Pulse & BP discrepancy suggesting CoA
- Tachycardia & tachypnea suggesting CHF
- Tachycardia & flushing suggests hyperthyroidism or pheochromocytoma
- Features suggesting syndromes including Turner, Noonan, Williams, or tuberous sclerosis
- Cafe au lait spots in neurofibromatosis
- Ambiguous genitalia suggests CAH
- An epigastric bruit suggests renal artery stenosis
- Abdominal mass with obstructive uropathy, polycystic kidney, or tumors
- Retinal fundoscopic exam for hemorrhages, arterial narrowing, exudates, & edema
- Thyroid exam for goiter

Laboratory

Routine blood & urine

- Urinalysis & culture
- CBC
- Electrolytes, calcium, BUN & creatinine

Directed investigations

Laboratory

- Plasma renin
- Thyroid studies
- Urine & serum catecholamines
- Aldosterone
- Cortisol

Imaging studies

- Chest X-ray
- Echocardiography
- Ultrasound for UPJ obstruction, renal vein thrombosis, & abdominal masses
- Voiding cystourethrogram (VCUG)
- Radionuclide renal imaging
- Magnetic resonance imaging (MRI)

Management

We provide medication-dosing information in Appendix C.

General

- Treat pain
- Correct volume overload
- Wean inotropic infusion
- Consider pediatric nephrology consult

Acute ℞ options

- IV nitroprusside
- IV esmolol

14 Hypertension

Chronic ℞ options

- Oral angiotensin-converting enzyme inhibitors (ACE inhibitors) such as enalapril or captopril
- No ACE inhibitors in renal RAS or renal failure
- Oral angiotensin II-receptor blockers (ARBs)
- Oral calcium-channel blockers like amlodipine, if normal LV function
- Oral hydralazine, if hyperkalemia and ACE inhibitors contraindicated
- Diuretics as adjunct therapy
- We rarely use beta-blockers as a first-line medical ℞

Interventional ℞ options

Surgery or catheter intervention can provide definitive treatment, but the patient may also need adjunct medical treatment.

- CoA repair
- UPJ obstruction relief
- Renal artery stenosis relief
- Nephrectomy for polycystic & multicystic kidney disease
- Tumor resection

OLDER CHILDREN & ADOLESCENTS

Hypertension in older children and adolescents may be from similar causes found in infants and younger children. However, the most common cause of "hypertension" in older children, especially those with large biceps, is an inadequate BP-cuff size. For accurate blood pressure measurements, the cuff's air-bladder should encircle or almost encircle the upper arm. Even a cuff with a bladder encircling about 75% of the upper arm may artificially elevate the systolic blood pressure reading. The cuff width should cover ⅔ of the upper arm. Large adult cuffs and thigh cuffs may be necessary for accurate blood pressure measurements in older children and adolescents with obesity or with muscular upper arms.

History

Important historical information includes illicit drug use, including anabolic steroids, energy drink use. Also, stress and anxiety are common in older children and adolescents. Family history may be positive for adult members with hypertension.

Exam

- Weight & BMI above the 95% tile
- Pulse & BP discrepancy suggests CoA
- Tachycardia suggests hyperthyroidism or pheochromocytoma
- An epigastric bruit suggests renal artery stenosis
- Retinal fundoscopic exam
- Features of Cushing syndrome
- Vasculitis findings such as rashes & arthritis

Laboratory

Examinations are similar to those in infants and children but may be less extensive.
- Urine analysis
- BUN & creatinine
- Drug screen
- Echocardiography for LVH or CoA
- Ambulatory blood pressure monitoring
- Sleep study for obstructive apnea
- Urine & serum catecholamines
- Additional testing, depending on the degree of HTN

Management

General

- Lifestyle modification & obesity ℞
- Stress management
- Consider pediatric nephrology consult

Chronic ℞ options

Chronic treatment is similar to younger patients.
- ACE inhibitors like enalapril
- ARBs like valsartan
- Calcium-channel blockers like nifedipine
- Occasionally hydralazine & beta-blockers

Other methods

- Catheter intervention or surgery for CoA
- Catheter intervention for renal artery stenosis

14 Hypertension

CLINICAL VIGNETTES

27. A 17-year old football player presents with a history of hypertension noted during a school screening exam. He is otherwise asymptomatic and he denies using any medications or illicit drugs, including steroids. He does not drink caffeinated beverages. On exam, his automated blood pressure with a standard adult cuff is 150/80 mmHg the right arm. With a thigh cuff, however, his blood pressure is 120/60 mm Hg in the right arm. His pulses and his cardiac exam are normal. His EKG is normal. Your recommendation:

a. Immediate hospitalization and IV antihypertensives
b. Restriction from all sports activities
c. Extensive blood work to rule a renal cause for HTN
d. Reassurance that his blood pressure is normal

28. A 3-year old presents with a history of hypertension. A previous doctor's office performed his blood pressure, and the family is now seeking a second opinion. He has been asymptomatic, and his past medical history is negative. He is not overweight. On exam, his blood pressure with appropriate size cuffs is 120/70 mmHg in the right arm and 60/50 mmHg in the lower extremities. His pulses are accentuated in the upper extremities and absent in the groin. His precordium is not hyperdynamic. There is no murmur, but an ejection click is present. His most likely diagnosis:

a. Renal artery stenosis
b. White coat hypertension
c. Coarctation of the aorta with a bicuspid aortic valve
d. Acute glomerulonephritis

REFERENCES

1 Blood pressure levels for boys and girls by age and height percentile. http://www.nhlbi.nih.gov/guidelines/hypertension/child_tbl.pdf

2 Moss AJ. Blood pressure in infants, children, and adolescents. West J Med 1981; 134: 296-314

3 Zinner SH, Rosner B, Oh W, Kass EH. Significance of blood pressure in infancy: familial aggregation and predictive effect on later blood pressure. Hypertension 1985; 7: 411-416

4 Zubrow AB, Hulman S, Kushner H, Falkner B. Determinants of blood pressure in infants admitted to neonatal intensive care units: a prospective multicenter study. Philadelphia Neonatal Blood Pressure Study Group. J Perinatol 1995; 15: 470-479

5 Kaelber DC, Pickett F. Simple table to identify children and adolescents needing further evaluation of blood pressure. Pediatrics 2009; 123: e972-e974

6 Hornsby JL, Mongan PF, Taylor AT, Treiber FA. 'White coat' hypertension in children. J Fam Pract. 1991; 33: 617-623

7 Tozawa M, Oshiro S, Iseki C, Sesoko S, Higashiuesato Y, Tana T, Ikemiya Y, Iseki K, Fukiyama K. Family history of hypertension and blood pressure in a screened cohort. Hypertens Res 2001; 24: 93-98

8 Podoll A, Grenier M, Croix B, Feig DI. Inaccuracy of pediatric outpatient blood pressure measurement. Pediatrics 2007; 119: e538-e543

9 Flynn JT, Meyers KEC, Net JP, de Paula Meneses R, Zurowska A, Bagga A, Mattheyse L, Shi V, Gupte J, Solar-Yohay S, Han G. Efficacy and safety of the angiotensin receptor blocker Valsartan in children with hypertension aged 1 to 5 years. Hypertension 2008; 52: 222-228

10 Brady TM, Feld LG. Pediatric approach to hypertension. Semin Nephrol 2009; 29: 379-388

11 Stergiou GS, Karpettas N, Kapoyiannis A, Stefanidis CJ, Vazeou A. Home blood pressure monitoring in children and adolescents: a systematic review. J Hypertens 2009; 27: 1941-1947

12 Lande MR, Flynn JT. Treatment of hypertension in children and adolescents. Pediatr Nephrol 2009; 24: 1939-1949

13 Flynn JT. Pediatric hypertension update. Curr Opin Nephrol Hypertens 2010; 19: 292-297

14 Hypertension

15 Obesity & Lipid Disorders

CONTENTS

BACKGROUND OBESITY	**189**
EVALUATION & ℞ OPTIONS	**190**
BACKGROUND LIPID DISORDERS	**192**
LIPID DISORDER WORKUP & ℞	**196**
CLINICAL VIGNETTES	**199**

15 Obesity & Lipid Disorders

gary mayman

OBESITY BACKGROUND

The definition of childhood overweight is a body mass index (BMI) > 85th percentile for age, and the definition of obesity is a BMI > 95th percentile for age. Childhood obesity is an epidemic disease that continues to worsen worldwide. Studies show 80% of children overweight at 10 to 15 years old are obese at age 25. Similarly, studies show 25% of obese adults were overweight as children. Despite compounding factors including family history, psychological issues, and genetics, most exogenous obesity results from excessive carbohydrate intake and a lack of activity. Childhood obesity can lead to metabolic syndrome, manifested by lipid disorders, hypertension, nonalcoholic steatohepatitis (fatty liver), and insulin resistance. [1-4]

15 Obesity & Lipid Disorders

PRIMARY CARE EVALUATION & ℞ OPTIONS

Busy primary care physicians have little time, and treating childhood obesity is a time-consuming endeavor. Primary care providers can initiate prevention by beginning with parental education during the first newborn visit. Subsequently, each well-child visit is a time to track weight, BMI, and emphasize healthy lifestyles along with other anticipatory guidance. When confronted with an obese child, the following steps may be achievable in a primary care setting.

Obtain Family History

- Ethnicity, as more common in Hispanics & African Americans than others
- Socioeconomical factors
- Diabetes mellitus, particularly type II
- Hypertension
- Lipid disorders
- Cardiovascular disease

Review of Systems

- Psychological problems
- Sleep problems suggesting obstructive sleep apnea
- Reactive airway disease
- Orthopedic problems

Exam

- Growth parameters

Plot height and weight on standard growth curves. Calculate body mass index or BMI, and plot the results on a BMI curve.

BMI = weight in kg ÷ (height in meters)^2
BMI = 703 × weight in lbs ÷ (height in inches)^2

- Note other abnormal findings

Measure blood pressure with appropriate-sized cuffs for accuracy. Note acanthosis nigricans and potential syndromes like Prader-Willi.

Laboratory Tests

- Standard fasting lipid panel
- Fasting blood sugar
- Liver enzymes
- Renal function
- Thyroid function
- Fasting insulin

A Primary Care ℞ Approach

The 5-2-1-0 + H$_2$O recommendations:

A primary care approach	
5	fruits & vegetables a day
2	hours of screen time or less a day
1	hour of physical activity a day
0	sugar sweetened beverages
H$_2$O	encourage water for fluid intake

Target Behaviors

- Eating breakfast daily
- Limiting eating out, especially fast food
- Encourage family meals
- Control portion size & number

Activity recommendations

- At least 1 hour a day.

Reasons for specialty referral

- For a comprehensive obesity ℞ program
- ℞ prediabetes or overt type II diabetes
- Evaluation & ℞ of lipid disorders
- Evaluation & ℞ of abnormal liver enzymes
- Evaluation & ℞ of metabolic syndrome
- ℞ with medications such as sibutramine or metformin
- Evaluation & ℞ with bariatric surgery

LIPID DISORDERS BACKGROUND

Lipid disorders arise from excessive exogenous carbohydrates and fats and from abnormalities of endogenous lipid metabolism. Endogenous metabolic abnormalities are likely genetic, which environmental factors can accentuate. [5-8]

Figure A on the facing page sketches out lipoprotein metabolism. Dietary fats consist of triglycerides, fatty acids, and cholesterol (fat contents of a cheeseburger). The intestinal cells absorb fats and emulsify them into chylomicrons. Chylomicrons also carry apolipoproteins (black deposits) and free cholesterol (orange deposits). Chylomicrons travel through the lymphatic system to blood vessels that carry them to the muscles and to adipocytes. In the muscles, lipoprotein lipase breaks down chylomicrons into free fatty acids and chylomicron remnants. The liver packages chylomicron remnants into very low density lipoproteins (VLDL). VLDL later transform to intermediate density lipoproteins (IDL) that further metabolize to low density lipoproteins (LDL).

Figure B on the bottom left shows a blowup of a chylomicron. A chylomicron is a "lipoproteins micelle," a combination of cholesterol, triglycerides, phospholipids (fatty acids and phosphate molecules bound together), and apolipoproteins (proteins bound to lipids).

Figure C on the bottom right shows the relative size of lipoprotein particles. Metabolism converts VLDL into IDL and LDL.

Returning to schematic of lipoprotein metabolism in figure A on the top of the facing page, LDL becomes oxidized and damages the vascular endothelium. Such damage eventually causes arterial plaques. The liver and intestinal cells produce high-density lipoprotein (HDL) *de novo*. HDL participates in the removal of cholesterol from arterial plaques (black arrows), and HDL also removes some cholesterol from LDL particles (long orange arrow). Further HDL transports the cholesterol back to the liver (short orange arrow). Because LDL participates in arterial plaque formation it is also called "bad," and because HDL helps remove cholesterol from LDL and arterial plaques is it called "good." A simple mnemonic: low for L = "bad," and high for H = "good."

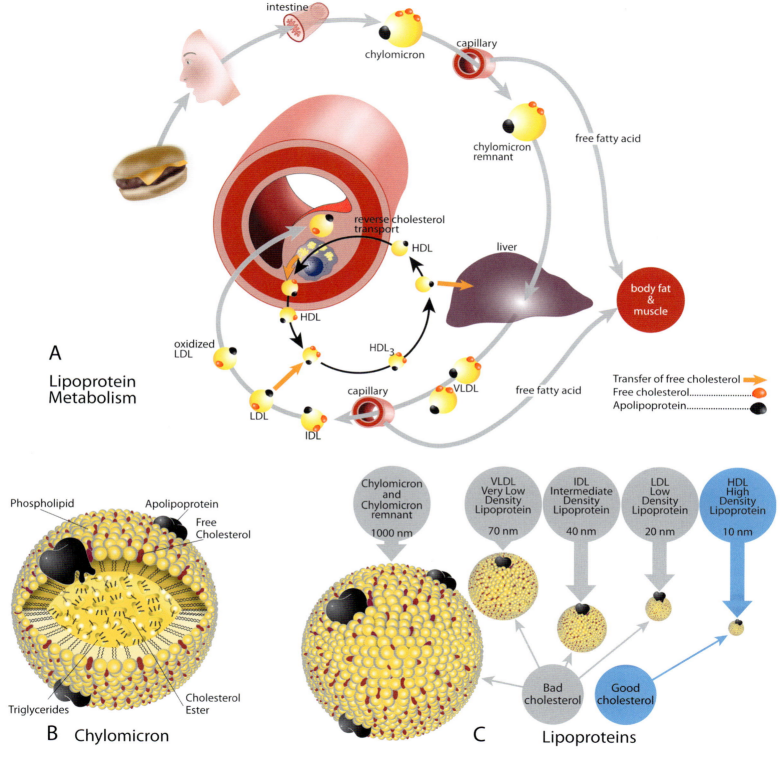

15 Obesity & Lipid Disorders

The liver synthesizes most of the body's cholesterol. The figure below left shows synthesis of cholesterol from acetoacetyl-CoA to mevalonate, a precursor of cholesterol. Mevalonate results via action of hydroxy-methyl-glutaryl-CoA reductase (HMG-CoA). Excessively high serum cholesterol rarely stems from diet alone. Rather, abnormalities in cholesterol metabolism are primarily responsible for total cholesterol values that exceed 300 mg/dL. As the figure below right shows, statins, which can significantly lower serum cholesterol, impair cholesterol synthesis by targeted action on HMG-CoA.

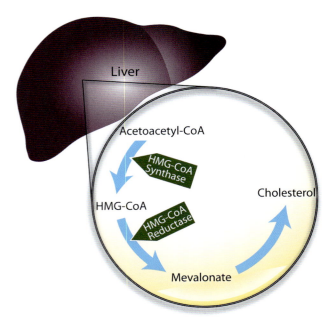

Cholesterol Production in the Liver

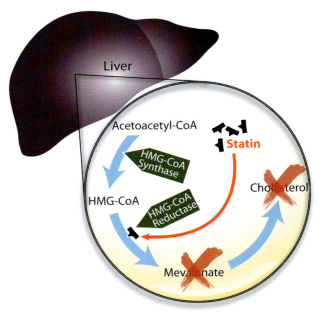

Cholesterol Production Blocked by Statin

Obesity is strongly associated with lipid disorders. The figure below displays a simplified schematic of metabolism. The simplified diagram demonstrates the relationship between excessive carbohydrates and lipogenesis, and it also clarifies why obesity has firm roots in excessive carbohydrate intake and reduced energy expenditure from lack of exercise.

With respect to food intake, most obese children and adults are obese from excessive carbohydrates rather than excessive fat or protein intake. The wide, dark-green arrow indicates the pathway taken by excess carbohydrates. If the body is inactive, excess carbohydrates lead to excess acetyl CoA that is not needed for energy, which is produced by the citric acid cycle and electron transport system. Rather, the body stores the excess acetyl CoA as fat through lipogenesis. From these pathways, it is clear why obesity can also contribute to lipid disorders.

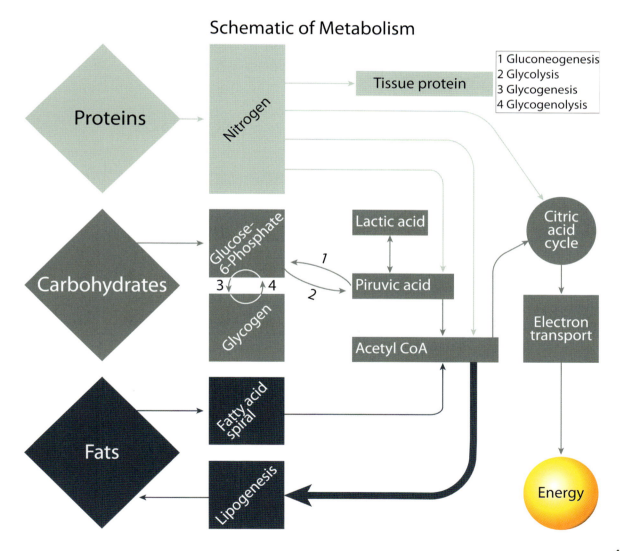

PRACTICAL APPROACH TO LIPID DISORDERS

A practical approach to lipid disorders includes a careful history, physical exam, laboratory testing, and treatment that consists primarily of nonpharmacological means.

History
- Family history of lipid disorders
- Family history of early myocardial infarctions
- The patient's dietary history
- Review of systems for comorbidities

Exam
- Growth parameters, including BMI
- Blood pressure
- Note acanthosis nigricans
- Note xanthomas

Laboratory
For normal values, see Appendix D.

- Lipid panel

A standard fasting lipid panel measuring total cholesterol (TC) and HDL cholesterol. Laboratories calculate an LDL cholesterol from the Friedewald formula:

$$\text{LDL cholesterol} = TC - (HDL\ cholesterol - triglycerides \div 5)$$

Most laboratories perform this calculation without a request. Alternatively, one can order a measured LDL (high cost), but a measured value is usually not needed. The Friedewald equation is inaccurate in the presence of a plasma chylomicrons or with plasma triglycerides > 400 mg/dL.

- Other laboratory tests

Include fasting glucose, fasting insulin level, thyroid function, liver enzymes, and renal function.

Practical Classification

Traditionally, the Fredrickson classification system categorizes lipid disorders as types I-IV. However, contemporary authors avoid this numerical system, as the Fredrickson classification adds little to clinical practice.

Most patients with hypercholesterolemia and hypertriglyceridemia do not have single gene abnormalities. Most develop lipid abnormalities in association with obesity. However, nonobese patients may have a hereditable cause from heterozygous or homozygous familial hypercholesterolemia or from polygenic factors.

A practical classification of lipid abnormalities includes: (1) High cholesterol and triglycerides with obesity, (2) Familial hypercholesterolemia, (3) Hypertriglyceridemias, and (4) Lipid disorders from medications or disease states. Treatment is similar regardless of the category.

1 - High cholesterol & triglycerides with obesity
- Most common form
- Possible family history, suggesting polygenic factors

2 - Familial hypercholesterolemia

This is the most common genetic type resulting in a hepatic LDL receptor abnormality. This abnormality causes a significant elevation in cholesterol, especially LDL-cholesterol. Inheritance can be heterozygous or homozygous.

- Heterozygous

Incidence is from 1:500 to as frequent as 1:250 in the general population. Young adults have significant risk for coronary artery disease and myocardial infarction.

- Homozygous

This condition is extremely rare. Homozygous incidence is about 1:1,000,000 in the general population. Even adolescents with homozygous familial hypercholesterolemia have severe coronary artery disease and early death.

3 - Hypertriglyceridemias

These consist principally of 2 rare conditions that have significant elevations in triglycerides with or without an elevation in cholesterol.

Lipoprotein lipase deficiency

- Increased chylomicrons
- No coronary artery disease

Familial hyperlipemia

- Abnormal triglycerides
- Increased VLDL
- Generally no coronary artery disease
- Some call the condition endogenous hypertriglyceridemia

4 - Diseases & medications

- Birth control pills, steroids, diuretics, beta-blockers, & retinoids
- Hypothyroidism
- Type I Diabetes
- Nephrotic syndrome
- Liver disease

℞ Options

Drug therapy, based on laboratory values, is controversial in children. Significantly elevated values may require medications, whereas mildly elevated values may respond to lifestyle changes alone. Risk factors including an elevated BMI, insulin resistance, type II diabetes, hypertension, and a strong family history of heart disease increase the need for lipid disorder treatment with both nonpharmacological and pharmacological means.

Indicators for ℞

Begin nonpharmacological treatment for children with abnormal fasting lipids. The decision to use pharmacological agents in children is difficult, and it may be best to refer patients for specialty evaluation before starting medications.

Nonpharmacological

Lifestyle modification

Includes increasing physical activity and altering diet. Nutrition recommendations follow on the next page.

- Physical activity

At least 1 hour a day.

- Nutrition

American Heart Association and National Cholesterol Education Program recommendations are in the table on the bottom of the following page. The Step I diet is for milder lipid abnormalities. Often we recommend starting with the Step II diet. When simultaneously treating obesity, attempt to lower carbohydrates to < 50% of caloric intake and raise low fat proteins to between 20-30% of caloric intake.

Pharmacological

Children have limited medication options.

15 Obesity & Lipid Disorders

- **Fish oil omega-3 fatty acids**

Small but significant lowering effects on triglycerides with minimal side effects.

- **Bile acid sequestrants like cholestyramine resin (Questran)**

For high cholesterol but not too effective. Also, compliance is poor.

- **Ezetimibe (Zetia)**

For high cholesterol, not as effective as the statins but less side effects.

- **Statins like atorvastatin (Lipitor)**

For high cholesterol, effective but controversial for prepubescent children. Treatment may cause significant side effects such as rhabdomyolysis and increased liver enzymes.

- **Gemfibrozil (Lopid)**

For high triglycerides but with significant side effects.

- **Nicotinic acid (Niacin)**

For high triglycerides. Less effect on cholesterol. However, nicotinic acid may cause significant side effects, limiting its use in young children.

Nutrient	Recommended Intake as Percent of Total Calories	
	Step I Diet	Step II Diet
Total Fat	30% or less	30% or less
Saturated	7 - 10%	Less than 7%
Polyunsaturated	Up to 10%	Up to 10%
Monounsaturated	Up to 15%	Up to 15%
Cholesterol	Less than 300 mg per day	Less than 200 mg per day
Carbohydrates	55% or more	55% or more
Protein	Approximately 15%	Approximately 15%
Total Calories	To achieve and maintain desired weight	To achieve and maintain desired weight

CLINICAL VIGNETTES

29. A 10-year old male presents with a lipid panel showing total cholesterol of 200 mg/dL, triglycerides of 175 mg/dL, an HDL-cholesterol of 35 mg/dL, and a LDL-cholesterol of 150 mg/dL. He has been asymptomatic, but there is family history of cardiac risk factors. On exam, his weight is above the 95th percentile and his height is at the 50th percentile. His BMI is above the 95th percentile. His blood pressure with an appropriate-sized cuff is 100/60 mmHg. His pulses and cardiac exam are normal. His most likely diagnosis:

a. Homozygous familial hypercholesterolemia
b. Lipoprotein lipase deficiency
c. Heterozygous familial hypercholesterolemia
d. High cholesterol and triglycerides related to obesity

30. A 15-year old Hispanic female presents with acanthosis nigricans. She is asymptomatic, but she has had a significant weight gain in the last 2 years. On exam, her blood pressure with an appropriate-sized cuff is 130/80 mmHg. Her weight is well above the 95th percentile and her height is at the 50th percentile, with a BMI well above the 95th percentile. Her pulses and cardiac exam are normal. Her laboratory tests show a fasting blood sugar of 100 mg/dL, mild elevation in SGOT and SGPT, and an abnormal lipid profile. Refer to treat:

a. Type II diabetes
b. Coarctation of the aorta
c. Liver transplantation
d. None, her exam and labs are within normal limits

REFERENCES

1 Spiotta R, Luma GB. Evaluating obesity and cardiovascular risk factors in children and adolescents. American Family Physician 2008; 78: 1052-1058

2 Latzer Y, Edmunds L, Fenig S, Golan M, Gur E, Hochberg Z, Levin-Zamir D, Zubery E, Speiser PW, Stein D. Managing childhood overweight: behavior, family, pharmacology, and bariatric surgery interventions. Obesity 2009; 17: 423

3 Epstein LH, Wrotniak BH. Future directions for pediatric obesity treatment. Obesity (Silver Spring) 2010; 18: S8-S12

4 Raghuveer G Lifetime cardiovascular risk of childhood obesity. Am J Clin Nutr 2010; 91: 1514S-1519S

5 Colletti RB, Neufeld EJ, Roff NK, McAuliffe TL, Baker AL, Newburger JW. Niacin treatment of hypercholesterolemia in children. Pediatrics 1993; 92: 78-82

6 Kwiterovich PO. Recognition and management of dyslipidemia in children and adolescents. J Clin Endocrinol Metab 2008; 93: 4200-4209

7 Maahs DM, Wadwa RP, Bishop F, Daniels SR, Rewers M, Klingensmith GJ. Dyslipidemia in youth with diabetes: to treat or not to treat? J Pediatr 2008; 153: 458-465

8 Clauss S, Wai KM, Kavey RE, Kuehl K. Ezetimibe treatment of pediatric patients with hypercholesterolemia. J Pediatr 2009; 154: 869-872

Part 2

Anatomy & Physiology

16 Cardiovascular Embryology

Contents

Background	205
Conception to heart tube	206
Ventricular Looping	207
Septation	208
Conotruncus	210
Aortic Arches	212
Systemic Veins	214

16 Cardiovascular Embryology

william evans

BACKGROUND

Cardiovascular embryology is a complex topic, but a basic understanding of events occurring during development can provide insight into the possible origins of malformations. The heart is the earliest embryonic organ. Its development begins at about 2 weeks post conception and is complete by approximately the end of the 2nd month of pregnancy.

The forces shaping cardiac development include the genome, blood flow patterns both embryonic (conception to 8 weeks) and fetal (after 8 weeks), and the intrauterine environment. Some cardiovascular defects relate to arrested stages in cardiovascular embryology like truncus arteriosus. For hypoplastic left heart syndrome (HLHS), however, fetal blood-flow patterns from a restricted foramen ovale may contribute to the malformation. Still, HLHS's etiology likely also resides in a genetic error, as HLHS can be familial and occur in conditions like Turner syndrome. In another example, the anatomical varieties of tetralogy of Fallot likely result from developmental errors in the outlet ventricular septum alignment, coupled with the downstream effects of reduced fetal flow to the branch pulmonary arteries. Further, the teratogenic effects of viruses like rubella, toxins, or maternal comorbidities may result in multifactorial effects on the developing embryo.

In large part, homeobox genes control the remarkable journey the single, fertilized cell travels to become a fully-formed individual. Homeobox genes are like genetic "boot programs" that are basic to a developing embryo. Researchers discovered homeobox genes in 1983. Since then, investigators have identified many cardiovascular developmental homeobox genes. Homeobox genes code for homeodomain-protein transcription factors that interact with the genome turning on and off genes, thereby controlling many aspects of the organism's development. The homeobox genes and the proteins they produce are evolutionarily conserved, meaning genes that control a fruit fly's cardiovascular development have similarities to genes in humans. Developmental processes are fundamental to an organism's survival during embryogenesis; thus, evolutionary forces have conserved vital functions like embryogenesis. [1-4]

The following sections outline the cardiovascular developmental stages. Nevertheless, we can not easily demarcate embryological stages into defined sequential steps, as many occur simultaneously. We list some cardiovascular malformations that likely arise from abnormal stages of cardiovascular development, but the actual mechanisms are far more complex than we represent in this brief outline. As we do not detail the development of the pulmonary arteries, the pulmonary veins, the semilunar valves, or the atrioventricular valves, the interested reader should consult comprehensive works on cardiovascular development.

16 Cardiovascular Embryology

SIMPLE SCHEMA

Fertilization to the Embryonic Disc

The blastocyst forms about 5 days after fertilization. The outer cell layer of the blastocyst is the cytotrophoblast, which implants on the uterine wall (figure below). The cytotrophoblast and the syncytiotrophobast ultimately develop into the placenta. The figure below shows the human embryo at about 15 days of development; and at this time, it exists as a flat cellular plate, the bilaminar embryonic disc. We illustrate the primitive steak (dorsal surface of the embryonic disc), which divides the embryonic disc into a right side and a left side. The primitive streak also defines the posterior part of the embryonic disc. Progenitor cardiogenic cells arise in the anterior part of the embryonic disc and organize into a "cardiac crescent," as we illustrate on the dorsal surface of the embryonic disc in the figure below left.

Embryonic Disc to Ventricular Looping

Beginning with the series of figures on the top of the facing page, figure 1 shows the ventral surface of embryonic disc with a ventral view of the early cardiac crescent (arrows). Figure 2 isolates the cardiac crescent and shows the developing paired heart tubes that fuse into a single heart tube shown in figure 3. Figures 4 and 5 show further development of the single heart tube.

The lower series of figures on the facing page show the progress of normal, rightward (dextro or D) ventricular looping from 21 to 35 days of development.

Possible related conditions

Errors in the cardiac crescent cells and ventricular looping many lead to the following cardiovascular malformations:
- Situs abnormalities
- Dextrocardia
- Unusual ventricular looping like left (levo or L) loop

16 Cardiovascular Embryology

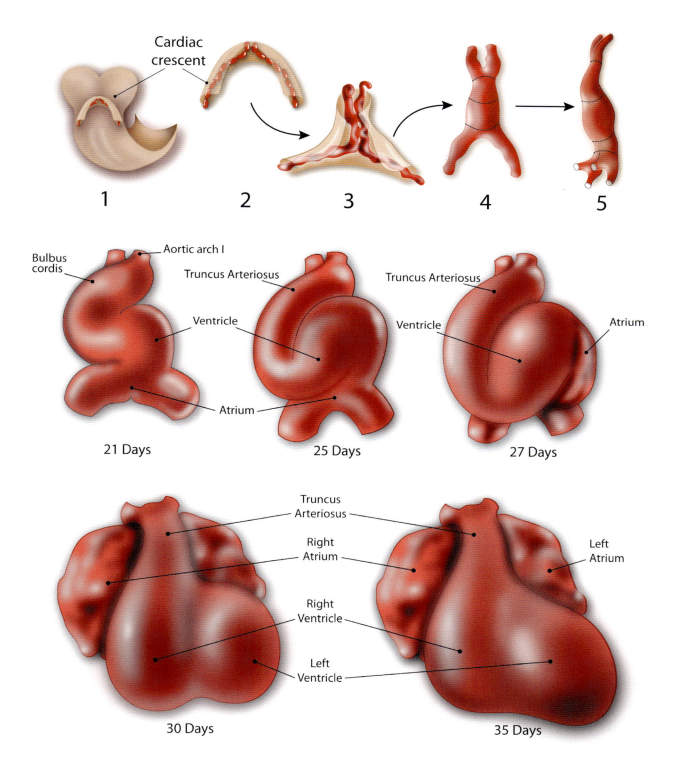

Septation of the Atria & Ventricles

On the facing page, figures 1 through 9 illustrate atrial and ventricular septation, which occurs approximately between 35 and 45 days of development. Even though we do not illustrate them, the atrioventricular valves (tricuspid and mitral) also form during the process of atrial and ventricular septation.

Figure 1 shows the embryonic heart at about 35 days, similar to the 35-day figure illustrated on the previous page; however, the image on the facing page is slightly rotated to expose the right lateral wall of the unseptated atrium and right lateral wall of the unseptated ventricle.

Figure 2 shows the interior of the unseptated embryonic heart. In figure 3, the black arrows indicate ingrowth of the superior and inferior endocardial cushions, as they grow towards each other to divide the single atrioventricular orifice into a right orifice (tricuspid) and left orifice (mitral). The white arrows in figure 3 show the initial growth of the atrial septum primum (the first atrial septum) and the muscular ventricular septum.

In figure 5, the septum primum has almost completely septated the atrium, except for a communicating orifice or foramen primum. Similarly, the ventricles are almost completely septated, except for the communication that will later be closed by the growth of the outlet septum, which develops during conotruncal septation (illustrated on the following pages).

In figures 6 and 7, perforations develop in the septum primum that lead to the foramen secundum. Figures 8 and 9 show the growth of the atrial septum secundum (second atrial septum). An opening persists in the septum secundum, the foramen ovale.

The atrial septation is particularly complex. The mammalian embryo, with the placenta as the organ of oxygenation, requires an opening between the right atrium and left atrium to bypass the right ventricle and the lungs to convey oxygenated fetal blood to the left heart, the coronary arteries, and the brain. For information on fetal physiology, see chapter 18.

Possible related conditions

Errors in atrial and ventricular septation may lead to the following cardiovascular malformations:
- Atrial septal defects both secundum and primum
- Ventricular septal defects of all kinds
- Possibly hearts with 1-functional ventricle

16 Cardiovascular Embryology

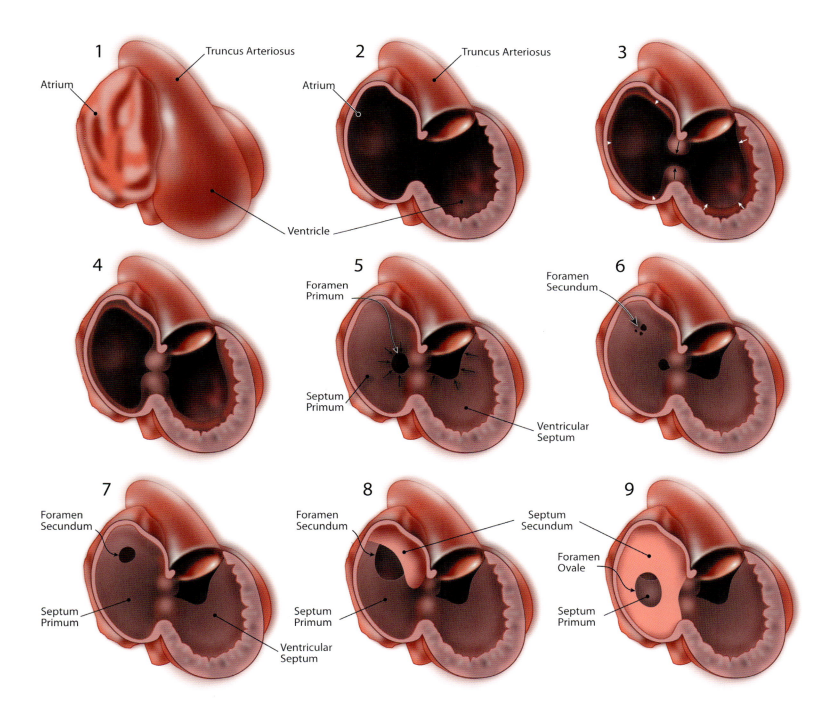

16 Cardiovascular Embryology

Conotruncus

Septation of the single truncal artery and development of the outlet or conal ventricular septum occur between about 35 and 50 days of development.

From figure 9 on the previous page, the large artery arising from the embryonic heart is a single trunk or truncus. Also in figure 9 from the previous page, an opening persists in the ventricular septum, which outlet septal growth closes during this phase of cardiac development. Some of the cells required to achieve truncal septation (into the pulmonary artery and the aorta), development of the outlet septum, and aortic arch development arise from migrating cells from the embryo's neural crest region, seen in the figure on the bottom right. Chromosome 22q11 deletion syndrome affects the neural crest cells, leading to various malformations that include the heart and the aortic arches. Conotruncal abnormalities result in the most common cyanotic conditions presenting in the newborn period, tetralogy of Fallot, transposition of the great arteries, and other complex malformations. For more information on chromosome 22q11 deletion, see Chapter 3.

Figure 1, of the series of figures 1 through 4 on the facing page, shows the embryonic heart (illustrated in figure 9 of the previous page) rotated towards the reader, thereby placing the ventricular septum on end.

Figures 2 through 4 show how the truncus septates and the outlet or conal septum completes ventricular septation; although we do not illustrate them, the semilunar valves also form at this time. In figure 4, the blue arrow indicates the path of the pulmonary outflow and pulmonary artery, and the red arrow shows the path of the systemic outflow and the aorta. Normally, the pulmonary artery becomes positioned over the right ventricle and anterior and to the left of the aorta, which becomes positioned posterior over the left ventricle and rightward with respect to pulmonary artery. See the section on transposition of the great arteries in Chapter 19, for a discussion on the abnormalities of the normal spiraling and positioning of the great arteries.

Possible related conditions

Errors in conotruncal development and septation may lead to the following cardiovascular malformations:
- Tetralogy of Fallot
- Transposition of the great arteries
- Double outlet right ventricle
- Truncus arteriosus
- Aortopulmonary window
- Interrupted aortic arch & ventricular septal defect

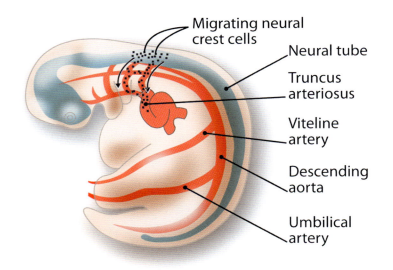

16 Cardiovascular Embryology

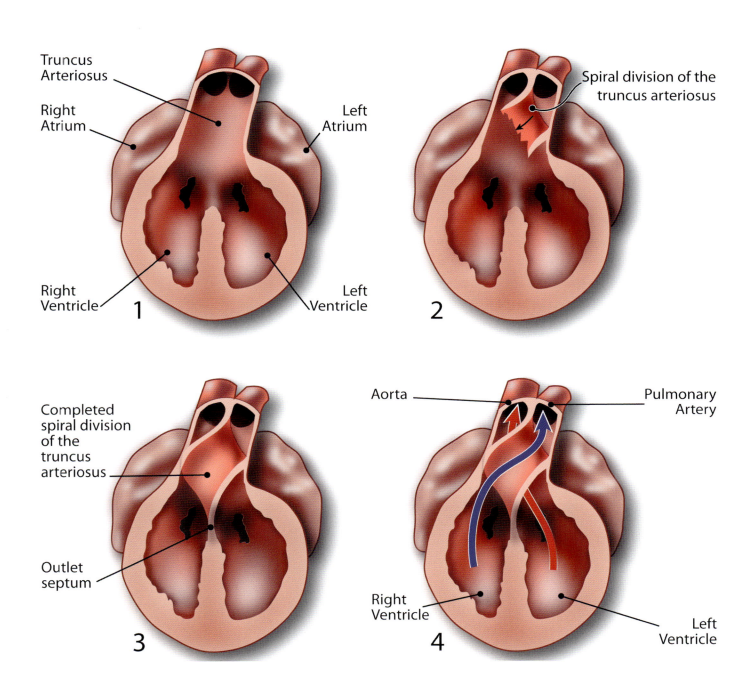

211

Aortic Arches

The aortic arches develop between approximately 28 and 35 days of development. Thus, the aortic arches develop during ventricular looping, which we illustrated previously.

In the figures on the facing page, aortic arch development usually results in a left aortic arch normal branching pattern (figure 1 at the bottom). The yellow segments are the parts of the embryonic arch that disappear during development, both in usual development and development that results in pathology. Normal aortic branching pattern includes the innominate artery, which is the proximal remnant of the right aortic arch. Another possibility is the development a right aortic arch and mirror image branching pattern (which we do not illustrate).

In figure 2, we illustrate a right aortic arch with an aberrant left subclavian that results in a vascular ring. In figure 3, we illustrate a double aortic arch that also results in a vascular ring. Vascular ring anomalies compress the trachea and the esophagus, as we illustrate in figure 2 and 3.

Possible related conditions

Errors in the aortic arch development may lead to the following cardiovascular malformations:
- Vascular ring as per above
- Coarctation
- Interrupted aortic arch

16 Cardiovascular Embryology

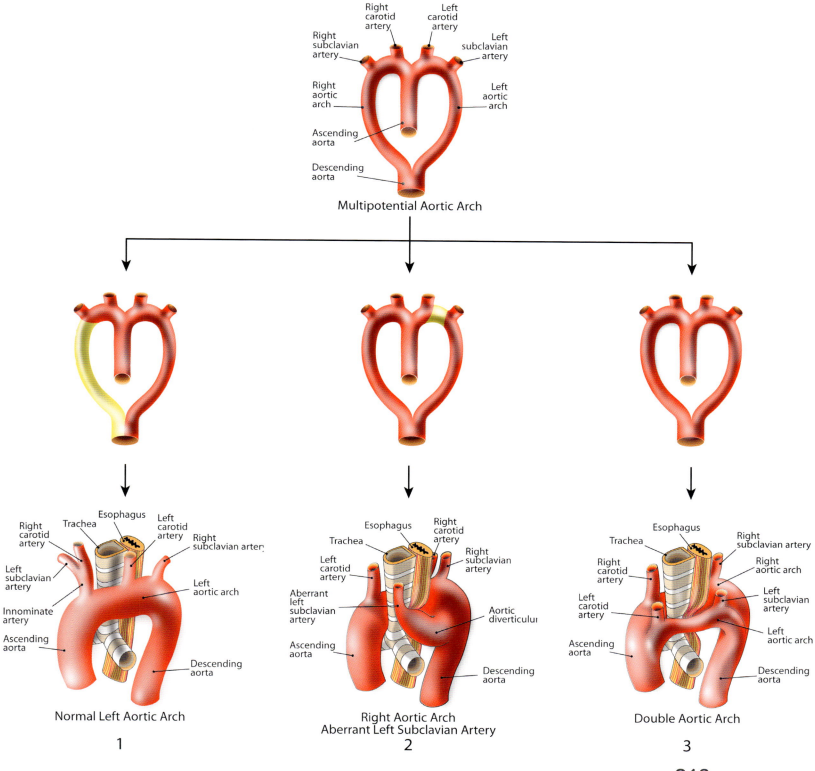

16 Cardiovascular Embryology

Systemic Veins

The figures on the facing page show the development of the proximal system veins as seen from the back of the heart; thus, left is on the reader's left. These figures trace development from 24 days to about 56 days. Figure 2, on the top right, shows the conclusion of usual development, which results in a single, right-sided superior vena cava (SVC).

Figure 4, on the bottom right, shows a common variant, a separate left SVC draining to the coronary sinus, which occurs normally in about 3 out of 1,000 births. However, a left SVC to the coronary sinus can also be associated with other congenital cardiovascular malformations in about 4 to 10 per 100 patients with congenital heart disease.

Figures 1 and 3 show the venous structures that involute, those outlined in light purple. Figure 1 also shows how the left superior cardinal vein normally involutes, while figure 3 shows how it persists, leading to the left SVC to the coronary sinus.

When placing a central venous line from above, consider the presence of a left SVC to the coronary sinus if a subsequent chest X-ray shows the radiopaque catheter near the left heart border rather than the right.

Possible related abnormalities

Errors in systemic vein development may lead to the following malformations:
- Persistent left SVC to coronary sinus as per above
- Interrupted inferior vena cava
- Other proximal system venous abnormalities

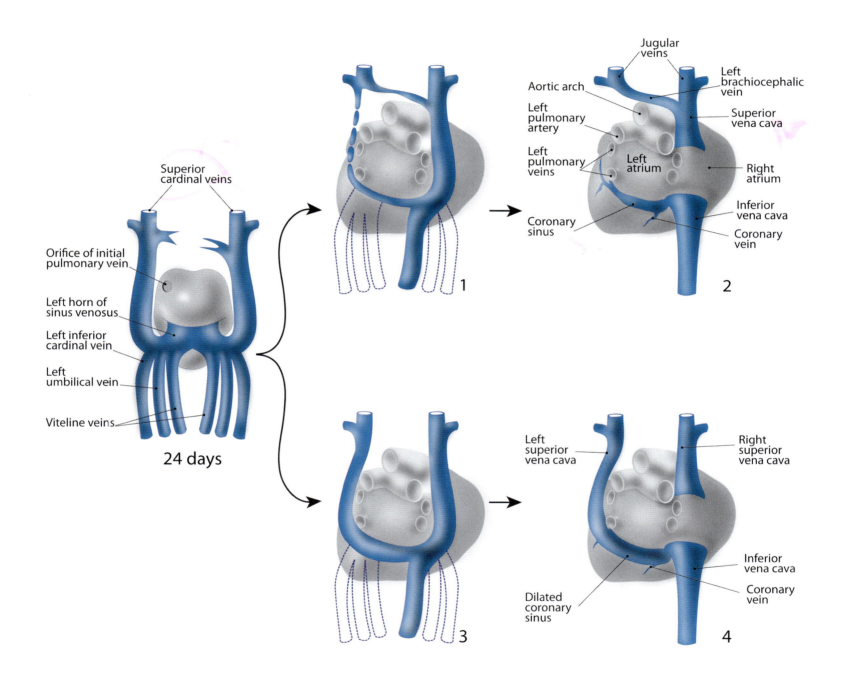

References

1 Angelini P. Embryology and congenital heart disease. Tex Heart Inst J 1995; 22: 1-12

2 Abdulla R, Blew GA, Holterman MJ. Cardiovascular embryology. Pediatr Cardiol 2004; 25: 191-200

3 Pelech AN, Broeckel U. Toward the etiologies of congenital heart diseases. Clin Perinatol 2005; 32: 825-844

4 Hu N, Christensen DA, Agrawal AK, Beaumont C, Clark EB, Hawkins JA. Dependence of aortic arch morphogenesis on intracardiac blood flow in the left atrial ligated chick embryo. Anat Rec (Hoboken) 2009; 292: 652-660

5 Rudolph, Abraham M. Congenital Diseases of the Heart: Clinical-Physiological Considerations. Chichester, Wiley-Blackwell, 2009

17 Situs & Cardiac Position

Contents

Background	219
Thoracoabdominal situs	220
Cardiac position	225
Segmental analysis	226

17 Situs & Cardiac Position

william evans

BACKGROUND

Embryogenesis most often results in situs solitus with levocardia, the usual position of the abdominal and thoracic organs. However, other situs arrangements and cardiac positions may occur. Alternate situses and cardiac positions have higher incidences of cardiovascular malformations. Unusual situs and cardiac position introduce complexity that even challenges pediatric cardiologists. Because of potential complexity, pediatric cardiologists developed the segmental approach for systematically describing situs, cardiac position, and cardiovascular anatomy.

Even though a chest X-ray may initially suggest an unusual situs (see Chapter 20), echocardiography (Echo), prenatally or postnatally, is the most common method we employ for anatomical diagnosis. Complementary tools include computed tomography (CT), magnetic resonance imaging (MRI), and angiography. [1-6]

The Segmental Approach

The segmental approach includes steps for evaluating anatomy in the following order:

- Thoracoabdominal situs
- Cardiac position
- Atrioventricular connections
- Ventriculoarterial connections
- Vena caval & pulmonary venous connections
- Additional cardiovascular malformations, if present

17 Situs & Cardiac Position

THORACOABDOMINAL SITUS

In segmental analysis, the first step determines the thoracoabdominal situs (the position of the liver, stomach, inferior vena cava, lung morphology, and atrial morphology). We establish thoracoabdominal situs independent of the cardiac position in the chest. Thoracoabdominal situs is solitus when the arrangement is usual.

Classification systems for thoracoabdominal situs are the subject of numerous reports, yet confusion persists, especially over the terms "heterotaxy" and "heterotaxy syndrome." We do not use the term "heterotaxy syndrome" as the wide-ranging forms of heterotaxy do not fit into the classic definition of syndrome. The term "syndrome" implies a collection of malformations that consistently occur together like Down syndrome. As heterotaxy simply means "other arrangement," we define heterotaxy as any situs other than the usual arrangement. The organigram on the facing page outlines thoracoabdominal situs variations.

17 Situs & Cardiac Position

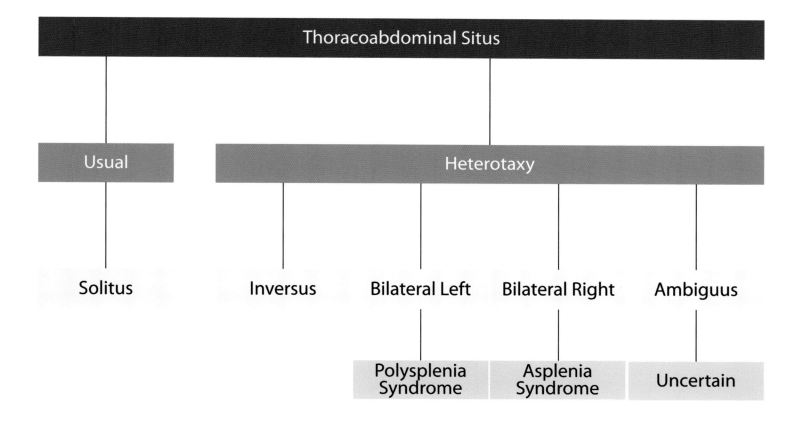

17 Situs & Cardiac Position

Usual Situs versus Heterotaxy

The figure on the facing page illustrates 4 possible situs arrangements.

Thoracoabdominal situs solitus (figure A) is usually associated with levocardia and normal atrioventricular and ventriculoarterial connections. There is a single, right-sided superior vena cava (SVC) and the inferior vena cava (IVC) in continuity with the right atrium. The pulmonary veins enter the left atrium. The right lung has 3 lobes (labeled 1 through 3). The left lung has 2 lobes. The liver is on the right. The stomach and single spleen are on the left.

Thoracoabdominal situs inversus (figure B) usually has dextrocardia and normal atrioventricular and ventriculoarterial connections, an arrangement usually resulting in normal organ anatomy and physiology just reversed. Note in figure B that the left lung has 3 lobes, the right lung has 2 lobes, the abdominal viscera and the atria are reversed, and the IVC and SVC are on the left. Nevertheless, thoracoabdominal situs inversus with dextrocardia has a higher incidence of cardiovascular malformations than thoracoabdominal situs solitus and levocardia. Past studies quote a 3-9% or higher incidence of significant cardiovascular defects in the former, comparing to an approximate incidence of 1% (excluding bicuspid aortic valve and patent foramen ovale) in the latter. In our review of dextrocardia, we found a 16% incidence of significant cardiovascular malformations in thoracoabdominal situs inversus with dextrocardia, and otherwise normal atrioventricular and ventriculoarterial connections. Also the immobile-celia, autosomal recessive Kartagener syndrome is associated with situs inversus, and the condition includes a triad of sinusitis, bronchiectatis, and situs inversus with dextrocardia.

Bilateral right-sidedness (figure C) occurs with a transverse liver; a stomach towards the midline; both lungs have right lung characteristics (3 lobes); both atria have right-atrium characteristics; bilateral superior vena cavas; the pulmonary veins usually drain abnormally; and no spleen exists. As normally there is no spleen on the right side, "bilateral right-sidedness" has no spleen at all—asplenia syndrome. Some refer to asplenia syndrome with complex cardiac malformation as Ivemark syndrome. An asplenic patient needs chronic prophylaxis, usually with penicillin, to reduce the chance of pneumococcal or meningococcal disease, against which the spleen normally guards.

Bilateral left-sidedness (figure D) also occurs with a transverse liver; a somewhat midline stomach; both lungs have left lung characteristics (2 lobes); both atria have left atrium characteristics; the presence of interrupted inferior vena cava with azygos continuation to the superior vena cava; and the presence of multiple spleens. As the spleen is normally on the left, "bilateral left-sidedness" logically has more spleens than normal—polysplenia syndrome.

If the situs arrangement does not fit into these categories, then the situs is ambiguus. Bilateral left-sidedness, bilateral right-sidedness, and situs ambiguus all have incidences of cardiovascular malformations approaching 100%.

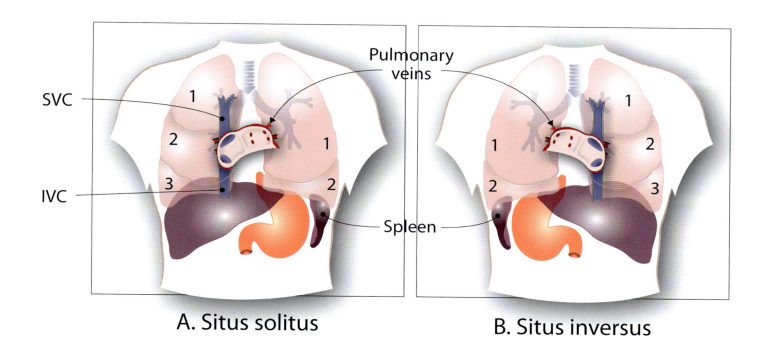

Summary of Polysplenia & Asplenia

The table below summarizes some salient features of bilateral left-sidedness (polysplenia syndrome) and bilateral right-sidedness (asplenia syndrome). Frequently, patients with asplenia and polysplenia syndormes have complex cardiac malformations. In addition, because the heart beat originates with the sinus node in the right atrium, patients with bilateral left-sided atria are more likely to have arrhythmias than those with bilateral right-sided atria. Also, those with bilateral left-sided atrial often have low atrial rhythms (see Chapter 21 for EKG interpretation).

	Polysplenia Bilateral Left-Sideness	Asplenia Bilateral Right-Sideness
Abdominal Situs	Unusual	Unusual
Inferior Vena Cava	Interrupted + azygos continuation	Same side of the aorta
Dextrocardia	Common	Common
Complex Heart Disease	Common	Common
Complete AV block	Common	Less common
Bradycardia 1:1	Common	Less common

CARDIAC POSITION

The cardiac base-apex axis defines dextrocardia, mesocardia, and levocardia. The figure below shows 3 cardiac base-apex axes; the arrows indicate the direction. The cardiac base-apex axis is not dependent on thoracoabdominal situs; although, the vast majority of those with thoracoabdominal situs solitus have levocardia. Nevertheless, thoracoabdominal situs solitus can also occur with dextrocardia or mesocardia.

Dextrocardia, mesocardia, and levocardia all result from cardiac embryology, whether usual or not. However, intrathoracic pathology, such as a diaphragmatic hernia or pneumothorax, can mechanically pull or push the heart to the right. Nevertheless, a patient does not suddenly develop dextrocardia just from mechanical rightward positioning of the heart. A chest X-ray demonstrating the heart in the right chest can be inconclusive for either a rightward position from mechanical factors or dextrocardia; however, an Echo can determine the difference.

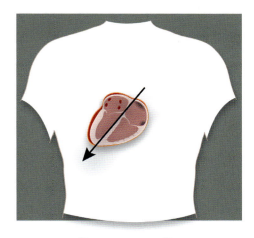 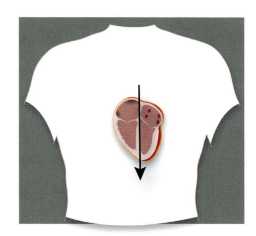 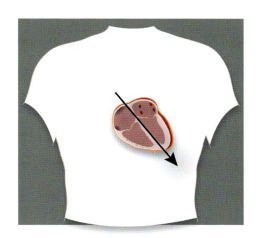

Dextrocardia Mesocardia Levocardia

17 Situs & Cardiac Position

ADDITIONAL SEGMENTAL ANALYSIS

Normally, the morphological right atrium on the right connects with the morphological right ventricle on the right. The right ventricle normally connects with the anterior pulmonary artery, which is normally anterior and left of the aorta. Further, the morphological left atrium on the left connects with the morphological left ventricle on the left. The left ventricle connects with the posterior aorta, which is normally to the right of the anterior pulmonary artery.

In segmental analysis, each relationship and connection requires definition. The thoracoabdominal situs predicts the atrial arrangements, as we outlined above. However, situs does not predict the ventriculoarterial arrangements or the cardiac position, as any combination can exist. Segmental analysis should also define the superior and inferior vena caval connections; the pulmonary venous connections; and other cardiovascular malformations including atrial septal defects, ventricular septal defects, valvular stenoses, abnormalities of the pulmonary arteries, abnormalities of the aorta, and others.

REFERENCES

1 Ellis K, Fleming RJ, Griffiths SP, Jameson AG. New concepts in dextrocardia. Angiocardiographic considerations. Am J Roentgenol Radium Ther Nucl Med 1966; 97: 295-313

2 Van Praagh R. The segmental approach to diagnosis in congenital heart disease. In: Bergsma D, editor. Birth defects original article series, VIII, No. 5. The National Foundation– March of Dimes. Baltimore: Williams and Wilkins; 1972, p 4-23

3 Fulton DR, Freed MD. The pathology, pathophysiology, recognition, and treatment of congenital heart disease. In: Fuster V, Alexander RW, O'Rourke RA, Roberts R, King SP, Prystowsky EN, Nash I (eds) Hurst's The heart 2. New York, McGraw-Hill, Medical Publishing Division, 2008, p 1830

4 Anderson RH, Shirali G. Sequential segmental analysis. Ann Pediatr Cardiol 2009; 2: 24-35

5 Evans WN, Acherman RJ, Collazos JC, Castillo WJ, Rollins RC, Kip KT, Restrepo H. Dextrocardia: practical clinical points and comments on terminology. Pediatr Cardiol 2010; 31: 1-6

6 Evans WN. Thoracoabdominal situs: a practical approach accompanied by a short history of descriptive terms. Pediatr Cardiol 2010; 31: 1049-1051

17 Situs & Cardiac Position

18 Fetal & Neonatal Cardiovascular Physiology

Contents

Background	231
Fetal Circulation	232
Fetal Adaptations	234
Changes at Birth	236

230

18 Fetal & Neonatal Cardiovascular Physiology

william castillo

BACKGROUND

Even though we celebrate current knowledge of fetal and neonatal cardiovascular physiology, centuries of investigation underlie contemporary comprehension. In Italy in 1600, Fabricius published his *De Formato Foetu,* which included illustrated plates of the foramen ovale and the ductus arteriosus. In England in 1669, Richard Lower published his *Tractatus de Corde* (Treatise on the Heart), which detailed fetal blood flow via the foramen ovale and ductus arteriosus with uncanny accuracy. In 1939 English physiologists, A.E. Barclay and Joseph Barcroft, confirmed Richard Lower's fetal flow description via experimental angiography in animal studies. By the mid-20th century at Oxford, Geoffrey Dawes elucidated the dramatic physiological changes occurring with birth.

The investigators, who followed, stood on the shoulders of giants while advancing scientific understanding of fetal and neonatal cardiovascular physiology. Over the past 50 years, most fetal cardiovascular research has occurred in sheep and other animals. During the last 25 years, however, researchers have gained considerable information from prenatal ultrasound. Such information has improved the understanding of cardiovascular physiology in human fetuses.

Cardiovascular malformations introduce additional factors affecting fetal and neonatal cardiovascular physiology, especially during the cascade of dramatic changes occurring with birth. Comprehensive texts of fetal and neonatal cardiology describe physiological mechanisms in abnormal cardiovascular states; thus, we do not discuss them in this brief summary. [1-8]

FETAL CIRCULATION

On the facing page, the figures display fetal circulation. The figure on the left shows the fetal heart a bit more posterior than the figure on the right. Hence, the figure on the left better demonstrates the foramen ovale's function, and the figure on the right is better for showing the function of the ductus arteriosus.

Deoxygenated fetal blood passes through the placenta's capillary bed and picks up oxygen from maternal blood. Deoxygenated fetal blood has a PaO_2 in the low 20s. However, the "oxygenated" blood in the umbilical vein conveys back to the fetal heart and has a PaO_2 of only about 35 mm Hg. The ductus venosus directs oxygenated blood from the placenta to cross the right atrium and enter the left atrium via the foramen ovale. Besides directing the blood from the umbilical vein to the heart, the ductus venosus restricts the volume of blood entering the fetal heart, preventing cardiac overload. The oxygenated blood in the left atrium then enters the left ventricle. From there, the left ventricle pumps the oxygenated blood principally to the brain and the coronary arteries. The fetal right ventricle primarily receives desaturated venous blood from the superior and inferior vena cavas. The fetal right ventricle pumps most of its blood to the lower body via the ductus arteriosus; a fraction of the blood from the right ventricle, however, enters the collapsed lungs. The desaturated umbilical arterial blood reenters the placenta for oxygenation via the umbilical arteries.

The placenta is more than the organ of oxygenation. Among other functions, the placenta also eliminates fetal CO_2; removes waste products; picks up nutrients from the mother's blood; and participates in hormonal and immunological regulation. [9,10]

18 Fetal & Neonatal CV Physiology

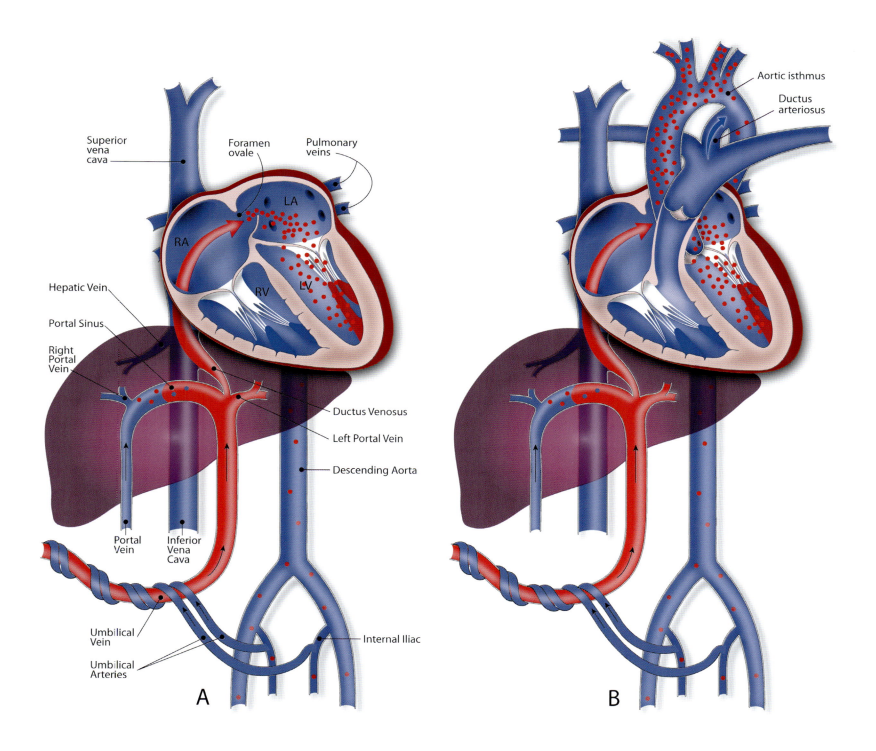

233

FETAL CARDIOVASCULAR ADAPTIVE MECHANISMS

Fetal Hemoglobin

Fetal hemoglobin binds oxygen better than adult hemoglobin. The enhanced binding property of fetal hemoglobin helps it take up oxygen from maternal blood, as maternal and fetal blood pass through the placenta separated by a thin, permeable membrane about 3.5 μm thick. As the figure below displays, a PaO_2 of about 19 mm Hg results in a fetal hemoglobin saturation of at least 50%. In contrast, it takes a PaO_2 of almost 27 mm Hg (> 40% higher) to produce a hemoglobin saturation of 50% for adult hemoglobin. The oxygen binding property of fetal hemoglobin allows adequate delivery to the fetal tissue, despite the relative hypoxic state of the fetus. [11]

Fetal Cardiac Output

The fetal heart has decreased reserve, compared with the hearts in infant and children, which limits adaptation to normal and abnormal physiological changes. The Frank-Starling law states that the heart, up to a point, increases its cardiac output as the diastolic blood volume increases. The fetal heart also increases cardiac output with increasing diastolic volume; however, the fetal heart has less ability to use this mechanism than the adult heart.

The fetal myocardium has structural differences from the adult myocardium. Noncontractile elements constitute 60% of fetal hearts. In contrast, noncontractile elements comprise 30% of adult hearts. This discrepancy partly

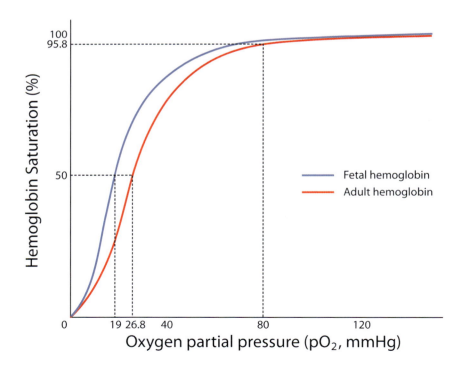

explains the fetal heart's limited ability to increase cardiac output.

The fetal cardiac output depends more on increasing heart rate than on the Frank-Starling mechanism. Nonetheless, an increasing heart rate is a less robust mechanism than the Frank-Starling law for increasing cardiac output. Additionally, the fetus's response to hypoxia is another adaptive mechanism related to cardiac output. This response undergoes change during gestation. Early in development, hypoxia causes fetal tachycardia but later in development, with maturation of the baroreceptors, fetal hypoxia results in bradycardia. [12-15]

NEONATAL TRANSITIONAL CARDIOVASCULAR PHYSIOLOGY

At birth, the lungs fill with air and the pulmonary arterial pressure decreases, the pulmonary blood flow increases, and the pulmonary vascular resistance (PVR) drops (figure on the right), reaching adult levels at about 2 months of age. The drop in PVR results from lung expansion and response to rising PaO_2, because oxygen is a potent vasodilator. As the PVR drops, the previous limited fetal-pulmonary blood flow acutely increases, increasing the pulmonary venous return and increasing the pressure in the left atrium. The placenta is an organ with low vascular resistance; thus, with clamping the umbilical cord, the systemic vascular resistance (SVR) goes up. Increasing SVR decreases flow into the right atrium, and decreasing flow decreases right atrial (RA) pressure.

Normally the ductus venosus, foramen ovale, and ductus arteriosus all close shortly after birth. The ductus venosus physiologically closes by about 4 to 6 days old; whereas, anatomical closure occurs between 15 and 20 days. Ductus venosus closure has practical implications when placing umbilical venous catheters (UVCs), because an open ductus venosus allows a UVC to pass into the right atrium. With a closed ductus venosus, the UVC becomes trapped in the liver. The ductus venosus closure mechanism is unclear but may result from a combination of lack of flow and other factors such as the effects from postnatal corticosteroid levels. A natural flap guards the foramen ovale. This flap allows fetal right-to-left shunting from the right atrium to the left. Postnatally, the left atrial pressure rises with increased pulmonary venous return and forces the foramen ovale flap to close against the interatrial septum.

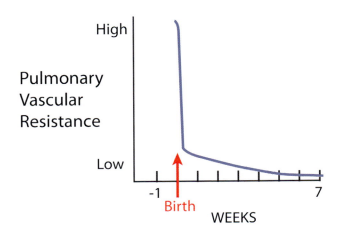

The drop in RA pressure augments foramen ovale flap closure.

Many have studied the ductus arteriosus closure in detail. During the last trimester of pregnancy, specialized smooth muscle develops within ductal walls. This specialized smooth muscle responds by contracting with oxygen and bradykinins. In contrast, certain prostaglandins cause ductal-wall smooth muscle to relax. With birth, the arterial PaO_2 rises, circulating bradykinins increase, and prostaglandin production decreases. All these factors promote physiological ductal closure. Anatomical closure occurs a few weeks later. The causes for the persistence of a patent ductus arteriosus (PDA) are complex and involve the autonomic nervous system, chemical mediators, and pathological changes to the musculature of the walls of the ductus arteriosus. [16-19]

References

1 Rosenberg SL. Hieronymus Fabricius Ab Aquapendente: parts I-III Cal West Med. 1933; 38: 173-176, 260-263, 367-370

2 Lowe R. Tractatus de corde, item de motu & colore sanguinis, & chyli in eum transitu. Amstelodami, Apud Danielem Elsevirium, 1671

3 Dawes GS, Mott JC, Widdicombe JG, Wyatt DG. Changes in the lungs of the new-born lamb. J Physiol 1953; 121: 141-162

4 Dawes GS. Foetal and Neonatal Physiology: A Comparative Study of the Changes at Birth. Chicago, Year Book Medical, 1968

5 Rudolph AM, Heymann MA. The circulation of the fetus in utero. Circ Res 1967; 21: 163-184

6 Friedman WF. The intrinsic physiologic properties of the developing heart. Prog Cardiovasc Dis 1972; 15:87-111

7 Lind J. Researches in perinatal circulation. http://www.neonatology.org/classics/mj1980/ch14.html

8 Yagel S, Silverman NH, Gembruch U. Fetal Cardiology: Embryology, Genetics, Physiology, Echocardiographic Evaluation, Diagnosis, and Perinatal Management of Cardiac Diseases. New York, Informa Healthcare, 2009

9 Acherman RJ, Evans WN, Galindo A, Collazos JC, Rothman A, Mayman GA, Luna CF, Rollins R, Kip KT, Berthoty DP, Restrepo H. Diagnosis of absent ductus venosus in a population referred for fetal echocardiography: association with a persistent portosystemic shunt requiring postnatal device occlusion. J Ultrasound Med. 2007; 26:1077-1082

10 Acherman RJ, Rollins RC, Castillo WJ, Evans WN. Stenosis of Alternative Umbilical Venous Pathways in Absent Ductus Venosus. J Ultrasound Med 2010; 29: 1227-1231

11 Adult versus fetal hemoglobin saturation curve. http://upload.wikimedia.org/wikipedia/en/f/fb/HbA_vs_HbF_saturation_curve.png

12 Gilbert RD. Control of fetal cardiac output during changes in blood volume. Am J Physiol 1980; 238: H80-H86

13 Thornburg KL, Morton MJ. Filling and arterial pressures as determinants of left ventricular stroke volume in unanesthetized fetal lambs. Am J Physiol 1986; 251: H961-H968

14 Artman M. Sarcolemmal sodium–calcium exchange activity and exchanger immunoreactivity in developing rabbit hearts. Am J Physiol 1992; 263: H1506-H1513

15 Mahoney L. Calcium homeostasis and control of contractility in the developing heart. Sem Perinatol 1996; 20: 510-519

16 Rudolph AM. Congenital Diseases of the Heart: Clinical-Physiologic Considerations in Diagnosis and Management. Chicago, Year Book Medical Publishers, 1974

17 Meyer WW, Lind J. The ductus venosus and the mechanism of its closure. Arch Dis Child 1966; 41: 597-605

18 Loberant N, Barak M. Closure of the ductus venosus in neonates: findings on real-time gray-scale, color-flow Doppler, and duplex Doppler sonography American Journal of Roentgenology 1992; 159: 1083-1085

19 Kondo M, Itoh S. Time of closure of ductus venosus in term and preterm neonates. Arch Dis Child Fetal Neonatal Ed 2001; 85: F57-F59

18 Fetal & Neonatal CV Physiology

19 Cardiovascular Malformations

Contents

Background	241
Physiological Concepts	244
Volume Overload	246
Pressure Overload	258
Cardiomyopathies	266
Presenting in Extremis	270
Low Oxygen Saturation	276
Vascular Rings	300

19 Cardiovascular Malformations

william evans • ruben acherman

BACKGROUND

Most references classify cardiovascular defects as acyanotic or cyanotic, but the basis for this classification system relies largely on cardiac anatomy defined by imaging or pathological exam. A patient symptomatic at presentation from a cardiac malformation may have medical history and physical exam findings consistent with heart failure or desaturation. However, clinicians do not initially know the complete anatomical details of a patient's cardiovascular defect. Although anatomical findings may be quite discrepant, clinical findings can overlap. As we point out in Chapter 7, some "cyanotic" heart defects do not present with visible cyanosis; rather, the first sign may be a low oximeter reading. Further, patients with large ventricular septal defects, heart failure, and pulmonary edema may present desaturated from intrapulmonary right-to-left shunts. Thus, we prefer to classify cardiovascular malformations clinically in a manner consistent with the Problems Chapters.

However, a clinical-classification approach also has limitations, as many malformations produce no overt symptoms or signs. Conditions with few symptoms include some atrial septal defects, patent ductus arteriosuses, valvular stenoses, coarctations, ventricular septal defects, and others. Even routine physical exam fails to detect some cardiovascular malformations. Newborns with complex ductal-dependent cardiovascular defects are especially at risk. Infants may go home from newborn nurseries and then present severely cyanotic or in extremis hours or days later when the patent ductus arteriosus closes. In an attempt to prevent the discharge of an infant with significant undiagnosed congenital heart disease, statements form the American Academy of Pediatrics and the American Heart Association have supported routine oximetry in asymptomatic infants prior to discharge from regular newborn nurseries. However, the same position papers note that oximetry's sensitivity for detecting serious congenital heart disease varies greatly, from 0-100%. Routine newborn oximetry is fraught with technical difficulties and false positives may result in unnecessary consultations, additional testings, and possible transports to cardiac centers. Along with preventing some discharges, significant increased healthcare costs will accompany universal newborn oximetry screening.

Routine prenatal fetal echocardiography (Echo) screening could identify the vast majority of fetuses with potential serious cardiovascular abnormalities that subsequent comprehensive fetal echocardiography could define in detail. Currently, however, standard obstetric ultrasound misses most cardiovascular malformations. Similar to oximetry, routine fetal echocardiographic screening studies will also increase healthcare costs. Nonetheless, evidence suggests that, in contrast to

19 Cardiovascular Malformations

oximetry's 0-100% sensitivity postnatally, fetal echocardiography is the best evidence-based method for detecting cardiovascular malformations antenatally. Antenatal detection allows advanced planning for delivery, a significant advantage over postnatal oximetry. Thus, when taking a medical history, always inquire about the findings from fetal ultrasound. However, short of pediatric cardiology oversight, a standard prenatal fetal ultrasound report usually does not contain complete cardiovascular anatomical details. For more on fetal Echo, see Chapter 23.

Defining the incidence of congenital cardiovascular malformations is difficult. In the general population, cardiovascular malformations occur in about 1% of live births (not including bicuspid aortic valve, which alone occurs in about 1-2% of the population). Ethnicity or changes that can occur in populations over decades can influence the incidence of cardiovascular defects. We reported such differences in Southern Nevada for D-transposition of the great arteries and tetralogy of Fallot [1]. Also, the chance of a child born with a cardiovascular defect increases following the birth of a previous child with a cardiovascular malformation. Familial incidence further increases when a parent, especially the mother, or other relatives have congenital heart disease. Reports provide approximate incidence numbers for familial factors. Syndromes have the highest incidence of congenital heart disease. For some syndromes, almost 100% have cardiovascular malformations. For more on syndromes with cardiac malformations, see Chapter 3. Clinicians should consult with geneticists or genetic counselors for more information about the incidence of cardiovascular defects.

Congenital heart disease complexity usually increases with unusual situs. A chest X-ray (CXR) showing an abnormal stomach bubble location or abnormal cardiac silhouette position or both suggests significant cardiac malformations. However, we use Echo, not CXR, to define situs and cardiac position (whether levocardia, dextrocardia, or mesocardia). For more on situs and cardiac position, see Chapters 17 and 20.

Cardiac malformations can occur in combination. Multiple defects may complicate treatment, as surgical risk may be low for individual lesions but high when in combination. Treating single or combined defects may include medications, catheter intervention, surgery, or multiple modalities. Also, other organ system abnormalities and comorbidities like pneumonia can complicate the clinical presentation. Regardless of the defect, the ultimate goal is to render a child's heart as normal as possible, using methods with the lowest risks.

For this chapter, we begin with the common defects frequently presenting with chronic heart failure. Next, we describe the abnormalities usually presenting in extremis. The 3rd group includes those presenting with low oxygen saturation, including the "5 Ts." We reserve a 4th group for vascular rings, as vascular rings usually have stridor or difficulty swallowing rather than heart failure or desaturation. Although, a vascular ring with severe airway obstruction may present with oxygen desaturation.

For each defect, we begin by briefly describing the malformation along with relevant Echo findings. We accompany each malformation's description with an anatomical illustration. The subsequent outline includes chief medical history points, physical exam positives or negatives, key CXR findings, and treatment options.

Other than occasionally, we do not include EKG findings, as EKGs provide little assistance in determining a complete structural diagnosis. Nonetheless, all patients

19 Cardiovascular Malformations

with cardiac malformations should have an EKG to assess electrical abnormalities and to check for any ST-T wave changes. ST-T wave changes occur with myocardial stress in severe pulmonary or aortic stenosis, and other defects causing significant pressure or volume overload.

Normal Anatomy

For orientation, the figures on the bottom of the page illustrate normal cardiac, great artery, venal caval, and pulmonary venous anatomy.

Figure A below is the 4-chamber view. Important features to note include the venal caval openings are posterior (not on the top and the bottom of the right atrium), 4 pulmonary veins open into the back of the left atrium, the tricuspid valve is slightly lower than the mitral valve, and the right ventricular (RV) walls are thinner and more trabeculated than the thicker and smoother left ventricular (LV) walls.

Figure B below is the left-ventricular outflow view, which is slightly anterior to the 4-chamber view. This view shows the trileaflet aortic valve, the coronary artery orifices, and the aortic arch to the left with its arterial branching pattern.

Figure C below is the right-ventricular outflow view, which is slightly anterior to the left-ventricular outflow view. This view shows the anterior pulmonary artery arising from the long, right ventricular outflow tract (or infundibulum), the trileaflet pulmonary valve anterior and to the left of the aorta, and the pulmonary artery branching to the right and left lungs. The aortic valve is in continuity with the mitral valve, but the pulmonary valve is distant from the tricuspid valve. [1-7]

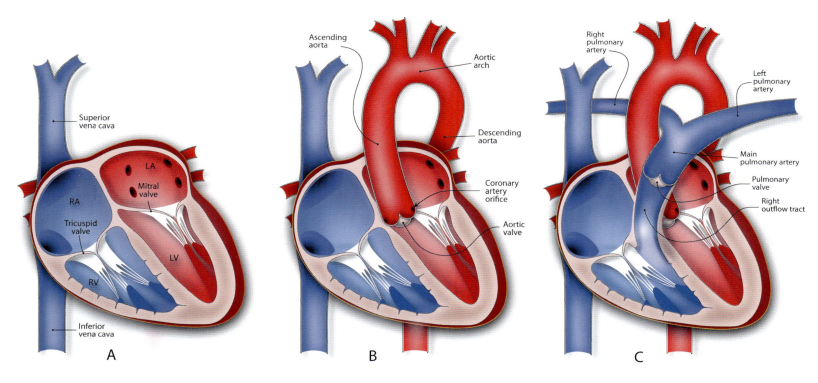

19 Cardiovascular Malformations

DEFECTS PRESENTING WITH CHRONIC HEART FAILURE

General Concepts

Symptoms and signs from a ventricular septal defect (VSD) or a patent ductus arteriosus (PDA) arise from left-to-right shunts that cause pulmonary overcirculation and from the systemic pressure the defect communicates to the lungs. In large VSDs and PDAs, both the increased flow and pressure contribute to long-term pulmonary vascular damage, leading to irreversible pulmonary hypertension or Eisenmenger syndrome. Early repair of these defects can prevent progressive pulmonary vascular pathology.

Although an atrial septal defect (ASD) increases flow to the lungs via a left-to-right shunt, no communication of high pressure exists. Nevertheless, when an ASD is present for many years the increased pulmonary flow often results in pulmonary vascular changes and pulmonary hypertension. Therefore, ASDs need early detection in childhood. Additionally, when an Echo reveals an atrial septal aneurysm in an infant, especially with a fenestrated ASD and several areas of left-to-right shunt, the patient needs followup with pediatric cardiology. These patients are at higher risk for persistent, significant atrial level shunts that usually need later closure.

A VSD or PDA's size determines the pulmonary arterial pressure. For example, if a defect is large then the pulmonary arterial pressure is equal to systemic arterial pressure. Nevertheless, left-to-right shunting depends on 2 additional factors, the systemic vascular resistance (SVR) and the pulmonary vascular resistance (PVR), with PVR playing the larger role.

Vascular Resistance

Vascular pressure and vascular resistance are not equivalent. Vascular resistance is a vessel's resistance to flow. We measure pressure in mm of Hg, but we use formulas to calculate vascular resistance. Flow is proportional to pressure (more pressure more flow), but flow is inversely proportional to resistance (more resistance less flow). The formulas below mathematically relate flow (Q), pressure (P), and resistance (R):

$$Q \text{ (flow)} = P \text{ (pressure)} \div R \text{ (resistance)}$$

Then solving for resistance (R):

$$R = P \div Q$$

A straightforward way to appreciate vascular resistance is imagine drinking a milkshake with a narrow straw versus a wide one. Flow (Q) increases if resistance (R) decreases and the mean pressure (P) remains unchanged. From the "milkshake experiment," the wider straw, with lower resistance, delivers higher flow. In blood vessels, each of the formula's variables or > 1 variable can change under both physiological or pathological states.

PVR & SVR calculation examples

We report vascular resistance in Wood units.
- Pulmonary vascular resistance (PVR)

Using a pulmonary flow (Qp) of 6 L/min, and a mean

pulmonary arterial pressure (mPAP) of 12 mm Hg:

> PVR = mPAP ÷ Qp or PVR = 12 ÷ 6
>
> PVR = 2 Wood units

- Systemic vascular resistance (SVR)

Using a systemic flow (Qs) of 6 L/min, and a mean systemic arterial pressure (mSAP) of 60 mm Hg:

> SVR = mSAP ÷ Qs or SVR = 60 ÷ 6
>
> SVR = 10 Wood units

➤For an explanation of "arteriolar vascular resistance," see Chapter 25, as we simplified the formulas in the above examples.

Volume Overload

Ventricular volume loading increases cardiac output, as per the Frank-Starling law, up to a point. Increased volume load from a left-to-right shunt or valvular regurgitation may eventually impair the heart's ability to perform optimally; thus, congestive heart failure ensues. The excessive volume loading stretches the cardiac fibers beyond their ability to recover, leading to ventricular dilation and eventual dysfunction.

Pressure Overload

Common cardiac malformations that cause pressure overload include pulmonic stenosis, aortic stenosis, and coarctation of the aorta. The increased ventricular wall stress first leads to hypertrophy, but ongoing pressure overload may lead to subendocardial ischemia that results in ventricular dysfunction and dilation.

Ventricular Systolic & Diastolic Dysfunction

Congestive heart failure associated with cardiomyopathies primarily results from either ventricular systolic or diastolic dysfunction. Hypertrophic cardiomyopathies cause heart failure principally through diastolic dysfunction, and dilated cardiomyopathies lead to heart failure mostly secondary to systolic dysfunction.

Next Section

In the following section, we subdivide conditions that can present with chronic congestive heart failure into 3 categories: (1) Volume overload including patent ductus arteriosus, ventricular septal defects, atrial septal defects, and valvular regurgitation; (2) Pressure overload including pulmonic stenosis (included but rarely presents with heart failure), aortic stenosis, and isolated coarctation of the aorta, and (3) Cardiomyopathies.

19 Cardiovascular Malformations

VOLUME OVERLOAD

Patent Ductus Arteriosus

Usually, the ductus arteriosus (DA) closes spontaneously by the 1st day of life. On occasion, a full-term infant's DA fails to completely close until 2 to 3 weeks after birth, or sometimes even longer. A pathological PDA is any PDA causing symptoms at any age, or a DA not closing spontaneously. The figure below shows a PDA with a left-to-right shunt. For PDAs in premature infants, see Chapter 6.

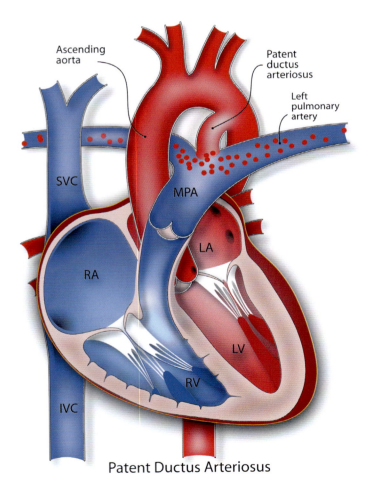

Patent Ductus Arteriosus

The normal DA's walls have spirally-arranged smooth muscle fibers that constrict in response to an increase in arterial oxygenation, which occurs with birth. The rising arterial oxygen levels inhibit the normal prostaglandin metabolism found in the cells of the DA's walls. During fetal life, high levels of normally occurring prostaglandins keep the DA relaxed and open. To maintain DA patency or to open a DA after closure, critical for ductal-dependent cardiovascular defects, we administer IV prostaglandin (PGE1).

Echo can determine the PDA size, the degree and direction of the shunt between the aorta and the pulmonary artery, presence of left atrial or left ventricular overload, and other defects. A PDA shunts left-to-right when the pulmonary vascular resistance is less than the systemic vascular resistance. Particularly in newborns, a PDA may be associated with a ductal aneurysm, possibly resulting from in utero ductal constriction. Ductus arteriosus aneurysms usually resolve spontaneously through constriction and thrombosis; nonetheless, extremely large ductal aneurysms pose some risk for thromboembolism and, in exceedingly rare cases, ductal aneurysm rupture. [8, 9]

PDA sizes

The table on the facing page top left lists PDA sizes in infants and young children. For older children and adolescents, double these diameters. These size values apply to direct measurements of the ductus. When the diameter is not measurable, we rely on other findings to assess the size of the PDA such as left atrial and left ventricular enlargement and the gradient across the PDA.

History

- Small PDA

19 Cardiovascular Malformations

PDA diameters infants & young children	
Small	< 3 mm
Moderate	3 - 5 mm
Large	> 5 mm

Usually, patients with small PDAs have negative medical histories.

- **Moderate to large PDA**

Moderate to large PDAs can cause failure-to-thrive, lead to congestive heart failure, or increase the risk for recurrent respiratory infections.

Exam

- **Small PDA**

A small PDA may produce no murmur or at most a grade II systolic murmur.

- **Moderate PDA**

A moderate PDA causes a hyperdynamic precordium and a grade III or louder continuous or machinery murmur.

- **Large PDA**

A large PDA causes a hyperdynamic precordium, a grade III or less systolic murmur, and a loud 2nd heart sound from pulmonary hypertension.

- **Peripheral pulses**

Pulses are usually bounding in moderate to large PDAs. Bounding pulses originate from a wide pulse pressure due to a low systemic arterial diastolic pressure, which results from diastolic run-off (left-to-right shunt) of systemic arterial blood flowing into the pulmonary arteries via the PDA.

CXR

- **Small PDA**

Small PDAs do not affect heart size or pulmonary vascular markings.

- **Moderate to large PDA**

A moderate to large PDA causes cardiomegaly with increased pulmonary vascular markings.

℞ options

- **Tiny PDA**

For tiny PDAs without murmurs found via Echo ("silent PDAs"), some suggest intervention while others suggest conservative followup or even no followup.

- **Small to moderate PDA**

Small to moderate PDAs are closable with embolization coils or vascular plugs via interventional cardiac catheterization.

- **Large PDA**

Large PDAs may undergo interventional cardiac catheterization; nevertheless, large PDAs usually need surgical ligation or division. Coils or vascular plugs may be too small to close a large PDA. Thus, these devices may embolize into the pulmonary or systemic circulations when attempting to place them through catheter intervention.

- **No interventional services**

If interventional services are not available, then surgical ligation is appropriate for small to moderate-sized PDAs.

19 Cardiovascular Malformations

Ventricular Septal Defect

VSD size

A VSD's size and location determine the pathological and clinical findings. Using Echo, we determine a VSD's size by comparing its dimensions with the aortic annulus's dimension, as the figure below and the tables on the right display. Echo can also determine left atrial (LA) enlargement, left ventricular (LV) enlargement, and associated abnormalities.

VSD Size	
Small	≤ 1/3 the aortic annulus
Moderate	1/3 - 3/4 the aortic annulus
Large	> 3/4 the aortic annulus

For an aortic annulus of 12 mm	
Small VSD	≤ 4 mm
Moderate VSD	4 - 9 mm
Large VSD	> 9 mm

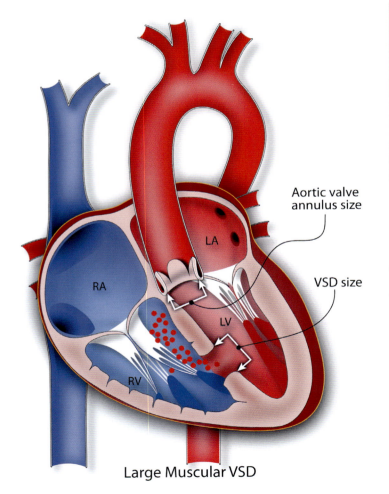

Large Muscular VSD

VSD location

VSDs can occur in 1 of 4 components of the ventricular septum: (1) Muscular (or trabecular) septum, (2) Perimembranous septum, (3) Inlet septum, and (4) Outlet septum. The following figures illustrate the location of these VSD types. We organize the VSD illustrations in order of occurrence from common to rare. The facing page displays figures for a muscular and a perimembranous VSD, and the following pages have illustrations of inlet and outlet VSDs.

Muscular septal defect

Figure A below.

- Most common VSD location in newborns
- Most small muscular VSDs close spontaneously
- May have multiple small VSDs
- Multiple muscular VSDs also called "swiss cheese" type
- Large defects often occur with other malformations, especially coarctation of the aorta

Perimembranous septal defect

Figure B below.

- Common
- Location is near the tricuspid valve (TV)
- Accessory TV tissue may promote closure
- Occasionally aortic regurgitation (AR) from aortic cusp prolapse
- Subpulmonic or subaortic stenosis occasionally develop

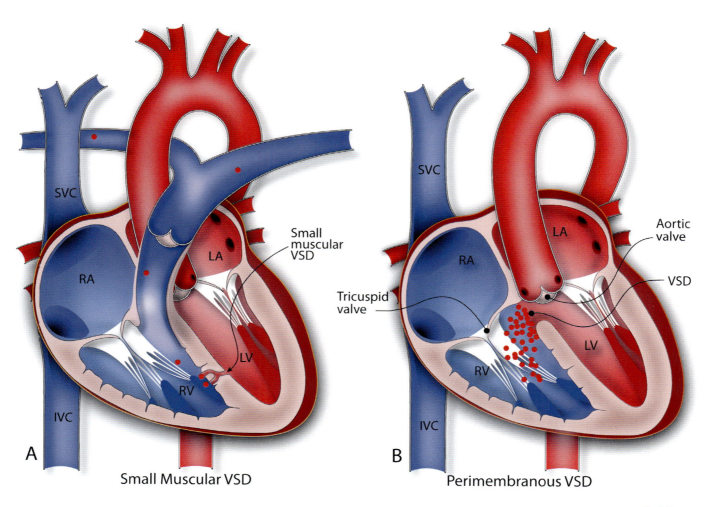

A Small Muscular VSD

B Perimembranous VSD

19 Cardiovascular Malformations

Inlet septal defect

An inlet VSD is often associated with a primum ASD (see next section), and the combination is an atrioventricular septal defect or an AVSD (figure below). AVSDs have a common atrioventricular valve, rather then distinct tricuspid and mitral valves (figures A and B on the right).

- Some call AVSDs atrioventricular canals or AV canals
- AVSDs are common in Down syndrome
- Common to have mitral regurgitation from a mitral valve cleft
- A negative QRS seen in lead aVF on the EKG

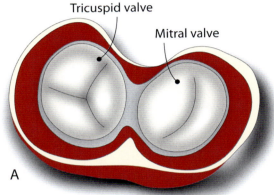

A

Normal Atrioventricular Valves

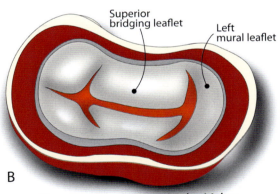

B

Common Atrioventricular Valve

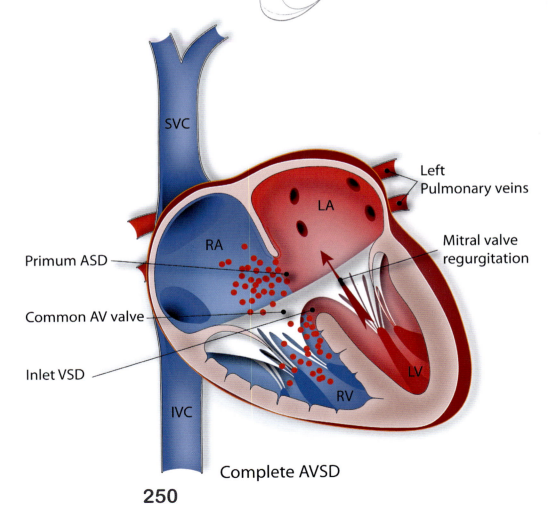

Complete AVSD

Outlet septal defect

Figures A and B below.

- Rare
- In the septum between the subaortic and subpulmonic areas
- Do not close spontaneously
- Location promotes aortic regurgitation (figure B below)

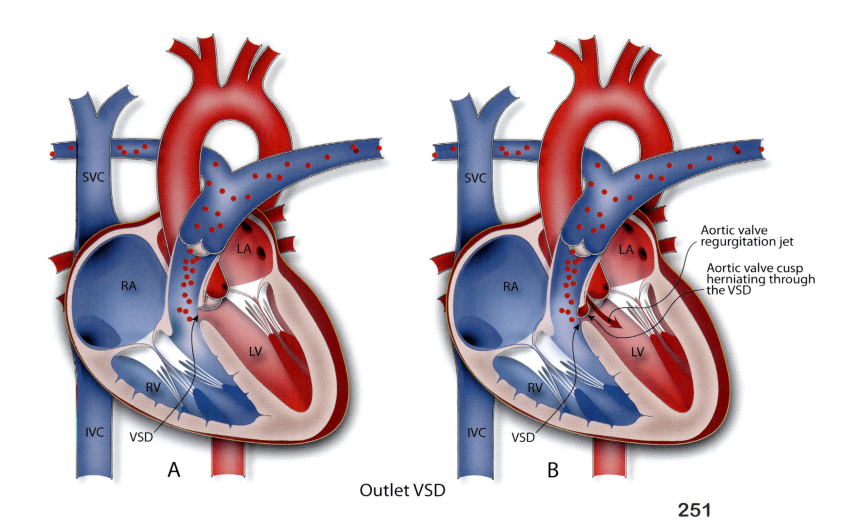

Outlet VSD

History

- **Small VSD**

A small VSD, without aortic regurgitation or other defects, produces no symptoms.

- **Moderate VSD**

Moderate-sized defects may cause chronic heart failure and failure-to-thrive. A left-to-right shunt causes pulmonary overcirculation with an increase in caloric expenditure and growth failure.

- **Large VSD**

Similar to a moderate-sized VSD, a large VSD often occurs with heart failure and failure-to-thrive.

- **Large VSD without growth failure**

A large VSD, without heart failure or failure-to-thrive, is a worrisome clinical problem. Such patients usually have high pulmonary vascular resistance, limiting the left-to-right shunt. A reduced left-to-right shunt results in less pulmonary overcirculation. Less pulmonary overcirculation results in less caloric expenditure. Less caloric expenditure allows normal weight gain rather than the poor weight gain usually associated with a large VSD. Therefore, a large VSD without growth failure is not reassuring. Such findings usually need further intervention, which likely includes cardiac catheterization and early surgical repair.

Exam

- **Dysmorphic features**

VSDs occur in many syndromes; thus, always note whether dysmorphic features are present.

- **Small VSD**

A small VSD creates a quiet precordium and a high-frequency grade III to IV holosystolic murmur from a high-velocity jet, generated by the transventricular-VSD blood flow from significant pressure differences between the LV and the RV. Occasionally, an Echo discovers a tiny VSD that does not produce an audible murmur.

- **Moderate-sized VSD**

A moderate-sized defect causes a hyperdynamic precordium, a lower frequency grade III to IV holosystolic murmur, and a grade I to II mid-diastolic murmur (diastolic rumble) from increased flow across the mitral valve. However, even expert auscultators have difficulty hearing diastolic rumbles.

- **Large VSD**

A large VSD causes a significantly hyperdynamic precordium. Pulmonary hypertension accentuates the 2nd heart sound. The murmur findings are usually a grade I to II low frequency systolic murmur from the minimal systolic pressure difference between the LV and RV. A grade I to II mid-diastolic murmur (diastolic rumble) may be audible.

- **Early-diastolic murmur**

For any size VSD, a high-frequency, early-diastolic murmur of aortic regurgitation (AR) may be an ominous finding requiring surgical closure of the VSD and also aortic valve repair or replacement. AR usually indicates aortic cusp prolapse through an outlet or perimembranous VSD. Pulmonary hypertension with a high PA diastolic pressure might also cause an early high-frequency early-diastolic murmur of pulmonary regurgitation (PR).

CXR

- **Small VSD**

Small VSDs, without aortic regurgitation, do not affect the heart size or the pulmonary vascular markings.

- **Moderate to large VSD**

A moderate to large VSD causes cardiomegaly and increased pulmonary vascular markings.

℞ options

• Small VSD

Small defects, without associated malformations or AR, require no intervention.

• Small VSD with AR

Small VSDs with AR usually require surgery, as AR can progress even when the defect is small.

• Moderate-sized VSD

Treating moderate-sized defects, especially in infants, includes maximizing nutrition, administrating diuretics plus afterload reduction agents, and early surgery when uncompensated heart failure or growth failure persists. Some perimembranous or muscular septal defects may spontaneously close or diminish in size. Thus, we may wait for them to decrease in size or close on their own; however, when surgical indications exist, we may still recommend early surgical closure. Inlet and outlet VSDs do not usually close spontaneously and protracted expectant care is not beneficial. Down syndrome patients are at higher risk of developing Eisenmenger syndrome at an earlier age than those without Down syndrome. Thus, Down syndrome patients need early surgical repair, usually before 6 months old. In other patients, moderate-sized defects usually require closure by about 2 years old or earlier if symptoms warrant.

• Large VSD

All the above points under moderate-sized VSDs pertain to large VSDs. Patients need surgical closure even at younger ages than those with moderate-sized VSDs. Without surgical repair, damaging pulmonary hypertensive changes may develop. Again, such changes are more likely to develop in patients with Down syndrome than those without Down syndrome. Occasionally, large muscular VSDs or multiple VSDs (swiss cheese type) usually require initial pulmonary artery banding that allows the patient to grow over several months, delaying a complete VSD closure to a later date when the risk of an open heart repair is reduced.

• Device closure

If the services are available. the device closure is an option for moderate to large-sized muscular VSDs.

Atrial Septal Defects & Partial Anomalous Pulmonary Venous Return

Atrial septal defects (ASDs) predominately occur in 3 locations, as we illustrate in the figures on the facing page: (1) Secundum (figure A), (2) Primum (figure B), and (3) Sinus venosus (figure C). ASDs may be multiple and include more than 1 type. Sinus venosus ASDs frequently occur with partial anomalous pulmonary venosus return (PAPVR), as figure C also shows. PAPVR may also occur without an ASD, as figure D shows. Figure D represents a particular type of PAPVR where the right pulmonary veins enter the inferior vena cava (IVC) with anatomy that resembles a scimitar sword.

ASDs allow left-to-right shunting from left atrium to right atrium, causing volume overload of the right atrium and right ventricle. Volume overloading produces chamber enlargement. Part of the left-to-right shunt, in a superior sinus venosus ASD with PAPVR, comes directly from the anomalous pulmonary veins. PAPVR usually involves the right pulmonary veins that enter the superior vena cava or the right atrium directly rather than entering the left atrium. The right ventricle pumps extra blood from the left-to-right shunt to the lungs. Over time, the left-to-right shunt leads to right atrial enlargement (RAE may cause arrhythmias), right ventricular enlargement, pulmonary overcirculation leasing to heart failure, and pulmonary vascular changes leading to pulmonary hypertension.

Echo can determine an ASD's location, size and other associated findings such as right atrial or right ventricular enlargement; presence of PAPVR (PAPVR may need MRI or CT to define the anatomy); the degree of left-to-right shunt; and the presence of a mitral valve cleft with regurgitation.

ASD size

We judge an ASD's size by measuring its diameter relative to the superior-inferior length of the interatrial septum (IAS), as we show in the table below [10]:

ASD size	% of the IAS
Small	< 30%
Moderate	30 - 60%
Large	> 60%

Several small ASDs may be equal to a moderate or large ASD, when adding the cumulative diameters of several small ASDs. From the newborn to about 3 to 5 years old, secundum ASDs can significantly decrease in size or even close. However, ASDs in other locations rarely close spontaneously.

Patent foramen ovale

A patent foramen ovale (PFO) is a persistent intrauterine pathway. Some refer to tiny secundum ASDs as PFOs. We prefer not to use the term PFO for a tiny secundum ASD that is not consistent with a persistent intrauterine pathway.

History

Even moderate to large ASDs may cause no symptoms; thus, an ASD may escape detection for years. Occasionally, however, newborns or infants may present with heart failure and failure-to-thrive, especially when an ASD occurs with a syndrome.

19 Cardiovascular Malformations

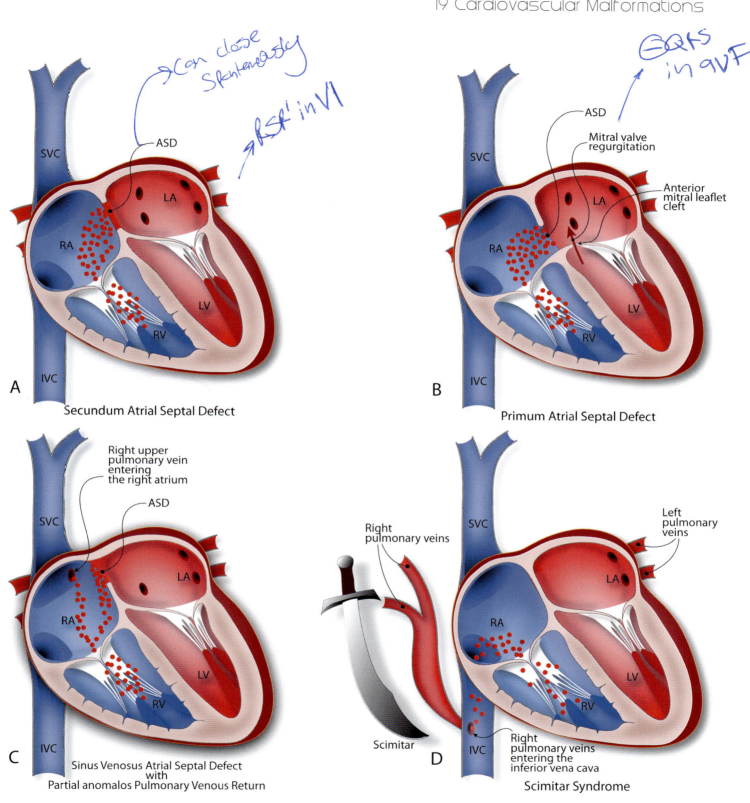

A Secundum Atrial Septal Defect
B Primum Atrial Septal Defect
C Sinus Venosus Atrial Septal Defect with Partial anomalos Pulmonary Venous Return
D Scimitar Syndrome

19 Cardiovascular Malformations

Exam

- **Dysmorphic features**

Syndromes occur with ASDs; note dysmorphic features.

- **Small to moderate ASD**

Despite past teaching, a small or even moderate-sized ASD may have minimal physical exam findings. A grade I to II systolic ejection murmur from increased pulmonary flow may be present. Nevertheless, a widely split 2nd sound may be absent. The lack of physical findings allows these defects to escape detection, sometimes for decades.

- **Large ASD**

With a large ASD, the findings usually include a hyperdynamic precordium; wide or fixed splitting of the 2nd heart sound; usually at least a grade II systolic ejection murmur from increased pulmonary flow; and a grade I low frequency mid-diastolic murmur (diastolic rumble) of increased TV inflow. Yet, even large ASDs can escape diagnosis for years.

- **Holosystolic murmurs**

A holosystolic murmur can arise from mitral regurgitation secondary to a cleft mitral valve in a primum ASD.

CXR

The CXR is normal with small ASDs. In moderate to large-sized ASDs, with or without PAPVR, the CXR shows cardiomegaly and increased pulmonary vascular markings.

As we illustrate in the previous figure D, a form of PAPVR, right-sided pulmonary veins that drain to the IVC, may create a an opacity in the right lung field that appears similar in shape to a a scimitar. The "scimitar syndrome" is also associated with pulmonary sequestration and a rightward displacement of the heart secondary right lung hypoplasia from the pulmonary sequestration.

EKG

- An RSR′ pattern in lead V1 in secundum ASDs
- A negative QRS in lead aVF in primum ASDs
- See Chapter 21 for EKG interpretation

℞ options

Unless contraindications exist for device or surgical closure, we rarely use only anticongestive therapy for ASDs.

- **Secundum ASD**

We observe asymptomatic newborns and infants with secundum ASDs, even moderately large ones, as these defects may diminish in size or close spontaneously over time. If clinically indicated, however, most secundum ASDs are amenable to device closure. Occasionally, defects too large for device closure need surgery.

- **Nonsecundum ASD**

Nonsecundum ASDs, including primum and sinus venous defects, do not close spontaneously. These defects usually require surgical closure, as nonsecundum ASDs are not easily amenable to device closure. Sinus venosus ASDs occur frequently with PAPVR, which usually also requires surgical repair. Primum ASDs frequently have associated cleft mitral valves. Mitral regurgitation results from a cleft mitral valve, which usually needs suture closure at the time of the primum ASD repair.

- **Patent foramen ovale**

Although the etiological connection is controversial, strokes or brain abscesses may occur with PFOs, even in children. Therefore, we may recommend device closure for a PFO in a child with a stroke or a brain abscess.

Valvular Regurgitation

Acute or chronic heart failure, from valvular regurgitation, is rare in children. Severe tricuspid regurgitation (TR), from a congenital tricuspid valve abnormality (excluding Ebstein anomaly), occasionally causes in utero heart failure. Pulmonary regurgitation (PR), apart from postoperative causes, also rarely causes cardiac volume overload and congestive heart failure. Congenital mitral valve regurgitation (figure below right) usually does not cause in utero heart failure but infants can present in the first few weeks or months after birth with symptoms and signs of CHF. Mitral valve regurgitation occurs with AVSDs, which may accentuate heart failure. Marfan syndrome may have aortic regurgitation (AR) associated with a dilated aortic root and mitral valve prolapse. Congenital AR, from aortic valve abnormalities or an aortic cusp prolapse from a VSD, progresses over time, resulting in left ventricular volume overload and CHF. Further, valve regurgitations can arise from acquired heart disease such as endocarditis or rheumatic fever.

Echo is especially sensitive for valve regurgitation and can even detect inaudible valve regurgitation. Severe TR causes right atrial and right ventricular enlargement. PR causes right ventricular enlargement and flow reversal in the pulmonary arteries. Severe MR causes marked left atrial and left ventricular enlargement (figure on the right). AR shows left ventricular enlargement and flow reversal in the aorta, detected by pulse-wave Doppler interrogation.

History

- May occasionally present at birth, especially TR
- Occasionally SVT from dilated right or left atria
- MR & AR may present with CHF
- May present with endocarditis

Exam

- Hyperdynamic precordium
- Early-diastolic murmurs of AR & PR
- Systolic or holosystolic murmurs of MR & TR

CXR

- Cardiomegaly with significant volume overload
- Pulmonary edema in MR

℞ options

- Treat endocarditis or endomyocarditis, if present
- Anticongestive medications
- Valve repair or replacement

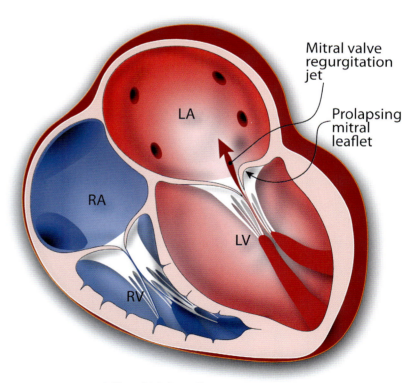

Mitral Valve Regurgitation

19 Cardiovascular Malformations

PRESSURE OVERLOAD

Pulmonic Stenosis

The most common cause of pulmonic stenosis (PS) is an abnormal pulmonary valve. However, PS can also occur as subvalvular, supravalvular, or a combination of subvalvular, supravalvular, and valvular abnormalities. PS can also include narrowing of the branch pulmonary arteries. Typical valvular pulmonic stenosis involves a doming valve, fusion of the leaflets, a normal pulmonary valve annulus, and post-stenotic dilation of the main pulmonary artery (figure A on the facing page). Figure B on the facing page demonstrates why we use the term "doming valve." Typical valvular pulmonic stenosis is amenable to balloon valvuloplasty.

Echo can determine whether stenosis is valvular, subvalvular, or supravalvular; evaluate for associated defects; and determine pressure gradients with continuous-wave Doppler (CW Doppler).

PS CW Doppler peak gradients

With respect to severity, multiple sources list various peak-Doppler gradient definitions. In the table above right, we list average values from multiple references and an average of our authors' opinions.

History

- Usually negative, even in severe PS
- Syncope may indicate a need for emergent intervention

Exam

- Noonan syndrome features suggest dysplastic valvular pulmonic stenosis
- Williams syndrome may have supravalvular PS & AS

Valvular Pulmonic Stenosis

Severity	Peak Doppler gradient
Mild	< 40 mm Hg
Moderate	40 - 70 mm Hg
Severe	> 70 mm Hg

- Ejection click in typical valvular PS
- Usually no ejection click in nonvalvular PS
- The louder the murmur often higher the gradient
- The murmur in critical valvular PS is often soft, as little blood crosses the valve

CXR

- Usually normal, even when severe
- Severe PS may have hyperlucent lungs fields
- Prominence of the main pulmonary artery from post-stenotic dilatation

℞ options

- PGE1

In neonates, with severe PS and inadequate pulmonary blood flow, we start PGE1 to maintain ductal patency or to open a closed ductus arteriosus.

- Catheter intervention

At any age, typical valvular PS is amenable to catheter intervention. Branch pulmonary artery stenosis may also respond to catheter intervention.

19 Cardiovascular Malformations

- Surgery

Subvalvular, supravalvular, dysplastic valvular pulmonic stenosis, and branch pulmonary artery stenosis often need surgery.

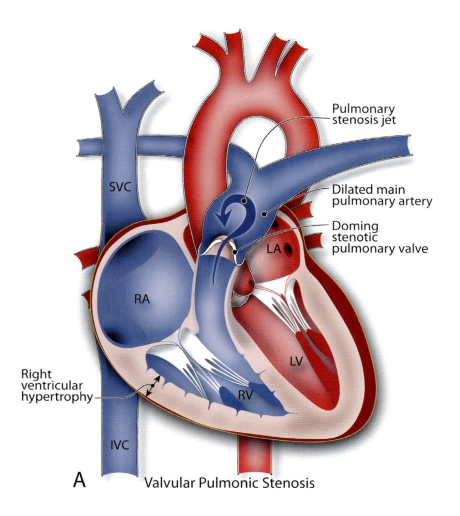

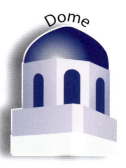

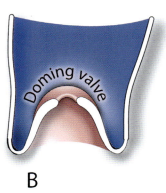

Aortic Stenosis & Bicuspid Aortic Valve

Aortic stenosis (AS) is less common than PS; however, similar to PS, AS can occur as a valvular, supravalvular, and subvalvular lesion. Also, similar to typical valvular pulmonic stenosis, valvular aortic stenosis with fused doming leaflets, a normal-sized aortic annulus, and post-stenotic dilation is the form most amenable to balloon valvuloplasty (figure A on the facing page). Occasionally AS eludes detection in infancy. Later, a clinician discovers AS on exam during childhood. Late discovery of AS is problematic, as a child may already be participating in sports. Restriction from sports, if indicated, can be psychologically devastating. Valvular aortic stenosis, more so than valvular PS, can progress. Rarely does AS improve.

Aortic obstruction can also occur as supravalvular aortic narrowing (figure B on the facing page) or as a subvalvular obstruction (figure C on the facing page). Supravalvular aortic obstruction occurs in Williams syndrome and autosomal dominant supravalvular aortic stenosis (SVAS). Subaortic obstruction can be discrete as in membranous subaortic obstruction (figure C). Subaortic obstruction can also be muscular as in hypertrophic cardiomyopathies (HCM), including muscular subaortic obstruction in infants of diabetic mothers (IDM), in syndromes, and in hereditary cardiomyopathies. Multiple levels of aortic stenosis can occur in Shone complex.

An isolated bicuspid aortic valve, without AS or significant AR, requires particular comment. As an isolated finding, bicuspid aortic valve (excluding a patent foramen ovale) is the most common congenital cardiovascular defect, present in about 1-2% of the population. Isolated bicuspid aortic valve may escape detection in infancy, childhood, or even adolescence. Because of the strong familial occurrence of bicuspid aortic valve, some recommend family screening. A patient with an undiagnosed bicuspid aortic valves can initially present with endocarditis. In later adulthood, the condition may promote aortic leaflet calcification, which may cause significant AS. Isolated bicuspid aortic valve may also have aortic root dilatation, which occasionally requires treatment with beta-blockers or angiotensin II-receptor blockers. On rare occasion, a bicuspid aortic valve and significant root dilation may require aortic root replacement.

Echo can determine whether stenosis is valvular, subvalvular, or supravalvular; evaluate for other defects; and determine pressure gradients with continuous-wave Doppler.

AS CW Doppler peak gradients

With respect to severity, multiple sources list various peak Doppler gradient values. In the table below, we list average values from multiple references and an average of our authors' opinions.

Valvular Aortic Stenosis	
Severity	Peak Doppler gradient
Mild	< 40 mmHg
Moderate	40 - 70 mmHg
Severe	> 70 mmHg

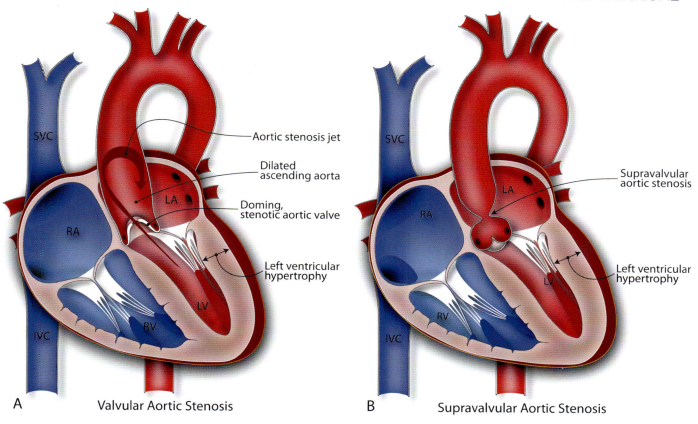
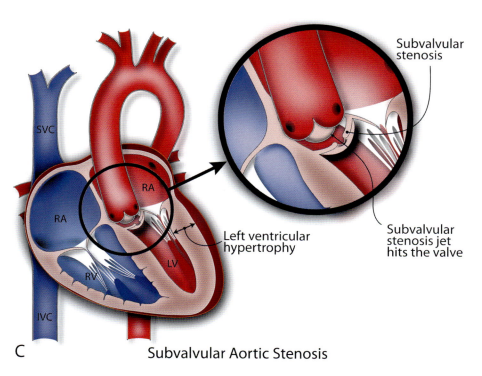

19 Cardiovascular Malformations

History

• Mild to moderate valvular aortic stenosis

Most often the history is negative. On rare occasion, patients may complain of chest pain with exercise or exercise intolerance if valvular stenosis is associated with moderate to severe aortic regurgitation.

• Severe valvular aortic stenosis

May present at any age with chronic or acute CHF. Patients may complain of chest pain. On rare occasion, patients with severe AS may present with syncope, which is an ominous symptom that usually indicates a need for immediate intervention.

• Supravalvular AS

History is usually negative other than possible concern over dysmorphic features.

• Subvalvular AS

Several congenital and acquired problems have subaortic obstruction. HCM can be familial, affecting multiple family members. Infants born to mothers with insulin-dependent or gestational diabetes may have mild, moderate, or severe IDM cardiomyopathy and subaortic obstruction. Subaortic obstruction, especially membranous-type obstruction, can cause aortic regurgitation and congestive heart failure.

Exam

• Syndromes

3 syndromes link to different AS types. Williams syndrome has supravalvular aortic stenosis. Turner syndrome frequently has bicuspid aortic valves, valvular aortic stenosis, coarctation of the aorta, and aortic root dilation. Noonan syndrome may have HCM with subaortic obstruction and also dysplastic valvular pulmonic stenosis.

• Large for gestational age (LGA)

Infants born to mothers with diabetes need an Echo to rule out HCM with subaortic obstruction.

• Systolic ejection murmur

Similar to PS, the louder the systolic ejection murmur, usually the higher the AS gradient.

• Early-diastolic murmur

An early-diastolic murmur is more common in AS than in PS. As the diastolic pressure in the aorta is higher than the pulmonary artery, AR generates more sound than PR.

• Ejection click

An ejection click may be the solitary auscultatory finding in isolated bicuspid aortic valve. Also, valvular stenosis may create an audible ejection click. Subaortic and supravalvular aortic stenosis produce no ejection clicks.

• Suprasternal notch thrill

A suprasternal notch thrill is common and may not correlate with severity, as a thrill may occur even with mild valvular AS.

CXR

Usually, the CXR is normal even in severe AS. Cardiomegaly, however, is possible in IDM cardiomyopathy, volume overload from AR, or in LV dysfunction secondary to severe AS.

℞ options

• Valvular AS

Newborns with critical valvular aortic stenosis usually need PGE1 to open a closed ductus arteriosus or maintain a PDA, which provides supplemental systemic blood flow. Most valvular aortic stenosis is amenable to balloon valvuloplasty at any age, unless significant aortic regurgitation exists. Complex valvular aortic stenosis may also involve aortic annular hypoplasia, which may require a surgical procedure to enlarge the annulus or Konno procedure.

Conservative followup is appropriate in mild to moderate valvular AS without symptoms, especially without syncope. Exercise restriction may be reasonable.

- **Supravalvular AS**

Supravalvular AS is common in Williams syndrome and requires surgical repair, when the aortic narrowing is significant.

- **Subvalvular AS & HCM**

Some hypertrophic cardiomyopathies with subaortic obstruction may benefit from beta-blockers or calcium-channel blockers acutely or chronically, while other subaortic obstruction types may need surgical resection with or without a Konno procedure, if aortic annular hypoplasia is present.

Coarctation of the Aorta

Coarctation of the aorta (CoA) may occur as a discrete narrowing of the proximal distal aortic arch or a diffuse process involving hypoplasia of the top of the aortic arch (transverse aortic arch) with or without further areas of discrete narrowing. In newborns, a coarctation of the aorta often occurs with a patent ductus arteriosus (figure on the facing page). Ductal closure may accentuate the coarctation. Because symptoms may be lacking, oximetry maybe normal, and positive physical exam features may be absent when the ductus arteriosus is open, a patient may go home from the newborn nursery and return in congestive heart failure when the ductus closes spontaneously. Occasionally, the aorta may be tortuous without narrowing creating a so-called "pseudocoarctation of the aorta" that needs no treatment. Coarctations are frequently associated with bicuspid aortic valves. Further, Shone complex (multiple left-sided abnormalities) may include mitral stenosis, subaortic obstruction, aortic stenosis, and CoA.

Echo can define the condition, image associated malformations, and determine a transcoarctation gradient. Coarctation gradients are less accurate than valvular pulmonic and aortic stenosis gradients. Nonetheless, upper and lower blood pressure differences can confirm Doppler-derived transcoarctation gradients. With left ventricular dysfunction, gradient measurements are unreliable. However, with inotropic support, ventricular function and cardiac output improves, which often increases the CoA gradient.

History

- History may be negative for older children
- Hypertension on exam may initiate referral
- Newborns may present in shock with ductal closure

Exam

- If female, then rule out Turner syndrome
- Diminished or absent femoral pulses
- A soft systolic murmur in the back
- Systolic ejection murmurs
- Ejection click, if an abnormal aortic valve

CXR

- May be normal
- May show cardiomegaly & pulmonary edema
- May show rib notching in older patients

℞ options

- **Emergent**

PGE1 for newborns presenting in shock. Also, we usually start PGE1 in asymptomatic newborns at the time of diagnosis and before ductal closure.

- **Catheter Intervention**

Neonatal, native CoA can undergo balloon angioplasty, but the procedure is controversial [11]. Older infants and children with discrete coarctation usually undergo balloon angioplasty. Older children and adolescents undergoing balloon angioplasty may also need a vascular stent.

- **Surgery**

Many centers perform surgical correction for discrete coarctations as the primary procedure. Coarctations with hypoplastic aortic arches likely need surgery rather than balloon angioplasty.

19 Cardiovascular Malformations

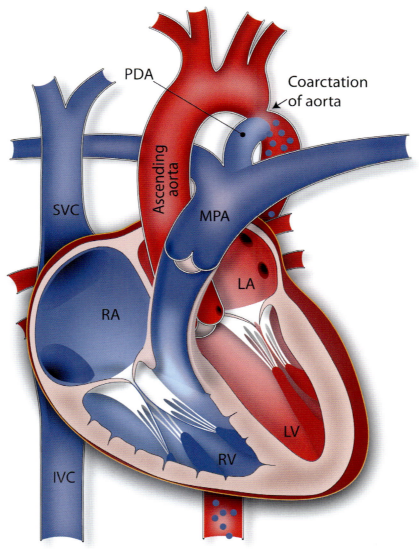

Coarctation of Aorta and Patent Ductus Arteriosus

CARDIOMYOPATHIES

Cardiomyopathies (CM) may cause ventricular systolic and diastolic dysfunction, leading to congestive heart failure (CHF). The facing page figures illustrate the principal CM subtypes. Most CM are either hypertrophic (figure A-asymmetric, B-concentric, and C-apical), dilated (figure D), or restrictive (figure E). Echo is the principal imaging tool; occasionally, diagnosis requires MRI and cardiac catheterization. For more on Echo, especially for diastolic function evaluation, see Chapter 22. [12 - 23]

Hypertrophic

Hypertrophic cardiomyopathy (HCM) is the most common type of CM. Beyond the newborn, most HCM results from gene mutations (see Appendix D). Thus, consider genetic testing with a positive family history. Further, all 1st-degree relatives require regular echocardiographic screening.

Symptoms and signs relate to decreased cardiac output and occasionally associated arrhythmias. Ventricular hypertrophy may result in: 1) Outflow obstruction that impairs cardiac output, and 2) Diastolic dysfunction that limits cardiac output by impeding ventricular inflow.

Maternal diabetes is the most frequent cause of neonatal ventricular hypertrophy in an infant of a diabetic mother (IDM). IDM HCM results from the trophic response to fetal hyperinsulinemia. IDM HCM is usually mild to moderate without hemodynamic impairment; although, severe cases may have left ventricular outflow obstruction and CHF. Hypertrophy resolves with time, which helps differentiate IDM HCM from other forms of HCM.

Asymmetric

- Asymmetric septal hypertrophy (ASH) commonest form
- ASH common also in IDM HCM
- Septal hypertrophy > ventricular free walls
- Frequently with subaortic obstruction
- Frequently mitral valve (MV) regurgitation by Echo
- Echo shows systolic anterior motion (SAM) of MV
- Usually normal or hyperdynamic LV systolic function
- Doppler can estimate subaortic gradients
- Ventricular diastolic dysfunction on Echo

Concentric

- Uniform ventricular wall hypertrophy
- May have hyperdynamic ventricular systolic function
- Ventricular diastolic dysfunction by Echo
- IDM HCM may also be concentric
- Glycogen storage diseases, including Pompe disease

Apical

- Left ventricular midcavitary obstruction with suprasystemic pressure at apex
- Suprasystemic apical pressure may lead to LV apical aneurysm
- The 4-chamber view is the best Echo view for diagnosis

History

- Family history
- Maternal diabetes
- Asymptomatic or history consistent with CHF
- May present with sudden cardiac death, see Chapter 9

Exam

- Large for gestational age (LGA) if IDM
- Features suggesting Noonan syndrome, see Chapter 3
- Tachypnea, tachycardia, hepatomegaly if CHF
- Systolic murmurs from outflow obstruction

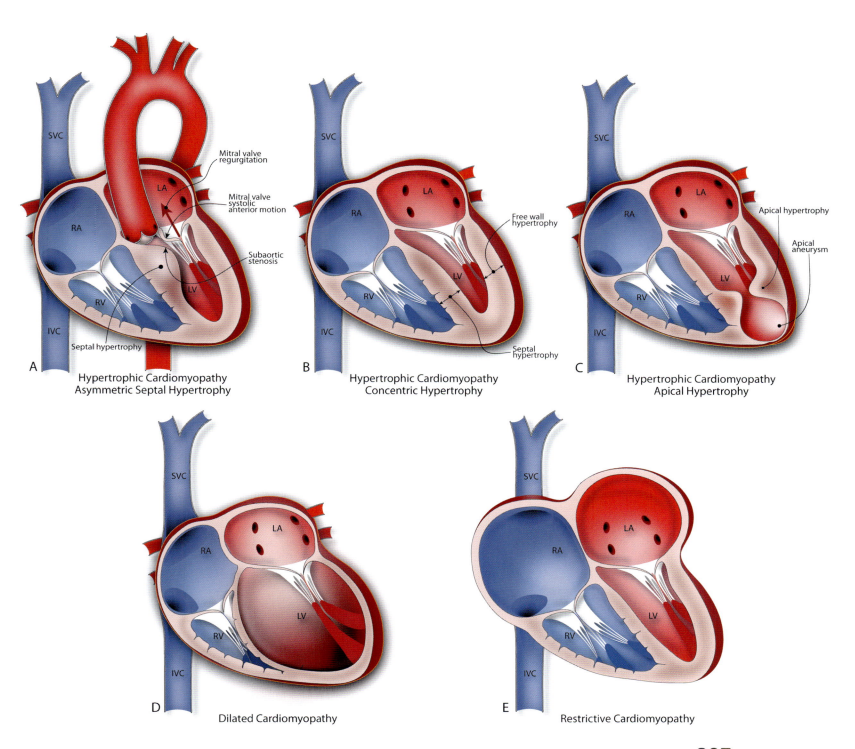

CXR
- May be normal
- Cardiomegaly & pulmonary edema

℞ options
- IV esmolol for significant outflow/inflow obstruction
- Avoid inotropes
- Oral beta-blockers
- Implantable cardioverter defibrillators (ICDs)
- Myectomy
- May need cardiac transplantation in severe cases

Dilated

Dilated cardiomyopathy (DCM) usually means systolic dysfunction and dilation of the LV (previous CM figure D); however, DCM can also involve the RV. Occasionally, a prenatal echocardiogram detects fetal-cardiac systolic dysfunction, accompanied by fetal CHF and hydrops.

Echo findings include increased LV end-systolic and end-diastolic diameters, resulting in a reduced shortening fraction. The LV acquires a globular-spherical shape. The atria may also dilate, especially with atrioventricular valve regurgitation. The mitral valve annulus dilates with progressive LV enlargement, leading to mitral valve regurgitation from poor leaflet coaptation.

Causes

Infections
- Viral
- Bacterial toxins with sepsis

Arrhythmias
- Principally tachyarrhythmias, see Chapter 4

Systemic hypertension
- Previous umbilical artery catheter
- Renal pathology

Cardiac malformations
- Aortic stenosis
- Coarctation of the aorta (CoA)
- Anomalous left coronary artery from the pulmonary artery (ALCAPA)

Familial dilated cardiomyopathy
- 20-50% of cases from gene mutations.
- 1st-degree relatives require regular Echos

Miscellaneous
- Perinatal asphyxia
- Toxins
- Immunological
- Endocrine
- Connective tissue & autoimmune diseases
- Metabolic, syndromes, & muscular dystrophy

History
- Growth failure
- Symptoms of CHF
- Abdominal pain
- Wheezing
- Palpitations
- Thromboembolic events, from LV mural thrombi

Exam
- Weight below the 5th percentile
- Signs of CHF
- Nonsinus tachycardias

CXR
- Usually cardiomegaly & pulmonary edema

℞ options

See Chapter 5 for the treatment of CHF. B-type natriuretic peptide (BNP) levels help guide treatment.

Restrictive

Restrictive cardiomyopathy (RCM) is rare, comprising 2 - 5% of pediatric cardiomyopathies. Diagnosis usually occurs beyond the neonatal period. Nevertheless, even a fetal diagnosis of RCM is possible by fetal Echo [16].

Echo findings include normal or near-normal ventricular systolic function with abnormal ventricular diastolic function. The atria are severely dilated, and the ventricles appear underfilled, giving the 4-chamber view a "Mickey mouse" appearance (previous CM figure E). Elevated venous pressure dilates the inferior vena cava and hepatic veins. Pericardial effusion may be present. Pulmonary artery hypertension may result from increased pulmonary venous pressure.

History
- May be negative
- May have symptoms of CHF

Exam
- May be normal
- May have signs of CHF

CXR
- Usually cardiomegaly from dilated atria
- Pulmonary edema

℞ options
- Only effective ℞ is heart transplantation

Other

Noncompaction and arrhythmogenic right ventricular cardiomyopathy (ARVC) are 2 CM types that are usually localized in the myocardium rather than occurring as a generalized myocardial processes such as hypertrophic, dilated, and restrictive CM.

Noncompaction is a developmental error in endomyocardial morphogenesis, and it occurs more often in the LV than the RV. Noncompaction may be sporadic or familial. Echo can image the deep ventricular trabeculations characteristic of noncompaction. Treatment includes management of CHF, associated arrhythmias, possible use of ICDs, occasionally anticoagulants, and occasional need for transplantation.

ARVC is a progressive fatty replacement of RV myocardium. Presentation includes ventricular arrhythmias, CHF, right bundle branch block, and sudden cardiac death including sudden infant death (SIDS). Diagnosis may require multiple modalities including EKG, Echo, MRI, myocardial biopsy, and electrophysiology testing. Management includes arrhythmia treatment, ICDs, and even heart transplantation.

Endocardial fibroelastosis (EFE) is not a form of CM; rather, EFE is an endocardial-cellular stress reaction primarily to pressure or volume overload and can be associated with CM [20]. EFE can be localized or generalized and is associated with a wide-range of cardiac malformations including, but not limited to, aortic stenosis, coarctation of the aorta, DCM, RCM, immunological reactions such a transplacental SSA/SSB antibodies, but surprisingly not HCM [21].

DEFECTS PRESENTING IN EXTREMIS

Hypoplastic Left Heart Syndrome

Hypoplastic left heart syndrome (HLHS) is a spectrum of malformations. The most characteristic findings are severe ascending aorta hypoplasia with or without aortic atresia, marked left ventricular underdevelopment, and severe mitral valve hypoplasia or atresia (figure on the facing page). A restricted atrial septum compounds the pathology, because a restricted atrial communications obstructs the pulmonary venous return. Normally, the pulmonary venous blood passes into the left ventricle without restriction; however, with small left heart structures blocking the return, the pulmonary venous blood must decompress across the atrial septum into the right atrium. With atrial septum restriction, decompression cannot occur. A restricted atrial septum results in severe pulmonary edema, pulmonary hypertension, and a sicker patient at presentation. HLHS can have a familial occurrence, including an increased risk for bicuspid aortic valve in family members. Therefore, family screening, is appropriate.

Echo can confirm the diagnosis, evaluate the right ventricular function, resolve atrial septal restriction, define other abnormalities, and visualize tricuspid regurgitation.

History

- Poor feeding, paleness, & lethargy
- Cardiovascular collapse with ductal closure

Exam

- Shock with poor pulses throughout
- Hyperdynamic precordium without loud murmurs

CXR

- CXR may be normal when clinicians detect HLHS before the onset of shock
- Cardiomegaly & pulmonary edema

℞ options

- Immediate PGE1 to open or maintain a ductus arteriosus
- Norwood palliation or hybrid procedures in newborns
- Later Glenn procedure around 6 months old
- Fontan procedure at 2 to 3 years old

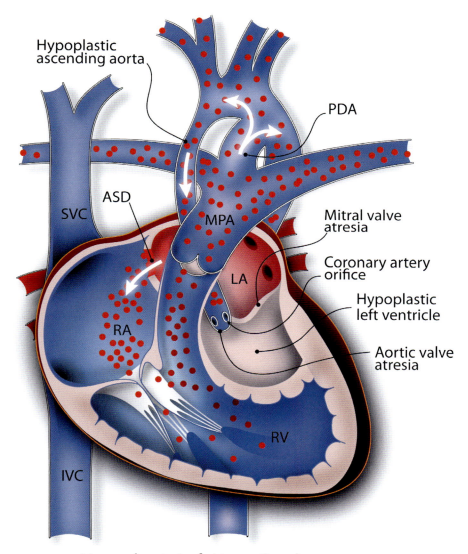

Hypoplastic Left Heart Syndrome

Coarctation with Large VSD

Although an infant with an isolated CoA may present in heart failure or extremis, an isolated CoA may produce no symptoms and escape diagnosis for years. An infant with a CoA with a large VSD (figure on the facing page), however, often presents in extremis once the ductus arteriosus closes. As the ductus closes, the ascending aortic pressure and left ventricular pressure rise. As the pressure rises, the left-to-right shunt through the VSD acutely rises, and marked pulmonary overcirculation, pulmonary hypertension, and pulmonary edema result.

Echo can confirm the diagnosis, determine the VSD location, aortic arch anatomy, and evaluate ventricular function.

History
- Frequently no symptoms or signs with an open ductus
- Poor feeding, paleness, or irritability as the PDA closes
- Increased work of breathing

Exam
- Note dysmorphic features as syndromes are common
- Absent femoral pulses
- Hyperdynamic precordium
- Low frequency systolic murmur or no murmur
- Shock

CXR
- Cardiomegaly
- Increased pulmonary vascular markings
- Pulmonary edema

℞ options
- PGE1 to open or maintain a ductus arteriosus
- Surgical aortic arch & VSD repair
- Hybrid procedure with later arch & VSD repair

19 Cardiovascular Malformations

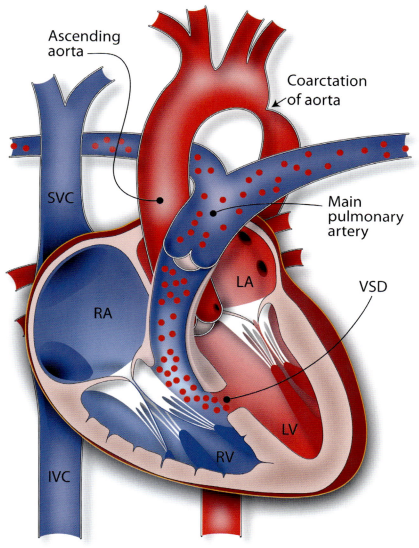

Coarctation of Aorta and Large VSD

Interrupted Aortic Arch with VSD

Interrupted aortic arch (IAA) with VSD is rarer than coarctation with VSD, but the consequences and presentations are similar. On the facing page, the figure displays the 3 forms of IAA: (1) "A" between the left subclavian and the descending aorta; (2) "B" between the left carotid artery and the left subclavian; and (3) "C" between the innominate artery and the left carotid. A, B, and C types are labeled in the opposite direction of blood flow. B-type is the most common. Chromosome 22q11 deletion is common with IAA. IAA usually occurs with a VSD, although there are rare case reports of isolated IAA.

Echo can determine the IAA type, presence of a PDA, other abnormalities, and ventricular function.

History

- The newborn history may be negative
- Cardiovascular collapse with ductal closure

Exam

- Chromosome 22q11 deletion is common
- Hyperdynamic precordium
- Nonspecific murmur or no murmur
- Absent lower extremity pulses
- Lower extremity saturations < upper extremities
- Shock

CXR

- Cardiomegaly
- Increased pulmonary vascular markings
- Pulmonary edema

℞ options

- PGE1 to open or maintain a ductus arteriosus
- Surgical aortic arch & VSD repair
- Hybrid procedure with later repair of arch & VSD
- Caution in chromosome 22q11 deletion, patients may have hypocalcemia & immune deficiency

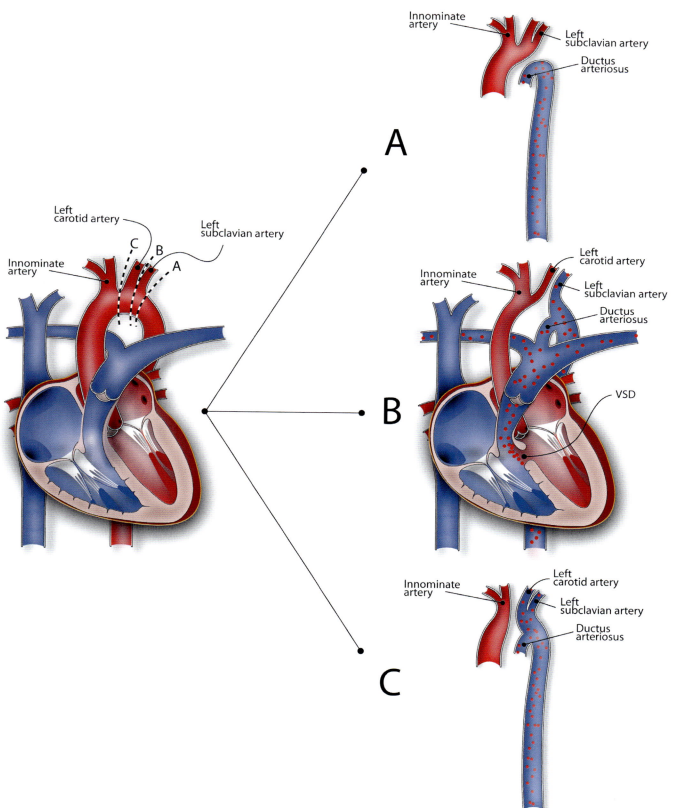

DEFECTS PRESENTING WITH OXYGEN DESATURATION

THE 5 "Ts"

For centuries, physicians have written about cardiovascular malformations with cyanosis. However, cyanosis is a sign visually obvious. Many "cyanotic lesions" have the potential, depending on anatomical variations, to appear "acyanotic," especially in newborns. Hence, without a prenatal diagnosis, and no demonstrable physical findings at birth, patients with "cyanotic" conditions may go home from the newborn nursery and present later, sometimes in extremis. Nonetheless, pulse-oximeter recordings usually demonstrate decreased oxygen saturation at any age, whether visually cyanotic or not, as all of these conditions have right-to-left shunts. Also, see Chapter 7. The following section includes the commonly taught "5 Ts":

Tetralogy of Fallot

Transposition of the great arteries

Total anomalous pulmonary venous return

Truncus arteriosus

Tricuspid atresia

Besides the 5 Ts, this section also includes descriptions for other defects presenting with oxygen desaturation including double outlet right ventricle (DORV), pulmonary atresia with intact ventricular septum, Ebstein anomaly of the tricuspid valve, hearts with 1-functional ventricle, and pulmonary arteriovenous malformations.

Tetralogy of Fallot

For decades, medical students have busied themselves with memorizing the "4 findings" comprising typical tetralogy of Fallot (figure below). Étienne-Louis Arthur Fallot described these 4 findings in 1888 [24]:

(**1**) Pulmonic stenosis
(**2**) Ventricular septal defect
(**3**) A rightward overriding aorta
(**4**) Right ventricular hypertrophy

Nevertheless, "tetralogy" of Fallot (ToF) probably results from 1 ("monology") primary developmental abnormality. During cardiovascular embryology, a portion of the ventricular septum—the outlet or infundibular septum—deviates towards the right ventricle and partially blocks blood flow to the lungs. The outlet septal deviation creates a hole in the ventricular septum (the VSD), creates the pulmonic stenosis (PS), and causes the aorta to move rightward and straddle the VSD (aortic override). One particular form, ToF with absent pulmonary valve (figure below) has markedly dilated main and branch pulmonary arteries. ToF also occurs with AVSDs (see above).

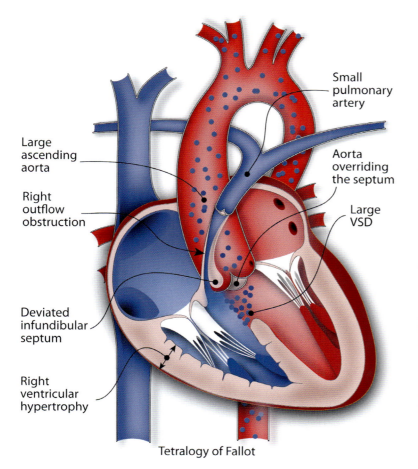

Tetralogy of Fallot

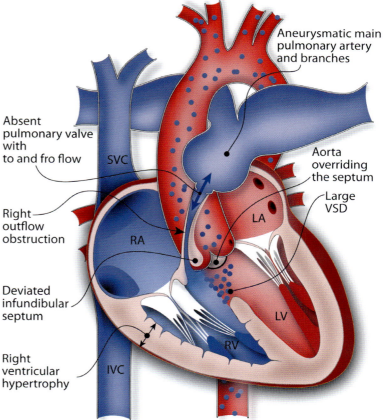

Tetralogy of Fallot with Absent Pulmonary Valve

19 Cardiovascular Malformations

Right ventricular hypertrophy stems from the systemic pressure the VSD communicates to the right ventricle, causing right ventricular pressure overload. The PS in ToF can be mild, moderate, or severe. Cyanosis equates to PS severity, with severe PS causing the lowest oxygen saturations. With an atretic right ventricular outflow to the lungs, the terminology changes to either ToF with pulmonary atresia or, preferably, pulmonary atresia with VSD.

Echo can define the anatomy and provide insight into the need for catheter interventional or surgical procedures. Diagnostic cardiac catheterization or other imaging studies are sometimes necessary.

History

- May be negative in newborns
- History of cyanosis and squatting in older children
- May present with a "Tet" spell, see Chapter 7

Exam

- **Dysmorphic features**

ToF is common in several syndromes.

- **Systolic ejection murmur**

The systolic ejection murmur emanates from PS not from the VSD. The PS murmur loudness increases as the obstruction increases, unless the obstruction becomes severe. With severe obstruction, the patient is profoundly cyanotic and has only a soft systolic ejection murmur, as little blood passes through the pulmonary valve. Also during a Tet spell, pulmonary blood flow is diminished, resulting in a previous loud systolic ejection murmur almost disappearing.

- **Clubbing**

Possible in older patients if presenting late.

CXR

- **Hyperlucent lungs**

Lung fields may be hyperlucent from decreased pulmonary blood flow.

- **"Boot-shaped heart"**

An upturned cardiac apex may give a wooden-shoe ("*coeur en sabot*") or boot appearance to the cardiac silhouette on CXR. However, this CXR finding is often absent in infants with ToF; thus, avoid such descriptors.

℞ options

- **Newborn without significant desaturation**

We may observe a patient with mild ToF and a predominant left-to-right shunt through the VSD ("pink Tet") without catheter intervention or surgery until a few months old, and then proceed with complete repair.

- **Newborn with desaturation or cyanosis**

Use PGE1 to maintain ductal patency. Interventional cardiac catheterization procedures may include ductal stenting, RV outflow tract stenting, or pulmonary valvuloplasty. Surgical palliation may include a systemic-to-pulmonary artery shunt or combination of surgery and catheter procedures. The anatomy and symptoms direct the timing of newborn palliative catheter intervention or surgery. With favorable anatomy (mild PS and normal PA branches), an initial complete repair may be possible. Palliation, with catheter intervention or surgery or both, allows time for infant growth before undergoing a complete repair.

- **Older patient**

Occasionally, older patients may present with Tet spells requiring emergency medical treatment before catheter intervention or surgery.

Transposition of the Great Arteries
Dextro (D) or D-TGA

Following the developing heart's single-tube phase, the heart tube loops normally to the right (dextro or D-looping). For more on embryology, see Chapter 16. D-looping places the right ventricle on the right and anterior to the left ventricle, which is left and posterior. Normally, the great arteries spiral while forming. The anterior pulmonary artery winds up over and connects to the anterior right ventricle. The posterior aorta winds up over and connects to the posterior left ventricle.

"Transposition" of the great arteries (TGA) means the aorta and pulmonary artery arise from the wrong ventricles; the aorta connects with the morphologic right ventricle; and the pulmonary artery connects with the morphologic left ventricle. For whatever reason, TGA arises in part because the normal spiraling of great arteries does not occur. Thus, the great arteries become parallel rather than spiral around each other. The lack of spiraling causes the aorta to become rightward and anterior rather than leftward and posterior, and the opposite occurs for the pulmonary artery. In this arrangement, the anterior rightward (dextro or D) aorta comes to lie over and connect to the right ventricle; hence, the term D-TGA arises from the aorta's rightward relationship with the pulmonary artery (figure on the right). Likewise, the pulmonary artery winds up posterior and connects to the left ventricle. D-TGA results in cyanosis because the desaturated systemic venous blood enters the normal right ventricle, which pumps blood to the body via the abnormally connected anterior-rightward aorta. The opposite is true for the pulmonary artery, which conveys oxygenated pulmonary venous blood from the lungs back to the lungs. Patients with D-TGA usually present desaturated shortly after birth.

In newborns, Echo can determine anatomical relationships and associated defects. Rarely does a newborn need MRI or CT scanning, which an older child may require. Newborns with D-TGA frequently undergo cardiac catheterization and balloon atrial septostomy (BAS). During cardiac catheterization, the coronary arteries usually undergo angiographic imaging, as coronary artery anatomy may influence surgical repair.

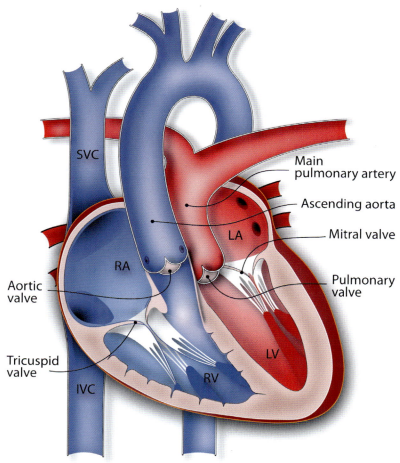

D-Transposition of the Great Arteries

19 Cardiovascular Malformations

History
- Usually negative in newborns other than cyanosis
- Rare to present beyond 1 week old

Exam
- Simple D-TGA usually not associated with syndromes
- Hyperdynamic precordium
- No loud murmur without PS or other defects
- Accentuated S_2, reflecting the anterior aortic valve

CXR
- Heart size usually normal
- Increased pulmonary vascular markings
- Narrow superior mediastinum from parallel great arteries

℞ options
- PGE1
- Atrial level mixing improves after BAS (figures below)
- Repair with an arterial switch operation (ASO)
- Repair of associated defects like VSDs with the ASO

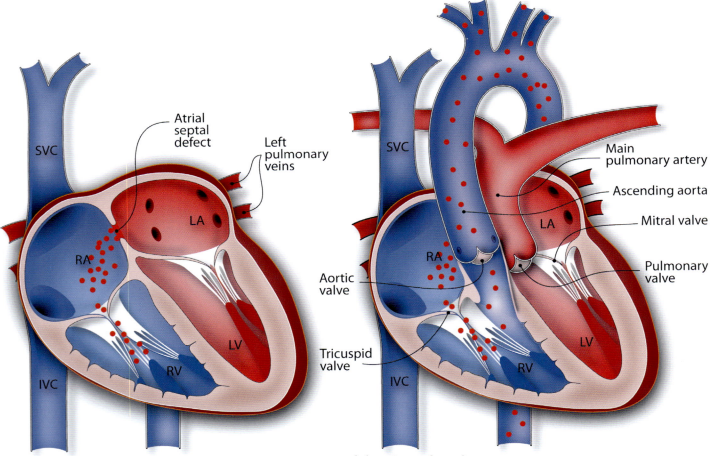

D-Transposition of the Great Arteries
The left to right atrial level shunt improves the systemic oxygen saturation

Levo (L) or L-TGA

We include L-transposition of the great arteries or L-TGA (figure below right) under this section on transposition; although, the condition usually does not cause desaturation. Some call L-TGA "corrected transposition." We avoid the term "corrected," because neither surgery nor nature has corrected L-TGA. L-TGA is a rare condition often associated with other cardiovascular malformations. L-TGA occurs from an embryological error causing the single cardiac tube to loop to the left rather than the right. Here, the morphologic "left ventricle" winds up on the right and side-by-side to the morphologic "right ventricle" on the left. Similar to D-TGA, spiraling of the great arteries is also abnormal in L-TGA. The aorta comes to lie anteriorly and leftward (levo or L) and connects to the leftward "morphologic right ventricle." In L-TGA, the pulmonary artery comes to lie posteriorly and rightward and connects to the rightward "morphologic left ventricle." In this arrangement, desaturated systemic venous blood enters the rightward ventricle, which pumps to the lungs, and the oxygenated pulmonary venous blood enters the leftward ventricle, which pumps to the body. The lack of cyanosis in L-TGA prompted the 19th-century pathologist Karl Rokitansky to coin the term "corrected transposition," later becoming "congenitally corrected transposition."

Because the conduction system is abnormal, L-TGA often presents with congenital heart block at birth. Additionally, if patients do not present at birth with heart block, then those with L-TGA are at risk to develop heart block later. Patients with L-TGA also frequently have VSDs or PS or both. Without these other defects, however, L-TGA can escape diagnosis for years. As the systemic ventricle is the morphologic right ventricle, patients are at risk for developing systemic ventricular dysfunction. Further, since the left-sided or systemic-atrioventricular (AV) valve is a morphologic tricuspid valve, this valve does not work well under systemic pressures. Hence, the left-sided AV valve frequently develops regurgitation.

Echo can identify the anatomy and determine associated abnormalities, especially the presence of a VSD, PS, and left-sided AV valve regurgitation.

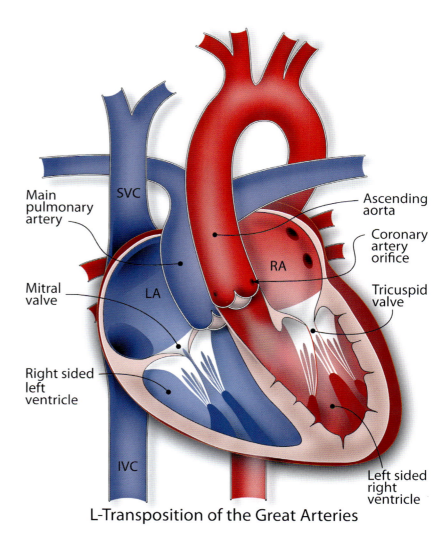

L-Transposition of the Great Arteries

History
- Depends on associated abnormalities

Exam
- Usually not found in syndromes
- Bradycardia from heart block
- Accentuated S_2 secondary to the anterior aortic valve
- Murmurs arise from associated defects

CXR
- Can be normal
- Abnormal left heart border from leftward aorta
- Increased pulmonary vascular markings if a VSD

℞ options
- Pacemaker for heart block
- When indicated, surgery for VSD or PS or both
- Medical or surgical ℞ for left AV valve regurgitation
- Occasionally, a "double switch operation" [25]

Alternate nomenclature

As a final comment about transposition of the great arteries, both D-TGA and L-TGA specify the relationship of the great arteries to each other. However, in both D-TGA and L-TGA these relationships do not always follow the above descriptions. Thus, some use an alternative nomenclature: (1) D-TGA, becomes atrioventricular concordance with ventriculoarterial discordance, and (2) L-TGA, becomes atrioventricular discordance with ventriculoarterial discordance. These later descriptions describe the connections between the atria and ventricles; and ventricles and the great arteries; and these descriptions do not rely on the rightward or leftward relationship of the aorta to the pulmonary artery.

Total Anomalous Pulmonary Venous Return

In total anomalous pulmonary venous return (TAPVR), all the pulmonary veins come to a confluence and then drain into the right atrium rather than the left atrium. Facing page figures A through C show structures behind the heart in the left figures and intracardiac anatomy in the right ones. White arrows show the path of pulmonary venous blood.

TAPVR types

- **Supracardiac**

Pulmonary veins enter the right atrium via an ascending vertical vein and the superior vena cava, as in figure A on the facing page.

- **Cardiac**

Pulmonary veins enter the right atrium directly via the coronary sinus, as in figure B on the facing page.

- **Infracardiac**

Pulmonary veins enter the right atrium via a descending vertical vein to the inferior vena cava, as in figure C on the facing page.

Frequently, the infracardiac type has obstructed pulmonary veins. The descending vertical vein from the pulmonary vein confluence dives below the diaphragm and enters the liver. The pulmonary venous return enters the inferior vena cava via the ductus venosus (left figure C). The ductus venosus closes after birth, creating obstruction to the pulmonary venous return. Supracardiac and cardiac types usually have no obstruction, although certain anatomic features can cause pulmonary venous obstruction in these types also.

Echo can define the TAPVR type and image associated malformations. MRI or CT-scanning may be needed also.

19 Cardiovascular Malformations

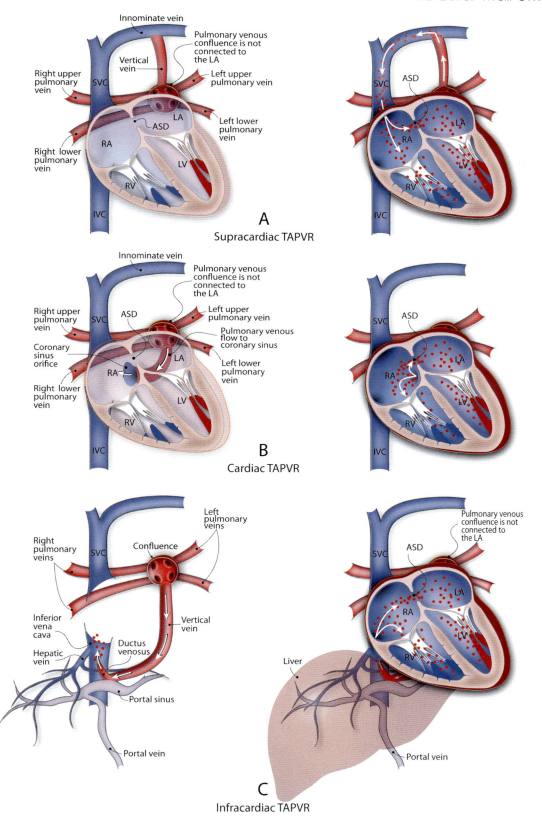

A Supracardiac TAPVR

B Cardiac TAPVR

C Infracardiac TAPVR

History

- History may be negative in unobstructed TAPVR
- Unobstructed TAPVR may present later with chronic CHF
- Obstructed TAPVR presents with distress at birth

Exam

- Dysmorphic features are usually not present
- Hyperdynamic precordium
- Murmur findings may be nonspecific
- Severe cyanosis and acidosis with obstructed veins

CXR

- **Unobstructed TAPVR**

TAPVR usually presents with cardiomegaly and increased pulmonary vascular markings. Supracardiac TAPVR may also have a wide mediastinum, creating the "snowman sign." Nonetheless, the snowman sign may be absent.

- **Obstructed TAPVR**

Typical CXR picture is normal-sized heart with "ground glass" appearing lung fields from pulmonary venous obstruction.

℞ options

- **Interventional cardiac catheterization**

When emergency surgery is impossible for patients with obstructed TAPVR—for whatever reason—temporizing vascular stents in obstructed pulmonary venous pathways may be life saving [26].

- **Surgery**

TAPVR frequently is a medical-surgical emergency requiring an emergent operation, especially for obstructed pulmonary veins. For patients with unobstructed veins, surgical repair is less urgent.

Tricuspid Atresia

Tricuspid atresia has 1-functional ventricle (figures on the facing page below). Hearts with 1-functional ventricle have a solitary effective pumping chamber and usually another hypoplastic ventricular chamber, too small to pump blood to the body or the lungs. Tricuspid atresia usually includes right ventricular hypoplasia with or without main and branch pulmonary artery underdevelopment. Often, however, the main and branch pulmonary arteries develop normally as the fetal ductus usually provides appropriate blood supply to developing pulmonary arteries. Also, the hypoplastic right ventricular chamber may communicate with the left ventricle via 1 or more ventricular septal defects, providing additional flow to the pulmonary arteries. Postnatal pulmonary blood flow determines symptoms that include cyanosis when the pulmonary valve significantly restricts flow; heart failure when the pulmonary valve does not restrict flow; and balanced physiology when the pulmonary valve moderately restricts flow.

Echo can define the anatomy, especially the pulmonary blood flow and whether the pulmonary blood flow needs augmentation or restriction. Echo can also determine whether the atrial septum is restrictive, as all the systemic return must bypass the right ventricle to enter the left atrium. Therefore, a restricted atrial septum significantly impairs systemic venous return and cardiac output.

History

- May be negative with balanced pulmonary blood flow
- CHF with pulmonary overcirculation
- Cyanosis with restricted pulmonary blood flow

Exam

- Hyperdynamic precordium

19 Cardiovascular Malformations

- Minimal murmur when no pulmonic stenosis
- Loud systolic murmur with pulmonic stenosis or VSD

CXR

- May be normal at birth
- Lungs are hyperlucent with PS
- Increased pulmonary vascular markings without PS

EKG

- Negative QRS in lead aVF

℞ options

- PGE1 for restricted pulmonary blood flow
- A restrictive atrial septum requires BAS
- Shunt for restricted pulmonary blood flow
- Possibly PDA stent for restricted pulmonary flow
- Pulmonary artery band when no PS
- Glenn procedure at about 6 months old
- Fontan procedure at about 2 to 3 years old

℞ approach to 1-functional ventricles

Hearts with 1-functional ventricle, such as tricuspid atresia, require a staged-palliation approach. A principal treatment decision involves the pulmonary blood flow status. On the following the pages, we have outlined the approach to patients without pulmonic stenosis that need restriction to flow via a pulmonary artery band (figures A and B), and those with restricted blood flow that need a reliable source of pulmonary blood flow via a systemic-to-pulmonary artery shunt (modified BT shunt as in figures D and E). The subsequent steps connect the systemic venous return (superior and inferior vena cava): first the superior vena via a Glenn shunt (figures C and F) and second the inferior vena cava via an extracardiac Fontan (figure G). For more information and an extensive discussion, see Chapter 27.

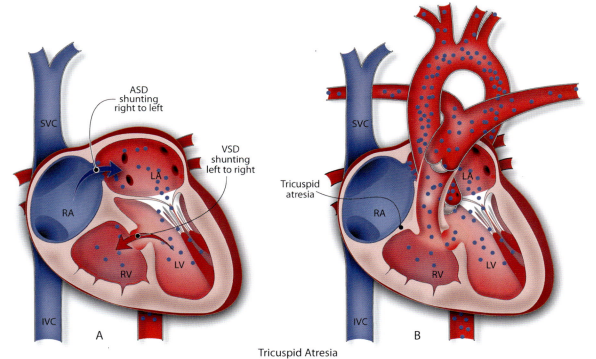

Tricuspid Atresia

19 Cardiovascular Malformations

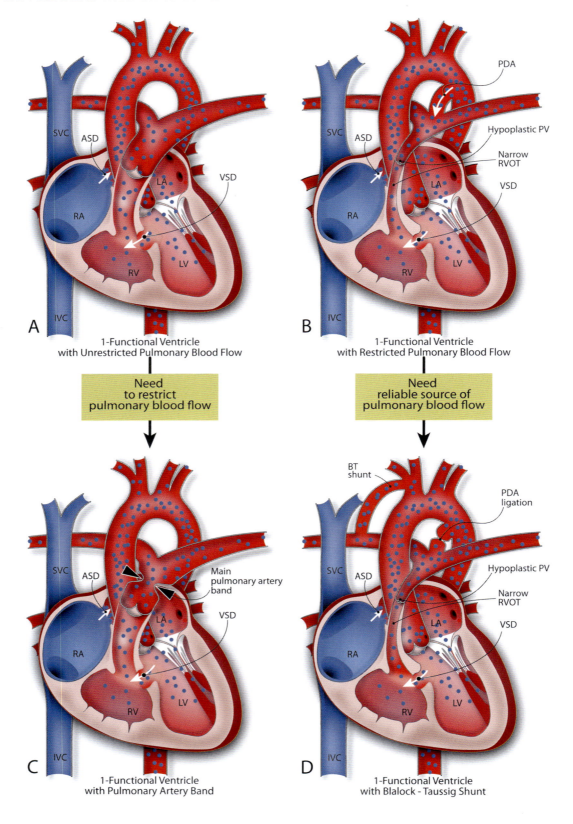

19 Cardiovascular Malformations

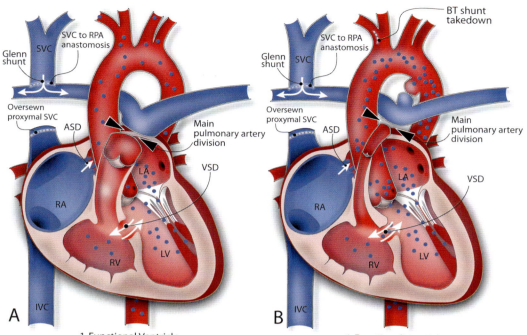

A
1-Functional Ventricle
with Unrestricted Pulmonary Blood Flow
Pulmonary artery division and Glenn shunt

B
1-Functional Ventricle
with Restricted Pulmonary Blood Flow
BT shunt takedown, pulmonary artery division
and Glenn shunt

Completion of Fontan

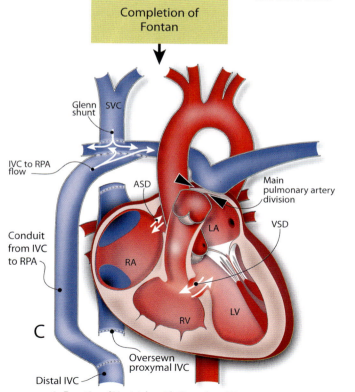

C
1- Functional Ventricle with Completed Fontan

Truncus Arteriosus

Truncus arteriosus has a single great artery and single semilunar valve. This defect arises from an embryological error in the septation process of the primitive truncus. For more on embryology, see Chapter 16. Truncus arteriosus is almost always associated with a VSD. The pulmonary arteries arise from the truncal artery without a pulmonary valve. The pulmonary artery branching patterns define truncus arteriosus variations. Type I truncus is present when a short, main pulmonary artery arises from the truncal artery (figure on the facing page); type II when the pulmonary arteries arise independently from the truncal artery but in proximity; and type III when the pulmonary arteries arise independently from the truncal artery but with more distance between them than type II. We no longer use the term "type IV truncus arteriosus." Patients often present with congestive heart failure and minimal oxygen desaturation because truncus usually has unrestricted rather than restricted pulmonary blood flow.

Echo can determine the truncus type and the presence of truncal valve stenosis or truncal valve regurgitation or both. Echo can also reveal an interrupted aortic arch, which occasionally occurs with truncus.

History

- Without newborn detection, may present in CHF

Exam

- Chromosome 22q11 deletion is common
- Hyperdynamic precordium
- Systolic ejection click
- Loud S_2
- Minimal murmur findings without truncal valve stenosis
- Systolic & diastolic murmurs with truncal valve stenosis & truncal valve regurgitation

CXR

- Usually cardiomegaly
- Increased pulmonary vascular markings

℞ options

- Early surgical repair with the Rastelli procedure
- Caution with chromosome 22q11 deletion, patients may have hypocalcemia & immune compromise

19 Cardiovascular Malformations

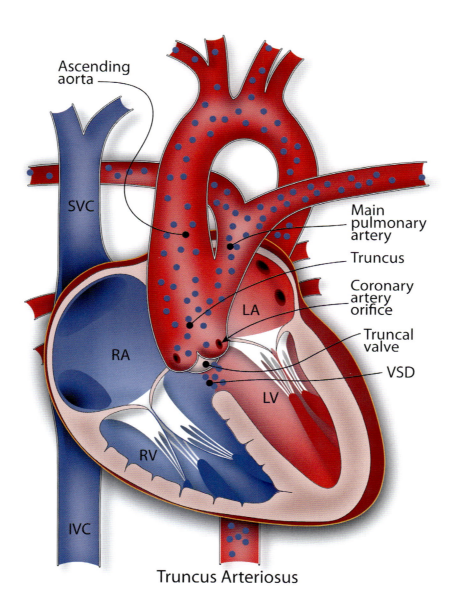

Truncus Arteriosus

19 Cardiovascular Malformations

MORE DEFECTS PRESENTING WITH OXYGEN DESATURATION

Double Outlet Right Ventricle

In double outlet right ventricle (DORV) (figure on the facing page), both great arteries arise from the morphologic right ventricle, and the left ventricle communicates with the right ventricle through a VSD. The great arteries can be abnormally related with an anterior-rightward aorta and a posterior-leftward pulmonary artery, as the figure on the facing page shows. Or the great arteries can be almost normal in their relationship. If the anatomy results in normally related great arteries, then surgical repair may simply entail a ventricular septal defect closure. However, a DORV often has abnormal aorta and pulmonary artery relationships. Further, DORVs often also have associated malformations such as pulmonary stenosis or coarctation. Symptoms and surgical-treatment complexity arise from the status of pulmonary flow, systemic flow, and other malformations. Those patients with near normal great artery arrangements and no pulmonic stenosis may have minimal to no oxygen desaturation. In contrast, those with abnormal great artery arrangements and pulmonic stenosis may be profoundly cyanotic.

Echo can evaluate the anatomical variations including the great artery relationships, the VSD's relationship to the aorta or pulmonary artery, and other defects such as pulmonic stenosis or a coarctation.

History
- Depends on anatomical variations

Exam
- Hyperdynamic precordium
- Murmurs from associated defects

CXR
- Can be normal
- Increased pulmonary vascular markings without PS
- Decreased pulmonary vascular markings with PS

℞ options
- PGE1 for severe PS or a CoA
- PA band for unobstructed pulmonary flow
- Shunt for restricted pulmonary flow
- Aortic arch repair for CoA
- Sometimes just VSD closure
- May need Rastelli procedure or arterial switch operation
- Possible hybrid procedure if severe arch obstruction

19 Cardiovascular Malformations

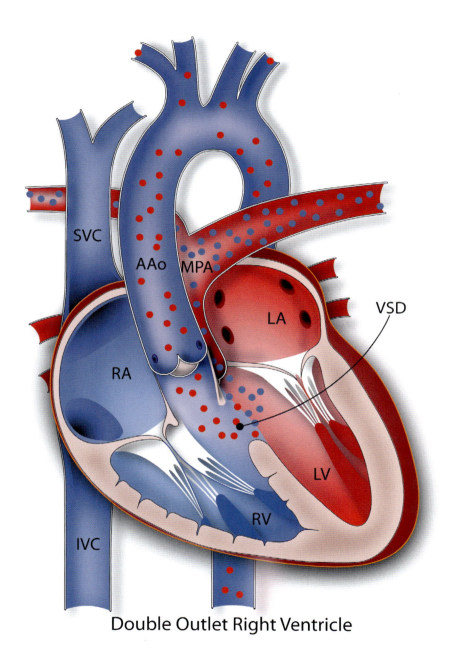

Double Outlet Right Ventricle

Pulmonary Atresia with Intact Ventricular Septum

This condition usually consists of a hypoplastic right ventricle (RV) and complete obstruction of blood flow to the lungs (figure on the facing page). A postnatal PDA is the sole supply of pulmonary blood flow. Further, the hypoplastic right ventricle is commonly hypertensive. Usually, the only decompression of the hypertensive RV comes from tricuspid valve regurgitation (TR). A hypertensive hypoplastic RV chamber may develop fistulous communications with the coronary arteries that can also partially decompress the high right ventricular systolic pressure. Further, coronary artery connections may result in coronary blood flow being dependent on the hypertensive RV chamber—"RV-dependent coronary artery circulation."

Echo can determine the RV size and the presence of RV fistulas. RV fistulas suggest RV-dependent coronary artery circulation. Cardiac catheterization and angiography, however, are necessary to conclusively determine whether the patient has RV-dependent coronary artery circulation. RV-dependent coronary artery circulation influences the treatment approach, because pulmonary valvotomy is contraindicated with RV-dependent coronary circulation. Opening an atretic pulmonary valve (PV) decompresses the RV, which and can lead to coronary insufficiency.

Echo can also determine the ductal patency, branch pulmonary artery sizes, and the status of the atrial septum. Similar to tricuspid atresia, all the systemic venous return bypasses the right ventricle through the interatrial septum and a restricted atrial septum can cause low cardiac output.

History
- Usually cyanotic shortly after birth

Exam
- May have no murmur
- May have holosystolic murmur from TR
- May have a systolic or continuous murmur from a PDA

CXR
- May be normal
- Hyperlucent lungs with ductal closure

℞ options
- PGE1 in every case
- RV-dependent coronary arteries influence ℞
- Catheter intervention possible for some atretic PVs
- Possible candidate for ductus arteriosus stent
- Possible candidate for surgical PV valvotomy
- May need shunt with or without PV opening
- Isolated shunt, if RV-dependent coronary circulation
- Glenn procedure at about 6 months old
- Fontan procedure at about 2 to 3 years old
- Occasionally the RV may be big enough for 2-ventricle repair
- Occasionally may need heart transplantation if severe coronary artery abnormalities

19 Cardiovascular Malformations

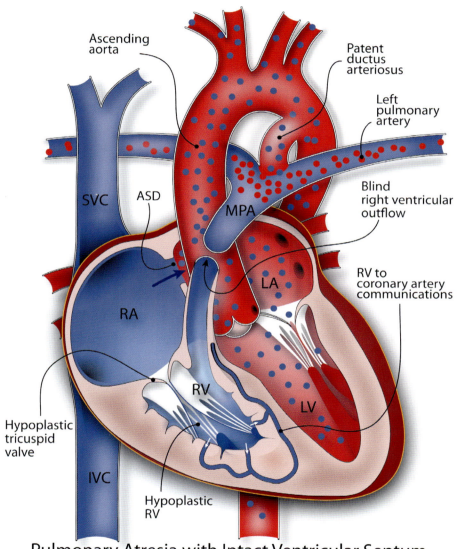

Pulmonary Atresia with Intact Ventricular Septum

Ebstein Anomaly

During cardiovascular development, the atrioventricular valve leaflets originate from an undermining process of the ventricular endocardial surface. A failure of the tricuspid valve (TV) to complete this undermining process causes Ebstein anomaly of the TV (figure on the facing page). A severe lack of undermining results in a severely abnormal TV, with marked displacement into the RV. The abnormal valve leaflets cause tricuspid regurgitation or tricuspid stenosis or both. The abnormal tricuspid valve leaflets can limit pulmonary blood flow.

At birth, cyanosis results from the large right-to-left shunt through an ASD. There are 2 main conditions that accentuate the atrial level right-to-left shunt: (1) A malformed TV that limits right atrial-to-right ventricular flow, and (2) The initial elevated neonatal pulmonary vascular resistance that prevents adequate pulmonary flow.

Echo can determine the Ebstein anomaly's severity by evaluating the tricuspid regurgitation or stenosis (TR, TS), the right-to-left shunting through the ASD, the antegrade pulmonary flow, and other defects.

History

- History may be negative in mild Ebstein anomaly
- May have preexcitation & SVT
- May have severe cyanosis & right heart failure

Exam

- Occasionally born with hydrops
- Multiple heart tones
- TR & TS murmurs
- Other murmurs from defects like VSDs

CXR

- May be normal in mild Ebstein anomaly
- Mild to moderate cardiomegaly in mild to moderate forms
- Classic finding of "wall-to-wall" heart in severe form

℞ options

- **Mild to moderate Ebstein anomaly**

Mild to moderate Ebstein anomaly may need no surgical or catheter interventional procedures. In some patients, residual atrial communications may be amenable to catheter device closure. In some patients, a tricuspid valve repair or replacement may also be necessary at some point.

- **Severe Ebstein anomaly**

In cyanotic newborns, allow time to pass for a fall in postnatal pulmonary vascular resistance. Lower PVR increases pulmonary blood flow and improves oxygenation. An improvement in oxygenation allows a delay in possible surgical intervention, sometimes for days or years. However, a newborn with severe Ebstein anomaly, who does not improve with a fall in pulmonary vascular resistance, may need an RV exclusion surgery (Starnes procedure). The RV exclusion surgery requires a systemic-to-pulmonary artery shunt. The RV exclusion surgery is the first step in staged palliation of hearts with 1-functional ventricle, culminating in a Fontan procedure.

19 Cardiovascular Malformations

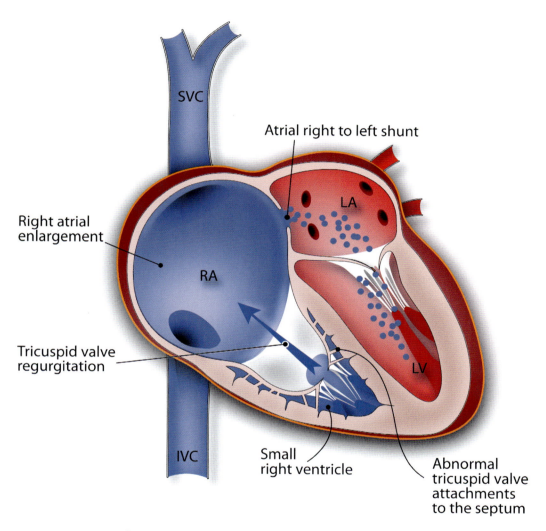

Ebstein Anomaly of the Tricuspid Valve

1-Functional Ventricles

Hearts with 1-functional ventricle have a solitary main ventricular chamber and either no additional ventricular chamber or an additional rudimentary ventricular chamber (figure on the facing page shows a hypoplastic right ventricle). Tricuspid atresia, hypoplastic left heart syndrome, and most pulmonary atresias with intact septums also have 1-functional ventricle. Various types of hearts with 1-functional ventricles occur with myriad anatomical variation. History, symptoms, signs, additional physical exam findings, and treatment most often depend upon the pulmonary and systemic blood flows, the pulmonary venous return, atrioventricular valve function, and the function of the main ventricular chamber.

Echo can determine the complex relationships between the atrioventricular valves and the ventriculoarterial arrangements. Echo can also determine the status of the systemic or pulmonary blood flow. Other pertinent findings include ventricular function, the status of the pulmonary and systemic venous returns, and the status of the interatrial septum.

History
- May be negative with balanced physiology
- Visible cyanosis with PS or transposed great arteries
- Desaturation & CHF without PS
- Possibly extremis with a CoA upon ductal closure

Exam
- Hyperdynamic precordium
- Murmurs depend on associated defects

CXR
- Can be normal
- Increased or decreased pulmonary vascular markings

℞ options
- PGE1 for severe PS or CoA
- PA band for unrestricted pulmonary flow
- Shunt for PS
- Possible CoA repair
- Catheter intervention for CoA or ductal stent
- Initial staged surgical palliation or hybrid procedure
- Glenn procedure at about 6 months old
- Fontan procedure around 2 to 3 years old

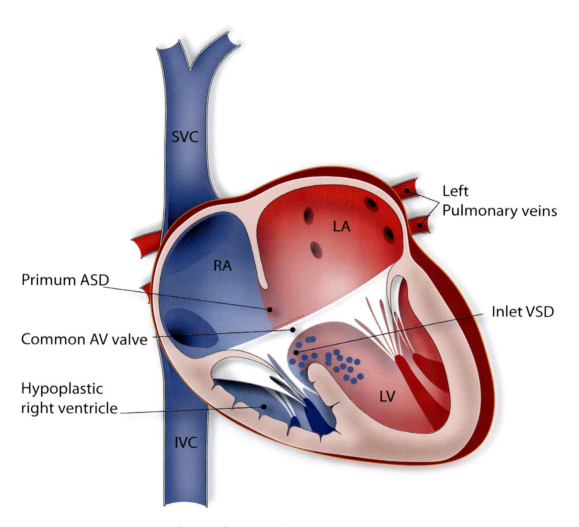

Complete, unbalanced AVSD

19 Cardiovascular Malformations

Pulmonary Arteriovenous Malformations

Pulmonary arteriovenous malformations (PAVMs) are rare direct, intrapulmonary connections between small and large pulmonary arteries and pulmonary veins, resulting in right-to-left shunts (figure on the facing page). Most PAVMs are congenital and occur more commonly in females. Some occur with hereditary hemorrhagic telangiectasia. Other conditions that may develop PAVMs include liver disease, trauma, and chronic pulmonary inflammatory problems.

Echo cannot image PAVMs, but a contrast Echo can demonstrate their pathology. Microcavitations appear rapidly in the left atrium, following an injection of agitated saline in a peripheral vein. Normally, with an injection of agitated saline, no microcavitations appear in the left atrium, as the lungs clear them. The microcavitations appear in the left atrium because of the direct pulmonary artery-pulmonary vein connections that bypass the alveoli. Anatomical imaging, however, is best with angiography, MRI, or CT scanning.

History
- Often negative
- May have history of cyanosis

Exam
- Physical exam may be negative
- May desaturate with exercise
- Clubbing in older children, example in figure on the right

CXR
- May be negative
- Large PAVM may produce mass-like lesion

℞ options
- Catheter embolization or surgical resection

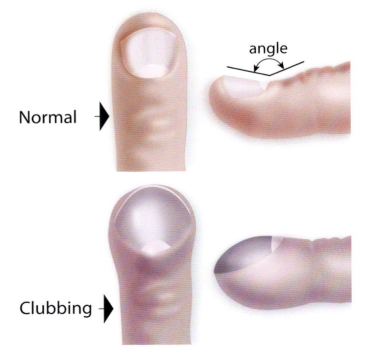

19 Cardiovascular Malformations

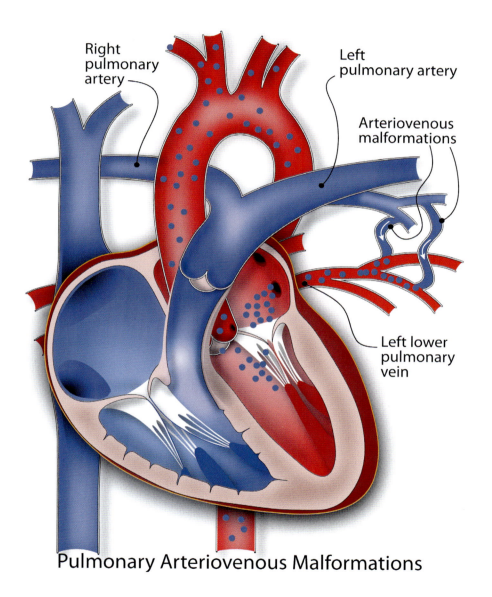

Pulmonary Arteriovenous Malformations

VASCULAR RINGS & SLINGS

Vascular rings and slings are abnormal aortic arch and pulmonary artery structures that cause airway and esophageal obstruction by encircling them. The 2 most common vascular rings are a right aortic arch with an aberrant left subclavian artery and a left-sided patent ductus arteriosus and a double aortic arch (figures B and C on the facing page). As seen in figure B, a right aortic arch and aberrant left subclavian from is usually associated with a an aortic diverticulum (Kommerell diverticulum), which often needs resection at the time of repair.

A rarer condition than the first 2 types is a pulmonary artery sling (figures A and B on the immediate right). In a pulmonary artery sling, the left pulmonary artery arises from the right pulmonary artery and passes behind the trachea and in front of the esophagus, resulting predominantly in airway obstruction.

Echo may not completely resolve the anatomy of vascular rings and slings. Barium swallows formerly played a role. However, MRI or CT scans provide for complete demonstration of the vascular anatomy, including the vascular ring's effect on the airway and esophagus.

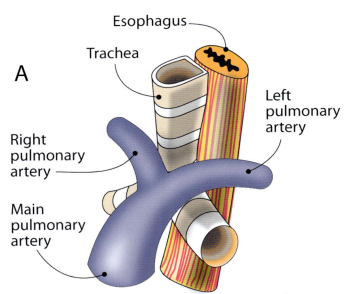

Normal Pulmonary Artery Branching

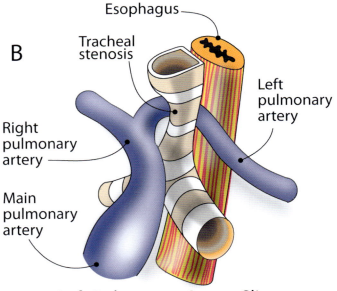

Left Pulmonary Artery Sling

History

- May have no stridor, but may prefer liquids & shun or choke on solid food
- Stridor or difficulty swallowing solid food or both
- Some patients present with exercise-induced asthma

Exam

- Dysmorphic features, as vascular rings may be associated with chromosome 22q11 deletion

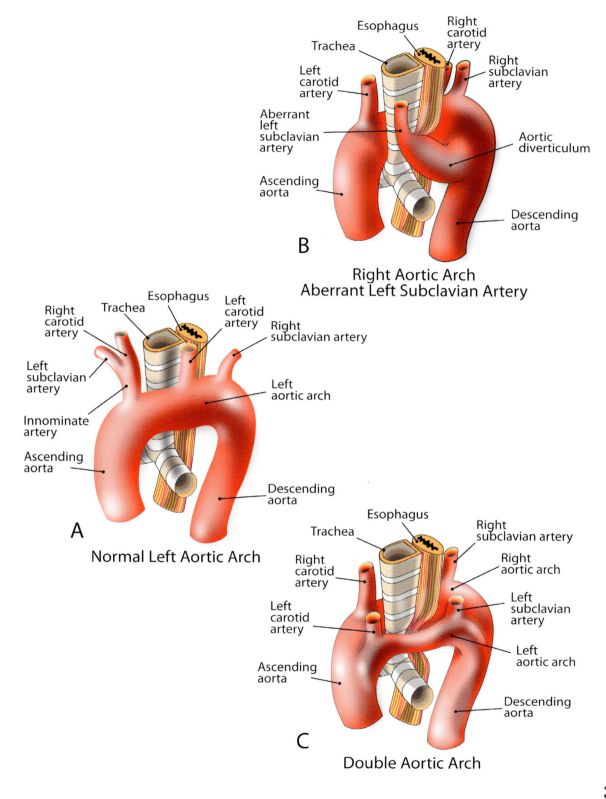

B Right Aortic Arch Aberrant Left Subclavian Artery

A Normal Left Aortic Arch

C Double Aortic Arch

- Usually normal cardiac exam

CXR
- Usually normal

℞ options
- Surgical relief of vascular ring
- Also may need airway repair procedures

References

1 Evans WN, Acherman RJ, Castillo WJ, Restrepo H. The changing occurrences of tetralogy of Fallot and simple transposition of the great arteries in Southern Nevada. Cardiology in the Young 2011; 21: 281-285

2 Garson, A. The Science And Practice Of Pediatric Cardiology. Baltimore, Williams & Wilkins, 2005

3 Moss, A. J., & Allen, H. D. Moss And Adams' Heart Disease In Infants, Children, And Adolescents Including The Fetus and Young Adult. Philadelphia, Lippincott Williams & Wilkins, 2008

4 Anderson, R. H. Paediatric Cardiology. Philadelphia, Churchill Livingstone/Elsevier, 2009

5 Mahle WT, Newburger JW, Matherne GP, Smith FC, Hoke TR, Koppel R, Gidding SS, Beekman RH 3rd, Grosse SD; American Heart Association Congenital Heart Defects Committee of the Council on Cardiovascular Disease in the Young, Council on Cardiovascular Nursing, and Interdisciplinary Council on Quality of Care and Outcomes Research; American Academy of Pediatrics Section on Cardiology And Cardiac Surgery; Committee On Fetus And Newborn. Role of pulse oximetry in examining newborns for congenital heart disease: a scientific statement from the AHA and AAP. Pediatrics. 2009; 124: 823-836

6 Walsh W. Evaluation of pulse oximetry screening in Middle Tennessee: cases for consideration before universal screening. J Perinatol; 2011; 31: 125-129

7 Acherman RJ, Evans WN, Luna CF, Rollins R, Kip KT, Collazos JC, Restrepo H, Adasheck J, Iriye BK, Roberts D, Sacks AJ. Prenatal detection of congenital heart disease in Southern Nevada: the need for universal fetal cardiac evaluation. J Ultrasound Med. 2007; 26: 1715-1719.

8 Oh SJ, Jeung IC. A case of isolated congenital ductus arteriosus aneurysm detected by fetal echocardiography at 38 weeks of gestation. J Clin Ultrasound 2011; 39: 530-533

9 Acherman RJ, Siassi B, Wells W, Goodwin M, DeVore G, Sardesai S, Wong PC, Ebrahimi M, Pratti-Madrid G, Castillo W, Ramanathan R. Aneurysm of the ductus arteriosus: a congenital lesion. Am J Perinatol 1998; 15: 653-659

10 Forfar JC, Godman MJ. Functional and anatomical correlates in atrial septal defect. An echocardiographic analysis. Br Heart J. 1985; 54: 193-200

11 Rothman A, Galindo A, Evans WN, Collazos JC, Restrepo H. Effectiveness and safety of balloon dilation of native aortic coarctation in premature neonates weighing < or = 2,500 grams. Am J Cardiol 2010; 105: 1176-1180

12 Richardson P, McKenna W, Bristow M, Maisch B, Mautner B, O'Connell J, Olsen E, Thiene G, Goodwin J, Gyarfas I, Martin I, Nordet P. Report of the 1995 World Health Organization/International Society and Federation of Cardiology Task Force on the Definition and Classification of cardiomyopathies. Circulation 1996; 93: 841-842

13 Wilkinson JD, Sleeper LA, Alvarez JA, Bublik N, Lipshultz SE; the Pediatric Cardiomyopathy Study Group. The Pediatric Cardiomyopathy Registry: 1995-2007. Prog Pediatr Cardiol 2008; 25: 31-36

14 Simpson KE, Canter CE. Acute myocarditis in children. Expert Rev Cardiovasc Ther 2011; 9: 771-783

15 Noori S, Acherman R, Siassi B, Luna C, Ebrahimi M, Pavlova Z, Ramanathan R. A rare presentation of Pompe disease with massive hypertrophic cardiomyopathy at birth. J Perinat Med 2002; 30: 517-521

16 Allanson JE, Bohring A, Dörr HG, Dufke A, Gillessen-Kaesbach G, Horn D, König R, Kratz CP, Kutsche K, Pauli S, Raskin S, Rauch A, Turner A, Wieczorek D, Zenker M. The face of Noonan syndrome: Does phenotype predict genotype. Am J Med Genet A 2010 ; 152A: 1960-1966

17 Russo LM, Webber SA. Idiopathic restrictive cardiomyopathy in children. Heart 2005; 91: 1199–1202

18 Sekar P, Hornberger LK, Smallhorn JS. A case of restrictive cardiomyopathy presenting in fetal life with an isolated pericardial

effusion. Ultrasound Obstet Gynecol 2010; 35:3 69-372

19 Nucifora G, Benettoni A, Allocca G, Bussani R, Silvestri F. Arrhythmogenic right ventricular dysplasia/cardiomyopathy as a cause of sudden infant death. J Cardiovasc Med (Hagerstown) 2008; 9: 430-431

20 Lurie PR. The perspective of ventricular noncompaction as seen by a nonagenarian. Cardiol Young 2008; 18: 243-249

21 Acherman RJ, Evans WN, Schwartz JK, Dombrowski M, Rollins RC, Castillo W, Haltore S, Berthody DP. Right ventricular noncompaction associated with long QT in a fetus with right ventricular hypertrophy and cardiac arrhythmias. Prenat Diagn 2008; 28: 551-553

22 Lurie PR. Changing concepts of endocardial fibroelastosis. Cardiol Young 2010; 20: 115-123

23 Pises N, Acherman RJ, Iriye BK, Rollins RC, Castillo W, Herceg E, Evans WN. Positive maternal anti-SSA/SSB antibody-related fetal right ventricular endocardial fibroelastosis without atrioventricular block, reversal of endocardial fibroelastosis. Prenat Diagn 2009; 29: 177-178

24 Evans WN. "Tetralogy of Fallot" and Etienne-Louis Arthur Fallot. Pediatr Cardiol 2008; 29: 637-640

25 Brawn WJ. The double switch for atrioventricular discordance. Semin Thorac Cardiovasc Surg Pediatr Card Surg Annu 2005: 51-56.

26 Rothman A, Galindo A, Evans WN. Temporary transumbilical stenting of the ductus venosus in neonates with obstructed infradiaphragmatic total anomalous pulmonary venous return. Pediatr Cardiol 2011; 32: 87-90

Part 3

Diagnostic & ℞ Methods

306

20 Chest X-ray

Contents

BACKGROUND	309
TECHNIQUE	310
ANATOMICAL STRUCTURES	313

20 Chest X-ray

carlos luna

BACKGROUND

In November 1895, Wilhelm Conrad Röntgen was experimenting with cathode-ray tubes at the University of Würzburg in Germany. Röntgen discovered certain objects he placed in the path of the cathode-ray tube's beam displayed different degrees of transparency. When he placed his wife's hand in the beam and a photographic plate below, Röntgen developed an eerie picture showing bones, her wedding ring, and transparent grayish flesh. This image became the first human X-ray. He designated the rays passing through objects as "X," because the "rays" were mysterious then. Contrary to other revolutionary moments in medicine, X-rays quickly became a hit, as physicians and laymen immediately recognized the power of X-rays to "magically" see inside the body.

Echocardiography has decreased chest X-ray's importance as a cardiac-assessment tool. However, a chest X-ray (CXR) is crucial for evaluating the symptoms and signs of respiratory disease or desaturation. In these cases, the CXR findings may provide clues for possible cardiovascular disease. A CXR for possible asthma or pneumonia may show cardiomegaly and vascular congestion, which, rather than asthma or pneumonia, suggests overcirculation from a large left-to-right shunt. Still, a CXR's sensitivity is low, as many cardiovascular conditions have no significant effect on the heart size or the prominence of the pulmonary vascular markings.

Nonetheless, an abnormally positioned heart or abdominal viscera on CXR likely indicates complex heart disease. Practically, the frontal view provides the most information; although, the lateral view may furnish complementary findings for some conditions.

CXR interpretation requires a stepwise approach. First, note the technique and film's quality, as these factors may affect how structures appear. Next, the assessment sequence can vary but should include evaluation of the heart's position; mediastinal and cardiac silhouette characteristics; pulmonary vascular markings and parenchyma; the airway and pleural space; and the spine and ribs. [1, 2]

CXR TECHNIQUE

Chest X-ray technique may influence the results. The key technical points include the film's projection, X-ray penetration, the depth of the patient's inspiratory breath, and whether the patient rotates with poor cooperation or poor positioning by the technician.

X-Ray Projections

Posteroanterior (PA projection)

The PA projection (figure A on the facing page) provides the best imaging for cooperative patients. A PA CXR places the film in front of a standing patient, and the X-rays penetrate from the back to the front or posterior to anterior.

Anteroposterior (AP projection)

The AP projection (figure B on the facing page) is better for infants, younger children, the sick, or older recumbent patients. An AP CXR places the film under the patient's back, while lying, and the X-rays penetrate from the front to back or anterior to posterior. The AP projection artificially creates "cardiomegaly" (a wider cardiac diameter on the X-ray film as compared to the thoracic diameter) as figure B on the facing page demonstrates.

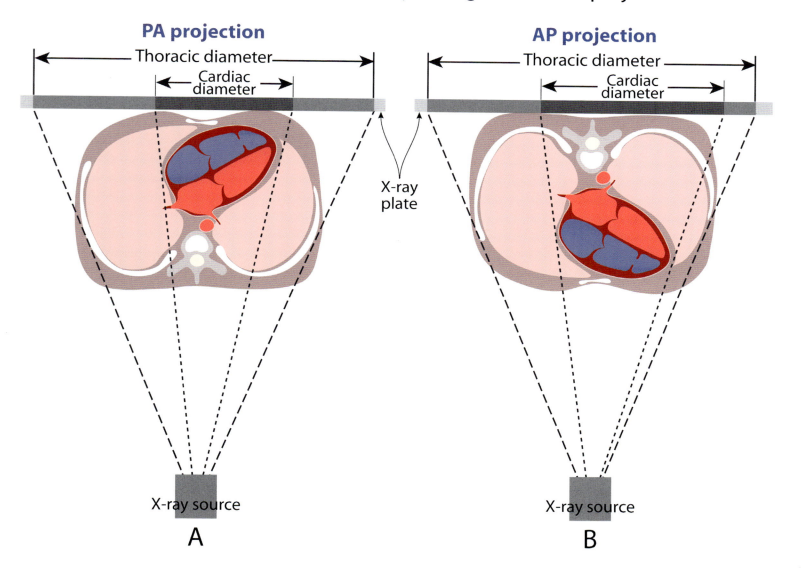

20 Chest X-ray

Optimizing the Image

The frontal (figure A on the right) and lateral (figure B on the right) films demonstrate correct X-ray penetration, inflation, and lack of rotation.

X-ray penetration

- Over penetration

This produces hyperlucent lung fields and the spine appears, through the cardiac silhouette, to have excessive boney detail.

- Under penetration

This produces hazy lung fields and the boney structures are especially white with few details.

- Correct penetration

With correct X-ray penetration, the spine has appropriate boney detail when we view the spine through the cardiac silhouette.

Inflation or inspiration

- Poor inspiration

Poor inspiration positions the top of the diaphragms higher than the 8th posterior rib, common in recumbent films.

- Over inflation

Over inflation pushes the top of the diaphragms below the 10th posterior rib.

- Proper inspiration

Proper inspiration places the top of the diaphragms between the 8th and 10th posterior ribs.

Absence of rotation

The frontal film (figure A on the right above) should show sternum-spine alignment and symmetric clavicles.

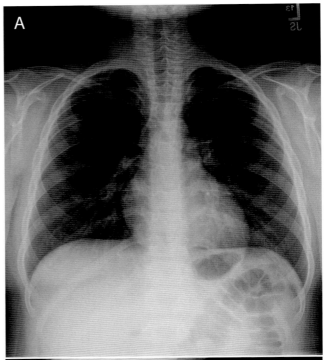
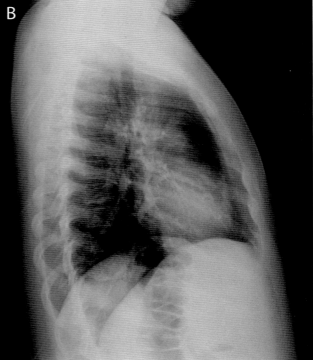

ANATOMICAL STRUCTURES

Heart & Stomach Bubble Positions

The heart's position can be on the left, right, or middle of the chest. A heart in the right chest may be from a process pushing or pulling the heart to right including right lung hypoplasia, a left-sided diaphragmatic hernia, chest masses, a unilateral pneumothorax, or a unilateral pleural effusion. Beware the occasionally mislabeled frontal film, if the technician inadvertently places the "L" marker (seen in the frontal film on the previous page) on the right. We prefer using the term "dextrocardia" for a heart in the right chest from an error in cardiovascular embryology resulting in a rightward base-apex axis, rather than using "dextrocardia" for a heart with a leftward cardiac base-apex axis that is mechanically positioned in the right chest [3]. Echo can determine the cardiac base-apex axis, but CXR cannot. Thus, for CXR, we prefer using the positional descriptors of left, right, or in the middle instead of levocardia, dextrocardia, or mesocardia. For more on thoracoabdominal situs and cardiac position, see Chapter 17.

Heart in the left chest

• Stomach bubble on the left

This is consistent with usual situs or "situs solitus."

• Stomach bubble on the right

This arrangement is consistent with an unusual situs and increases the risk of heart disease.

Heart in the right chest

• Stomach bubble on the right

This suggests dextrocardia with complete abdominal situs inversus, most commonly associated with a normal heart; although, the incidence of cardiovascular defects is somewhat higher than with situs solitus and levocardia. Lung pathology consistent with bronchiectatis suggests Kartagener syndrome.

• Stomach bubble on the left

This may represent situs solitus with the lung or other pathology pushing or pulling the heart rightward such as a right lung sequestration (scimitar syndrome - see Atrial septal Defects & Partial Anomalous Pulmonary Venous Return in Chapter 19), right lung hypoplasia, a left-sided chest mass, or left lung emphysema.

This arrangement may also be consistent with dextrocardia and an unusual abdominal situs, which significantly increases the chance of heart disease.

Heart in the middle of the chest

• Stomach bubble on the left

This is most likely consistent with situs solitus and a normal heart

• Stomach bubble on the right

This is most likely consistent with unusual situs and possible heart disease.

Cardiac Silhouette

Figure A below illustrates and labels the components of the cardiac silhouette, and the figure B on the facing page shows a labeled X-ray film. The superior vena cava and the lateral wall of the right atrium form the cardiac silhouette's right heart border. Part of the right ventricular wall forms the inferior border. However, we can evaluate the right ventricle better from the lateral view than the frontal view. The left ventricle, main pulmonary artery, and aortic arch form the left heart border.

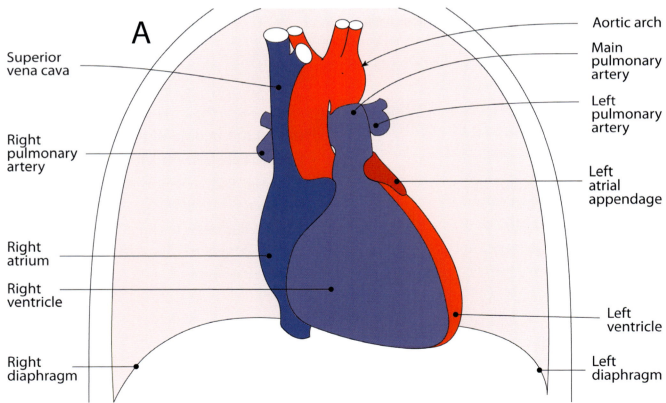

Posteroanterior projection of the normal cardiac silhouette

20 Chest X-ray

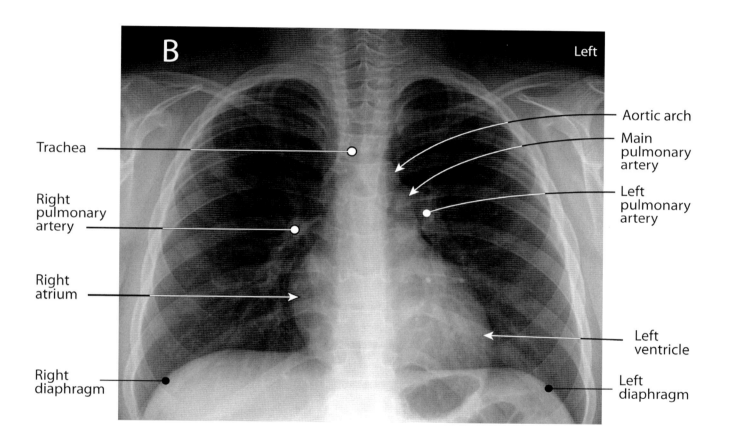

Cardiomegaly

Causes include cardiac volume overload, myocardial dysfunction, and especially pericardial effusions.

• Subjective

Cardiomegaly is subjectively assessable without objective measurements. However, exercise caution with a recumbent film; because, as we described on the previous page, the heart may appear artificially enlarged in an AP projection.

• Objective CT ratio

A cardiothoracic (CT) ratio (figure A and figure B on the right) compares the diameter of the cardiac silhouette with the diameter of the chest in the frontal view (cardiac diameter ÷ the thoracic diameter). Normal CT ratios are about 0.5 in a PA CXR, and about 0.6 in an AP CXR.

The mediastinum

The superior mediastinum (labeled in figure B on the right) contains the thymus, trachea, esophagus, central airways, central veins, and the great arteries. The mediastinum may be normal, wide, narrow, or show air.

Wide

- Thymus shadow in newborns & young infants
- Masses like neuroblastoma
- Supracardiac total anomalous pulmonary venous return
- Dilated aorta or central pulmonary arteries

Narrow

- Thymus absent or hypoplastic as in chromosome 22q11 deletion
- Neonates with transposition of the great arteries

Pneumomediastinum

- Radiolucent border with air leak

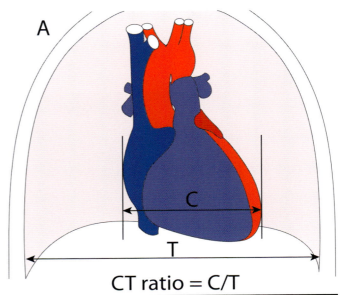

CT ratio = C/T

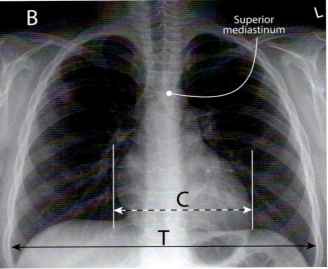

Cardiothoracic Ratio

Specific structure enlargement

- Right atrial enlargement (RAE)

RAE bulges the right border of the cardiac silhouette.

- Right ventricular enlargement (RVE)

A lateral film below best displays RVE with filling of the retrosternal space (white arrows).

- Right ventricular hypertrophy (RVH)

RVH tips the cardiac silhouette's apex upwards.

- Left atrial enlargement (LAE)

LAE may lift the left main bronchus, or widen the angle of the carina (normal up to 90°), or appear as a double density within the cardiac silhouette. Extreme LAE may cause prominence of the left atrial appendage in the left border of the cardiac silhouette, below and to the left of the main pulmonary artery segment.

- Left ventricular enlargement (LVE)

LVE increases the global cardiac silhouette size and displaces the apex leftward and inferiorly.

Pulmonary Vasculature

Vascular markings

Vascular markings in lung parenchyma may be arterial or venous or both.

- Arterial markings

As the film below shows, increased size of the pulmonary arteries with cardiomegaly may represent a left-to-right shun, increased right-ventricular stroke volume in pulmonary regurgitation, or pulmonary hypertension. Although, severe pulmonary hypertension decreases distal vascular markings, the hilar pulmonary arteries may be prominent. Cyanotic congenital heart defects with obstruction to pulmonary arterial flow usually have decreased pulmonary arterial markings, rendering hyperlucent lung fields.

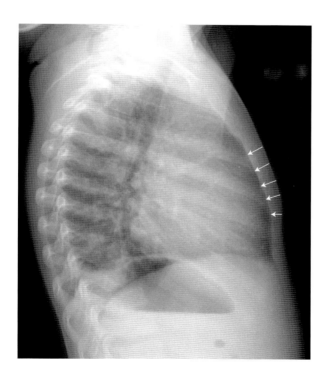

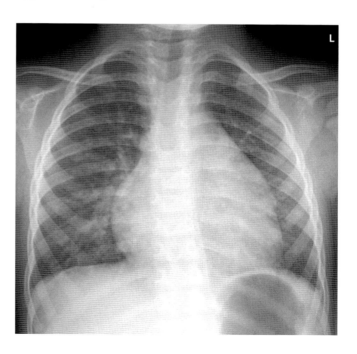

20 Chest X-ray

- **Venous markings**

Venous markings are near the heart and directed towards the left atrium. These markings are prominent in pulmonary venous congestion with left ventricular failure, pulmonary venous obstruction with obstructed TAPVR, pulmonary vein stenosis, obstructive cor triatriatum, and mitral valve stenosis. Kerley lines are engorged lymphatics from venous congestion. In an upright PA CXR, gravity accentuates vascular markings in the lung bases. In a recumbent AP CXR, vascular markings are more homogeneous from apex to base than a PA CXR.

Main pulmonary artery segment

The main pulmonary artery segment forms part of the upper left border of the cardiac silhouette (see previous labelled cardiac silhouette figures).

- **Enlarged**

The main pulmonary artery segment may enlarge with left-to-right shunts, pulmonary hypertension, valvular pulmonic stenosis with post-stenotic dilation, and severe pulmonary valve regurgitation.

- **Small or absent**

The main pulmonary artery segment is small or absent in tetralogy of Fallot (ToF), this feature contributes to the appearance of the cardiac silhouette as "boot shaped." However, avoid this term, as this sign may not be present in ToF.

Pleural Space

The pleural space is virtual space, but visible when fluid or air occupies it.

Pneumothorax

- Radiolucent separation of lung from chest wall
- Upright PA CXR, the air moves up
- Recumbent AP CXR, the air moves anteriorly

Pleural effusion

- Moderate effusion obliterates the costophrenic angle
- Large effusion creates a meniscus separating the lung from the pleural cavity
- Massive effusions cause whiteouts & shift the heart

Lung Parenchyma & Infiltrates

Infiltrates originate from edema, consolidation, or atelectasis. Sometimes infiltrates localize such as lobar consolidation or atelectasis, or the infiltrates may be diffuse such

as hyaline membrane disease or viral pneumonia.

Interstitial infiltrates

- Reticular pattern
- Usually in perihilar areas
- With viral pneumonitis

Alveolar infiltrates

- More dense than interstitial infiltrates
- Have air-bronchograms

Atelectasis

- May be linear or triangular densities
- From mucous plugs or external airway impingement
- Complete atelectasis of 1 lung shifts the heart

Spine & Ribs

Skeletal anomalies occur with congenital heart defects.

- Discordant rib number & hemivertebrae
- Scoliosis
- Fusion or duplication of ribs
- Rib notching from coarctation of the aorta

Postoperative Cardiac Surgery

The film below shows a typical postoperative cardiac surgical film. Important findings include:
- Endotracheal tube position
- Central intravascular catheters
- Pacemaker wires
- Surgical clips & sternal wires

Other postoperative findings

Although not seen in the film below, other findings may include the presence of the following:
- Pleural & mediastinal tubes
- Metallic valves, or other metal appliances
- A pneumothorax or pneumomediastinum
- Pleural effusions or infiltrates

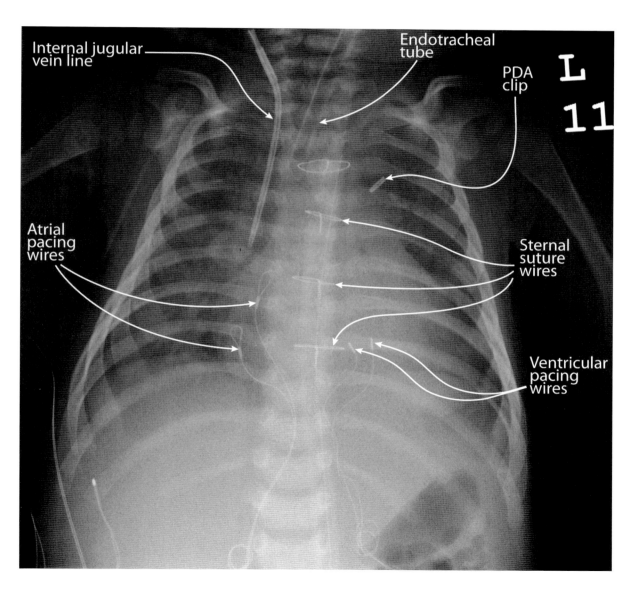

REFERENCES

1 Arthur R. Interpretation of the paediatric chest X-ray. Current Paediatrics 2003; 13: 438-447

2 "Wilhelm Conrad Röntgen" http://en.wikipedia.org/wiki/Wilhelm_Conrad_Röntgen

3 Evans WN, Acherman RJ, Collazos JC, Castillo WJ, Rollins RC, Kip KT, Restrepo H. Dextrocardia: practical clinical points and comments on terminology. Pediatr Cardiol 2010; 31: 1-6

21 Electrocardiogram

Contents

Background	323
EKG leads	324
Heart rate & rhythm	327
PR, QRS, QT intervals	335
P-wave & QRS axis	340
Hypertrophy Rules	343

21 Electrocardiogram

william evans

BACKGROUND

EKG is easier to say than ECG. In the hospital, confusion with EEG is less likely with EKG than ECG either verbally or in the medical record. Some hospitals require their staff use EKG for this reason. Willem Einthoven first used the abbreviation "EKG" in a 1912 report composed in English, not German. Thus, in this book, we use EKG rather than ECG.

Most nonpediatric cardiologists lack instruction in pediatric EKG interpretation. Computer EKG interpretation printouts frequently have inaccuracies, resulting in unnecessary concerns for clinicians and families.

Our method for simplified EKG interpretation requires 4 short steps and just a few memorized rules. With these 4 steps and condensed rules, any healthcare provider can provide an initial interpretation for most pediatric EKGs. Always follow the 4 steps in strict order for every EKG. All pediatric EKGs, however, should be sent to a pediatric cardiologist for confirmatory interpretation. [1-6]

21 Electrocardiogram

EKG LEADS

Lead placement is the basis for a proper EKG. The operator simply places the limb leads on the right and left arms and the right and left legs; however, the precordial leads are more difficult to place accurately. The figure below displays the proper positions for Leads V1 through V6.

➤ Beware of arm lead reversal, as this causes false P-wave abnormalities.

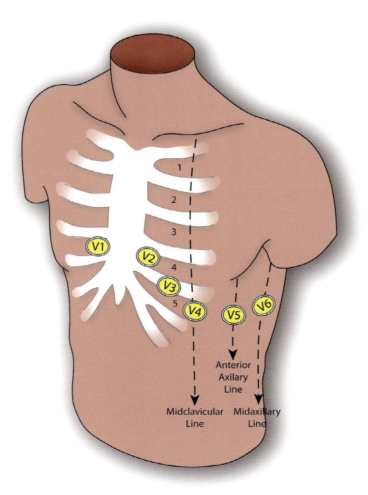

EKG COMPLEX & STANDARD EKG RECORDING PAPER

The figure below shows a blowup of a single EKG complex. The P-wave represents atrial contraction, the QRS results from ventricular contraction, and the T-wave is from ventricular repolarization (time for the heart to reset for the next heartbeat).

A 25 mm/sec imprint on the tracing indicates that the EKG paper is running at normal speed. At this speed, 1 small box represents 0.040 sec (40 msec), and 1 large box (5 small boxes) represents 0.20 sec (200 msec).

A 10 mm/mV imprint on the tracing indicates that the technician correctly ran the EKG at "full-standard." Full-standard results in the height of 1 large box equal to 5 mm, and 2 large boxes equals 10mm or 1 mV. Beware of EKGs that technicians perform at ½ standard. A 5 mm/mV imprint is present on a ½ standard EKG. In most settings, technicians should perform EKGs at full-standard settings.

In the figure below, we also indicate the beginning and ending measurement points for the PR, QRS, and QT intervals.

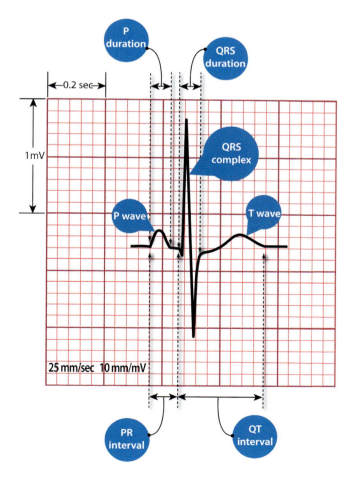

21 Electrocardiogram

4 STEPS

Before interpreting any EKG, first check the patient's age. Then check if the technician performed the EKG at a paper speed of 25 mm/sec and at full standard or 10 mm/mV, by noting that the machine imprinted these values on the strips. The 4 steps:

1 - Determine Heart Rate & Rhythm

2 - Measure PR, QRS, QT Intervals & Inspect ST-T Waves

3 - Check Frontal P-Wave Axis & QRS Axis

4 - Evaluate for RVH or LVH

STEP 1

Determine the Heart Rate & Rhythm

Heart Rate

Using lead II or the lead with the least artifact, calculate the approximate heart rate by counting the large boxes between 2 QRSs and divide into 300 (figure below left).

Rhythm

Ultimately, the rhythm is either normal sinus or not. Normal sinus rhythm variations are common including "sinus arrhythmia" (a misnomer and not a pathological arrhythmia), sinus bradycardia, and sinus tachycardia. All nonsinus rhythms require pediatric cardiology arrhythmia analysis. Leads aVR, aVL, aVF stand for "augmented vector" right (R), left (L) and foot (F). (figure below right)

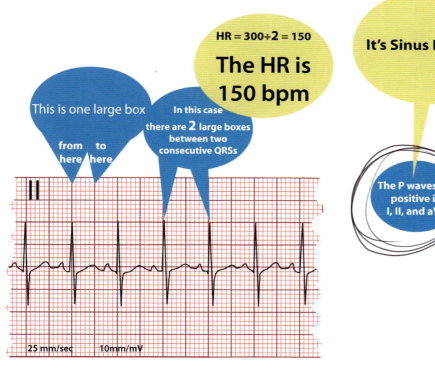
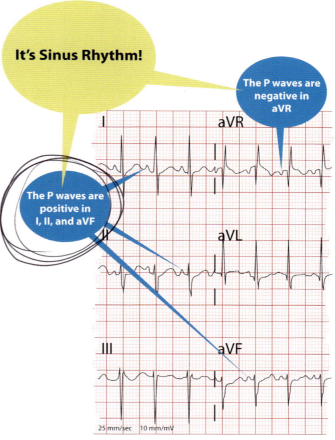

21 Electrocardiogram

Sinus rhythm variations

Sinus arrhythmia

Sinus arrhythmia (figure below) is more noticeable in young children as compared to infants or older children.

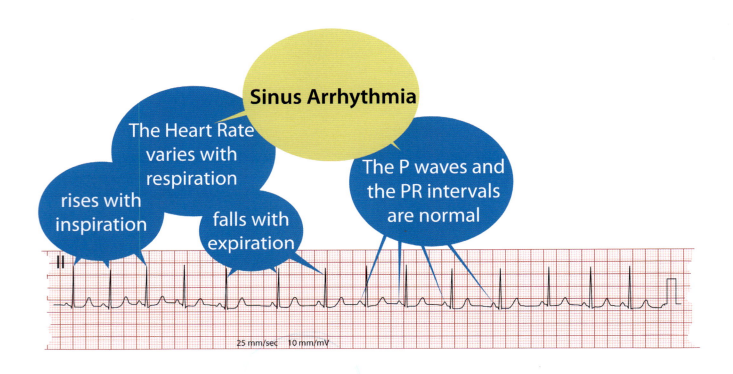

Sinus bradycardia

Sinus bradycardia (figure on the top of the facing page) is common in aerobically trained individuals. Sinus bradycardia may also be from hypothyroidism or long QT syndrome.

Sinus Tachycardia

Sinus tachycardia (figure on the bottom of the facing page) commonly results from pain, anxiety, crying, anemia, hyperthyroidism, congestive heart failure, and others.

21 Electrocardiogram

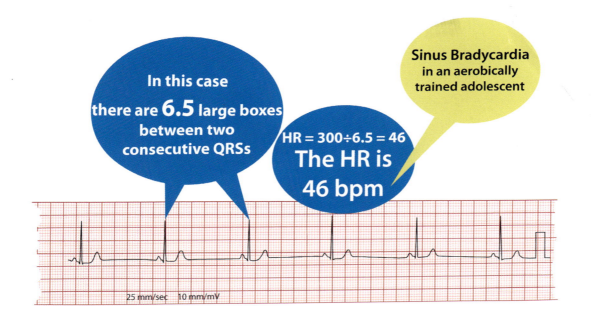

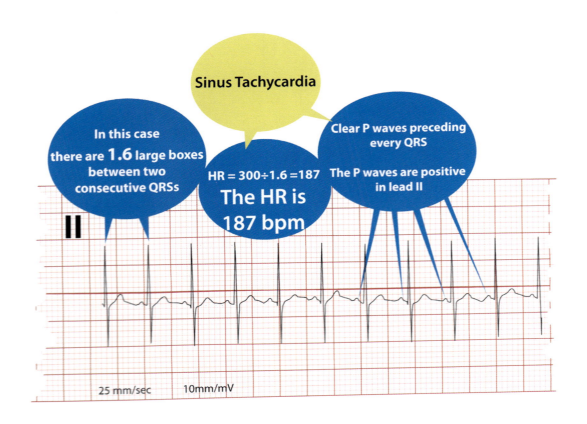

Common nonsinus rhythms

Low atrial rhythm

With a low atrial rhythm (figure below), the intrinsic cardiac pacemaker is in the low right atrium or in the left atrium. Contrary to normal sinus rhythm, the P-wave is negative in lead I, II, and aVF, but positive in aVR.

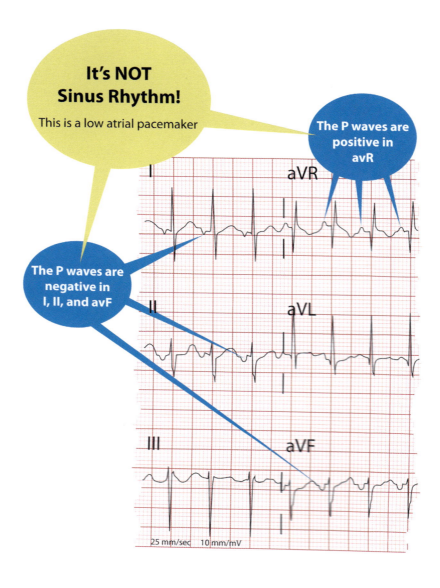

Nonsinus tachycardia

Supraventricular tachycardia

A narrow-QRS tachycardia, with P-waves or without, is usually SVT (figure top right).

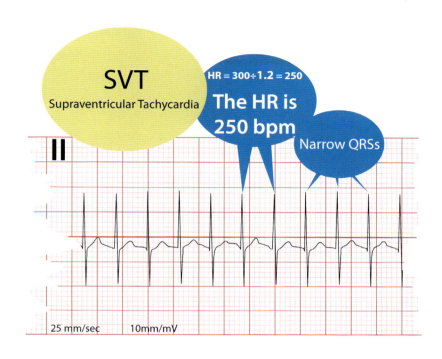

Ventricular tachycardia

A wide-QRS tachycardia is usually ventricular tachycardia (VT) (figure bottom right)

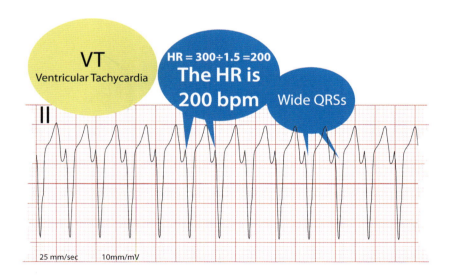

21 Electrocardiogram

Nonsinus bradycardia

If a QRS does not follow a P-wave or PR intervals are inconsistent, then atrioventricular (AV) block is often the cause. For our simplified method, recognizing AV block is more important than specifying the degree of block.

Nevertheless, figure A on the right shows 2nd-degree AV block with a progressive lengthening of the PR interval before a dropped QRS or Mobitz type I, also called Wenckebach rhythm. Figure B below shows Mobitz type II 2nd-degree AV block, and figure C below right shows 3rd-degree AV block.

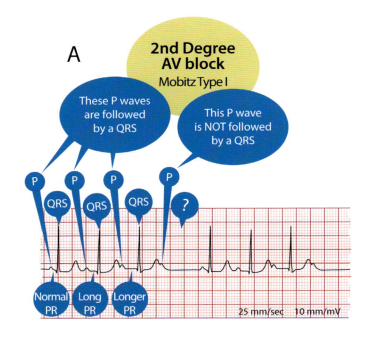

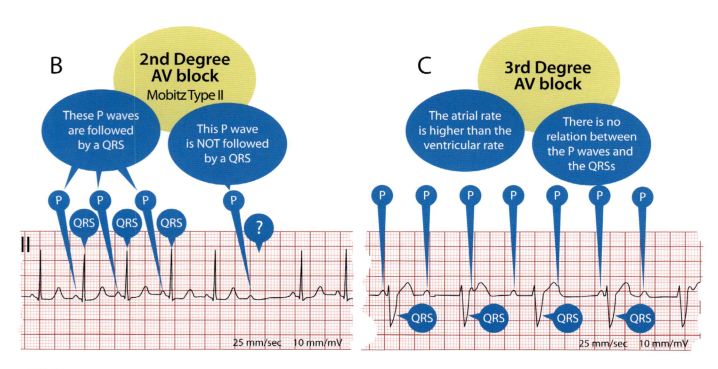

Ectopics

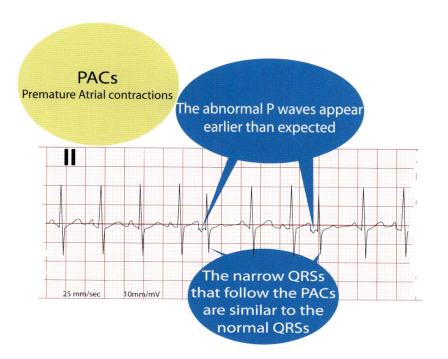

PACs

Infrequent or frequent narrow-QRS ectopics are usually premature atrial contractions (PACs). (figure top right).

PVCs

Infrequent or frequent wide-QRS ectopics are usually premature ventricular contractions (PVCs). (figure bottom right).

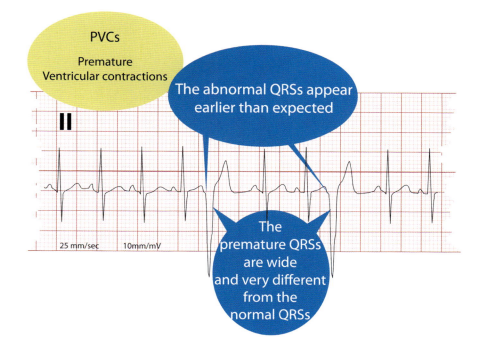

Mechanical pacemaker

Sharp, narrow pacemaker spikes appear before P-waves or the QRS or both. When a pacemaker spike occurs in front of a QRS, a wide complex follows (figure below).

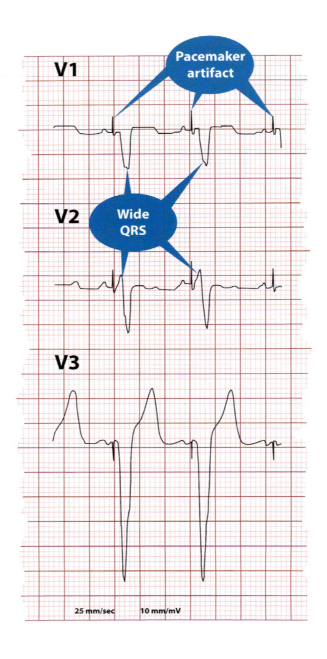

STEP 2

Measure the PR, QRS, QT Intervals & Inspect ST-T Waves

Using lead II or the lead with the least artifact, inspect the PR, QRS, and QT intervals. Interval measurements may appear in sec or msec. For example, PR intervals are often in sec and QT intervals in msec. We include both values.

PR interval

The PR interval can be normal (figure A), long, or short.
- In infants and young children, normal is < 0.16 sec, or 160 msec, or < 4 small boxes. Long (figure B)
- In older children and adolescents, normal is < 0.2 sec, or < 200 msec, or < 1 big box. Long (figure C)

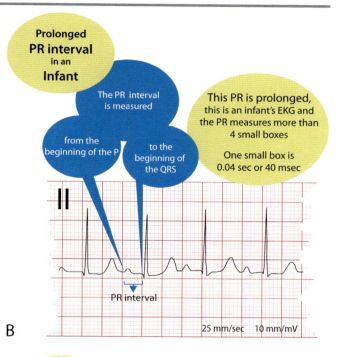

B

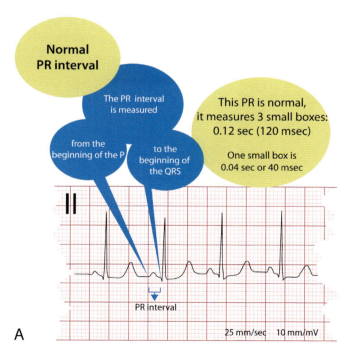

A

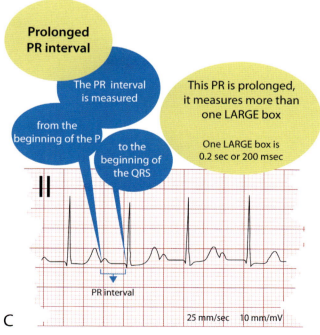

C

Short PR interval

A short PR can be normal when the P-wave adjoins a narrow QRS, or a short PR may be consistent with preexcitation or Wolff-Parkinson-White (WPW) syndrome when the QRS base is wide (figure on the right).

➤WPW's widened QRS is from a characteristic upstroke or downstroke (depending on the lead) forming a "delta wave." The "delta wave" term originates from the Δ shape the upstroke or downstroke makes with the vertical part of the QRS. The figure on the right demonstrates both upstrokes and down strokes. The EKG appearance of preexcitation arises from early ventricular excitation via congenital bypass tracts, as the figure below shows. Preexcitation occurs with SVT and on rare occasion sudden death. For more information, see Chapter 4.

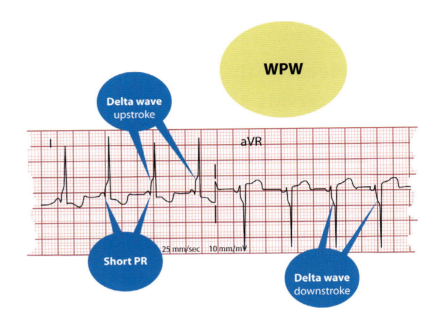

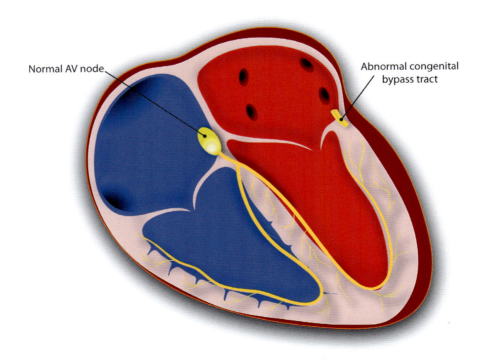

QRS interval

The QRS can be normal (figure left below) or wide (figure right below).

Normal

The normal QRS is about 1 small box wide (0.04 sec or 40 msec).

Wide

A wide QRS is 2 small boxes or more (≥ .08 sec or ≥ 80 msec). A wide QRS occurs in PVCs, bundle branch blocks, WPW, ventricular rhythm, hyperkalemia, hypercalcemia, or with a pacemaker.

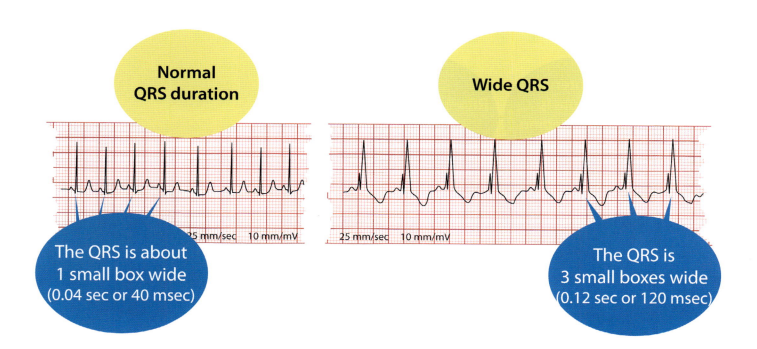

STEP 3

Check Frontal P-Wave Axis & QRS Axis

Simply use aVF to evaluate the P-wave and QRS axis. Determining the degrees of axis usually adds little information to an EKG's interpretation. The P-wave in aVF may be positive (figure below left) or negative (figure below right), while the QRS direction may be positive, negative, or biphasic.

P-wave axis

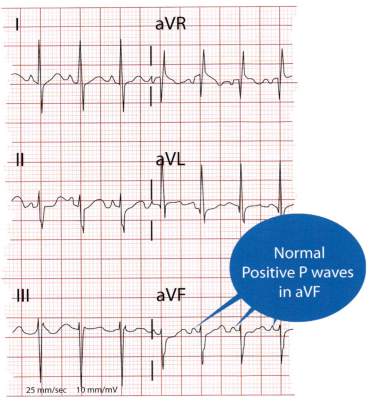
Normal Positive P waves in aVF

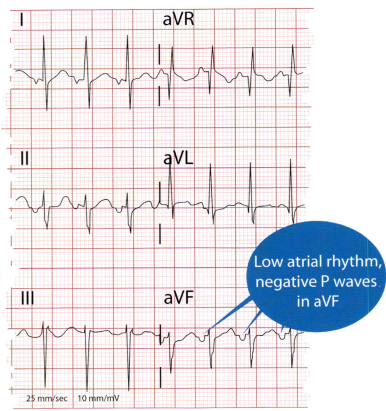
Low atrial rhythm, negative P waves in aVF

Rule 2

RSR′ in V1, if the R′ (2nd R-wave) is taller than the 1st R (figure below left).

Rule 3

Pure R-wave in V1 after about 6 months old (figure below right).

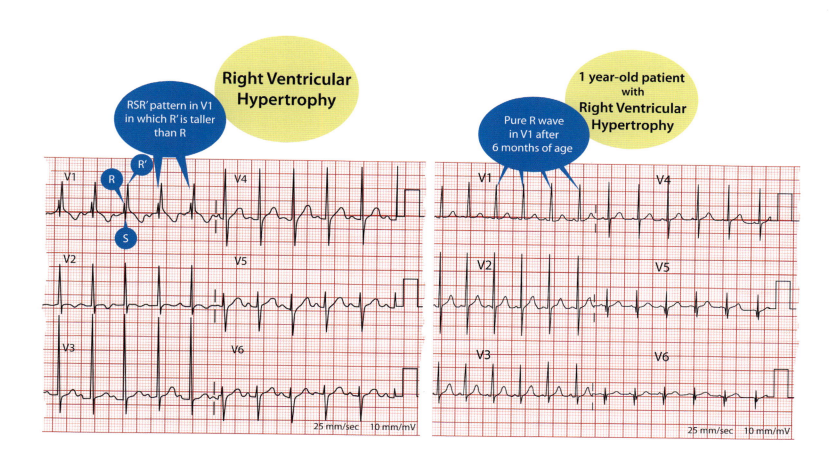

21 Electrocardiogram

Left ventricular hypertrophy

Simply use lead V6 to determine LVH. The EKG machine's computer interpretation is frequently incorrect for LVH, as the computer algorithms use the midprecordial leads. In children with thin chest walls, the midprecordial leads may be unreliable. The 4-step method uses just 1 rule for LVH:

Rule 1

LVH is present when the R-wave of V6 intersects the baseline of V5, in a full-standard, 4-channel EKG recording (figure below).

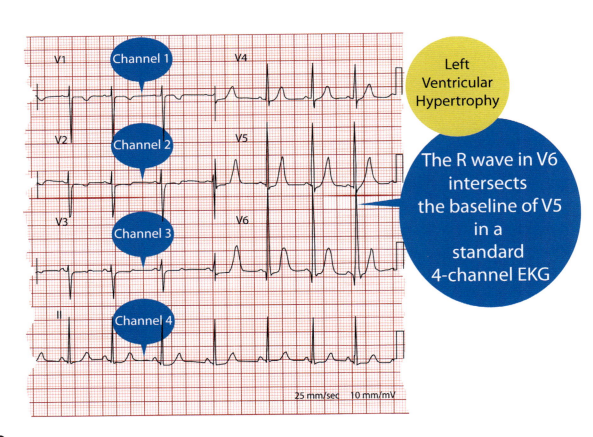

References

1 Evans WN, Acherman RJ, Mayman GA, Rollins RC, Kip KT. Simplified pediatric electrocardiogram interpretation. Clin Pediatr (Phila) 2010; 49: 363-372

2 Grier JW. eHeart: an introduction of ECG/EKG http://www.ndsu.edu/instruct/grier/eheart.html

3 Cardiology Department, Sunrise Hospital and Medical Center, Las Vegas, NV

4 Einthoven, W. The different forms of the human electrocardiogram and their signification. Lancet 1912; 1: 853-861

5 Goodacre S, McLeod K. Clinical review: ABC of clinical electrocardiography, paediatric electrocardiography. BMJ 2002; 324: 1382-1385

6 Chiu CC, Hamilton RM, Gow RM, Kirsh JA, McCrindle BW. Evaluation of computerized interpretation of the pediatric electrocardiogram. J Electrocardiol 2007; 40: 139-143

21 Electrocardiogram

22 Echocardiogram

Contents

Background	351
Transthoracic	352
Other Methods	365

22 Echocardiogram

carlos luna

BACKGROUND

Echocardiography (Echo) is the primary method for noninvasive cardiovascular imaging. Ultrasound originated in 1880 with 2 French scientists, Pierre Curie (spouse of Marie—famous for radium), and his brother Jacques. Together, the Curie brothers discovered the piezoelectric effect. The piezoelectric effect is a physical property found in certain naturally occurring crystals. These crystals emanate a minute electrical current when one physically deforms them. Further, when investigators applied electrical currents to piezoelectric crystals the crystals deformed. Researchers also found that, upon applying a repetitive electrical current, the crystals vibrated like a tuning fork. Vibrating piezoelectric crystals create "ultrasound" (sound inaudible to the human ear).

In 1954, Swedish doctor Inge Edler and a University of Lund physics student Carl Hellmuth Hertz were the first to employ reflective ultrasound for human, noninvasive cardiovascular evaluation. Edler and Hertz developed a machine, based on submarine sonar technology that sent high-frequency sound waves through a patient's chest. The equipment captured the reflected sound (or echo) from cardiovascular structures, generating an image. Edler and Hertz named their first ultrasound recordings "ultrasonic cardiograms or UCGs." These recordings, made on photographic paper, were similar to current M-mode (or motion-mode) recordings.

Our 21st-century echocardiogram machines stem from the 19th-century discovery of the piezoelectric principal, and current machines conform to the mid 20th-century foundations laid by Edler and Hertz.

Current image quality depends on the transducer's sound wave frequency in megahertz (MHz), and how fast the echocardiographic machine delivers the pulses (pulse repetition frequency). High frequencies (8 to 12 MHz) have better resolution, but the sound waves do not penetrate the chest far. However, lower frequencies (3 to 8 MHz) have more penetrance but less resolution. The transducer frequencies for pediatric echocardiography range from 3 to 12 MHz. Low frequencies are more effective in older children and adolescents, and higher frequencies are better for neonates and infants. [1-3]

Current Echo modalities include: (1) M-mode, which produces an icepick view of heart structures that we now use for structure dimensions and systolic ventricular function evaluation; (2) 2-D, which uses a "fan" of ultrasound energy to produce 2-dimensional cardiac images via several echocardiographic windows and views; and (3) 3-D, which renders 3-dimensional images of the heart. Although 3-D is still in a development phase, this modality may become the standard echocardiographic imagining modality in the future.

TRANSTHORACIC ECHO WINDOWS & VIEWS

We perform Echo imaging of the heart vial "ultrasound windows." Ultrasound windows allow the passage of ultrasound energy through the chest wall to "view" the heart. The chest figure on the facing page demonstrates, with the dotted black and solid white lines, the position of the Echo transducer for resolving the 6 primary cardiac ultrasound views: (1) Parasternal long axis, (2) Parasternal short axis at the level of the aortic valve, (3) Parasternal short axis a the level of the mitral valve, (4) Apical, (5) Subcostal, and (6) Suprasternal.

The following pages describe and illustrate each ultrasound view of the heart. In the figures that follow, each has 3 renderings: (1) A 3-D illustration of the heart showing a representation of the transducer and the alignment of its "fan" of ultrasound energy "cutting" the heart, (2) A labeled sketch of the anatomical findings resolved by a particular view, and (3) An actual Echo image. Experienced pediatric echocardiographers may employ several variations to the basic views. For those who wish additional information about other Echo views and findings, please consult reference 1 or other textbooks of echocardiography.

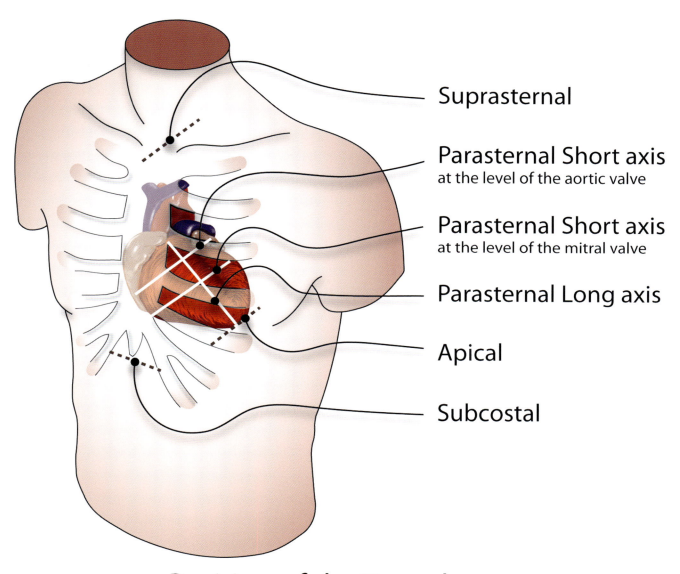

Position of the Transducer
for the Echocardiographic Views

Parasternal Long Axis View

Figure A on facing page shows the parasternal long axis view. This view images the heart in a plane cutting the heart in its long axis, from the apex of the ventricles to the roof of the atria. This view can define the anatomy and relationships of the mitral valve (MV), aortic valve, the ventricular septum, and the right and left ventricles.

Parasternal Short Axis View at the Mitral Valve

Figure B on the facing page shows the parasternal short axis view at the mitral valve (MV). This view produces a transverse imaging cut of the heart. The view further defines the anatomy of the mitral valve and the size relationship between the right and left ventricles.

22 Echocardiogram

Parasternal Long Axis View

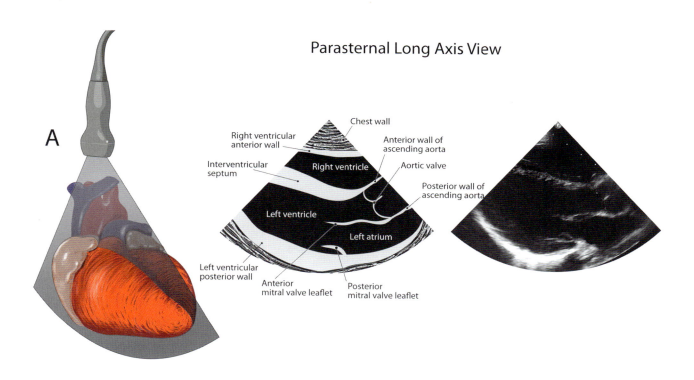

Parasternal Short Axis View
at the level of the mitral valve

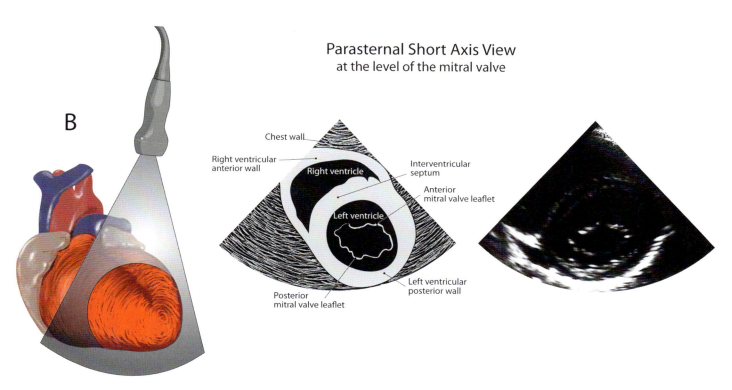

Parasternal Short Axis at the Aortic Valve

Figure A on the facing page shows the parasternal short axis view at the aortic valve. This view produces a transverse imaging cut of the heart. This view allows imaging of the aortic valve leaflets, especially important to rule out bicuspid aortic valve. A normal aortic valve is trileaflet and produces an image similar to a Mercedes-Benz logo. This view also allows further evaluation of the right ventricle and the relationship between the right and left atria.

Apical 4-Chamber View

Figure B on the facing page shows the apical 4-chamber view. This view simultaneously displays both atria and both ventricles. Imaging in this view allows evaluation of the size and function of the right and left ventricles, the relative sizes of the right and left atria, and the positions and appearance of the tricuspid and mitral valves. This view is also excellent for evaluating pericardial effusions.

22 Echocardiogram

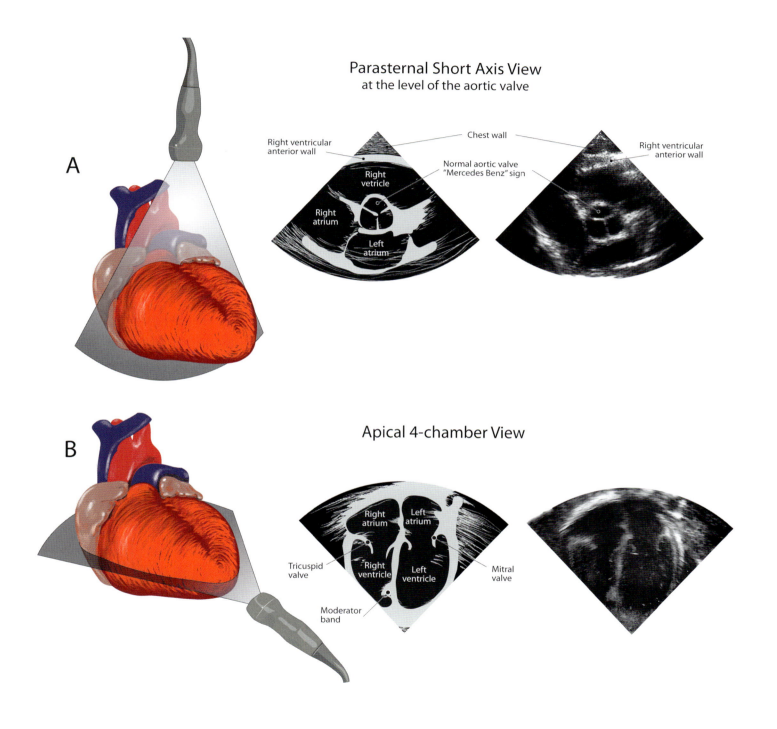

Subcostal View

Figure A on the facing page shows the subcostal view. This view allows a comprehensive evaluation of cardiovascular anatomy including cardiac position, venous return, atrioventricular and ventriculoarterial connections. The view is especially good for determining the presence and size of atrial septal defects.

Suprasternal View

Figure B on the facing page shows the suprasternal view. This view allows evaluation of the aortic arch, superior vena cava, and cross-section of the right pulmonary artery. The suprasternal view helps rule in or rule out a coarctation of the aorta.

22 Echocardiogram

Subcostal View of the Atria

Suprasternal Aortic Arch View

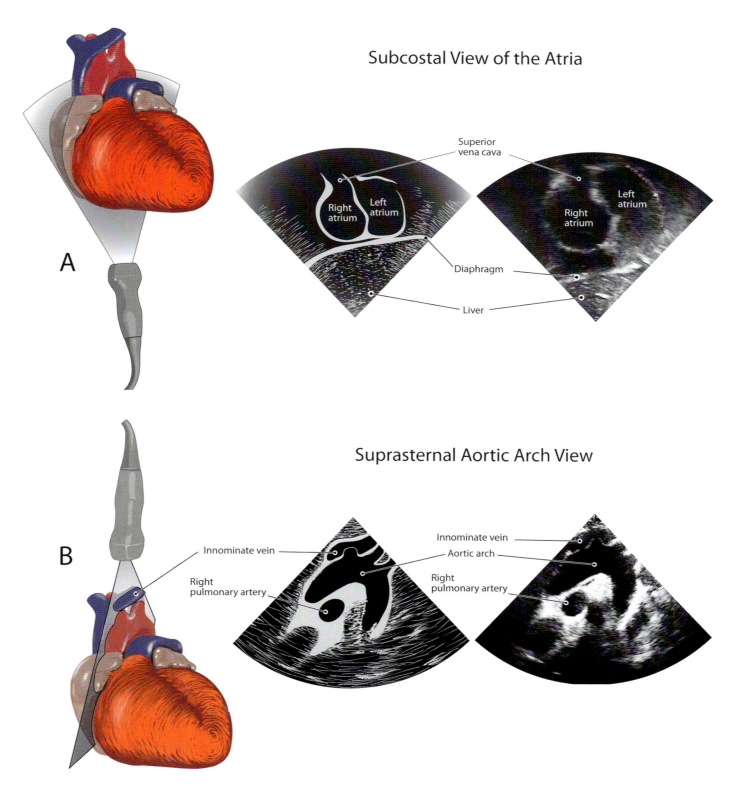

22 Echocardiogram

Echo Imaging

Anatomy

Comprehensive cardiovascular imaging requires a stepwise segmental approach that includes evaluating visceral situs; atrioventricular and ventriculoarterial connections; systemic and pulmonary venous return; aortic arch and neck vessels; pulmonary arteries; integrity of atrial and ventricular septums; the presence of a ductus arteriosus; and abnormal aortopulmonary connections

Thorough evaluation requires multiple echocardiographic views. In complex cases, the subcostal views may provide the best look at anatomical details. Parasternal, apical, and suprasternal views complete the echocardiographic evaluation. Sometimes we use non-conventional views with abnormal positioning of the heart or other complex cardiovascular malformations.

LV Ventricular systolic function

Qualitative assessment

With experience, a clinician can qualitatively assess ventricular function as normal, mildly, moderately, or severely reduced. Controlled studies show strong correlation between qualitative and quantitative assessment. Decreased ventricular function can be global or isolated to a ventricular wall or ventricular segment.

Quantitative assessment

Left ventricular shortening fraction (SF) and ejection fraction (EF) are the indices we commonly use in clinical practice for assessing cardiac contractility. These indexes are easy to obtain but are preload and afterload dependent.

Left ventricular SF

Using an M-mode long-axis view of the left ventricle

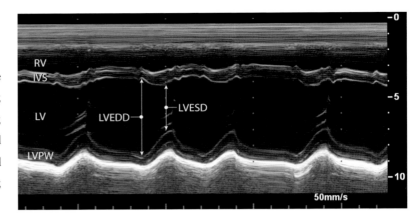

(figure above), we can measure the LVEDD (left ventricle end-diastolic dimension) and LVESD (left ventricle end-systolic dimension). The figure also displays the right ventricle (RV), interventricular septum (IVS); the left ventricle (LV) left ventricular posterior wall (LVPW).

Shortening fraction (SF) formula below:

$$SF = [(LVEDD - LVESD) \div LVEDD] \times 100$$

SF values expressed as %
- Normal   29% - 40%
- Abnormal   < 29%
- Hypercontractile > 40%
- Abnormal septal motion prevents SF calculation

Left ventricular EF

Using 2-D echo images of the left ventricle frozen in end-systole and end-diastole, the Echo machine calculates LVEDV (left ventricular end-diastolic volume) and LVESV (left ventricular end-systolic volume).

Formula for ejection fraction (EF) follows:

$$EF = [(LVEDV - LVESV) \div LVESV] \times 100$$

EF Values expressed as %
- Normal ≥ 60%

Right ventricle assessment
Right ventricular diastolic area index

The right ventricle dilates from volume loading, predominantly via atrial level left-to-right shunts or pulmonary valve and tricuspid valve regurgitation. The decision to treat abnormal RV volume overload rests partly on serial measurements of RV size and function. Because the RV geometry is tricky, quantitative RV volume methods are time-consuming and include angiography, cardiac magnetic resonance imaging (MRI), radionuclide ventriculography, and 3-dimensional echocardiography. Our group reported a simplified approach to assessing RV size semiquantitatively [4]. In a small patient sample, we found the right ventricular diastolic area index (RVDAI) correlated with MRI RV diastolic volumes (RVEDV). For the RVDAI, we obtain area measurements from frozen 2-D Echo images that show the largest diastolic excursions. We obtain right ventricular end-diastolic dimension (RVEDD) and LVEDD from M-mode measurements. Formula below:

$$RVDAI = [(RVDA\ cm^2\ parasternal\ short\ axis + RVDA\ cm^2\ apical\ view) \div 2] \div BSA \times [(RVEDD \div LVEDD)^3]$$

RVDAI values expressed as a unitless index

As the RVDAI is a new method for evaluating the RV morphometrics, current values come from our preliminary studies. However, from our study, we found the following RVDAI values for patients with BSAs ≥ 0.5 m²:

- Normal   ≤ 1
- Mild to moderate RV dilation   1-5
- Moderate to severe RV dilation   5-10
- Severe RV dilation   > 10

Echo Doppler

Christian Doppler (1803-1853) was a professor of mathematics and physics in Prague and Vienna. He discovered the frequency of waves (water, sound, or light) increase or decrease depending on whether the waves move towards or away from an observer (the Doppler effect). The best example is a rapidly moving train blowing its whistle. The whistle's sound pitch rises (increasing frequency) as the train speeds toward the observer; the sound pitch falls (decreasing frequency) as the train speeds away. [5]

Ultrasound equipment uses the Doppler effect to evaluate blood flow, moving toward or away from the ultrasound transducer. Reflective ultrasound demonstrates anatomy and Doppler ultrasound provides physiological information based on moving blood or moving cardiac structures. Doppler ultrasound modalities are color flow, spectral, and tissue Doppler.

Doppler modalities
Color flow Doppler

By convention, color Doppler usually displays flow velocities as spectrums of red or blue. Echo machines display flow moving towards the transducer in red, and flow moving away from the transducer in blue. Zones of turbulence show a speckled or mosaic pattern of different colors. Color Doppler provides a qualitative appraisal of blood flow velocity. Color Doppler can detect intracavitary, outflow, or vessel obstruction; intracardiac or extracardiac communications including ASDs, VSDs, or

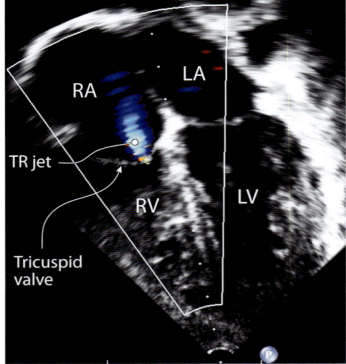

Tricuspid Valve Regurgitation
4-chamber view

PDAs; and valvular stenosis or regurgitation (tricuspid regurgitation jet or TR jet noted in figure above). However, color Doppler cannot provide precise velocity information. Nevertheless, color Doppler provides positional guidance for pulsed and continuous-wave spectral Doppler interrogation.

Spectral Doppler

There are 2 spectral Doppler modalities: (1) Pulsed Doppler (PD), and (2) Continuous-wave Doppler (CWD). We use PD for evaluating blood flow velocity at a specific point within the heart or a vessel. PD is suitable for measuring lower velocity flows. However, CWD is the best method for high flow velocities. Echo machines display spectral Doppler flow in cm/sec or m/sec. Echo machines display flow on the monitor above or below a reference baseline.

The figure on the top left of the facing page shows a continuous-wave recording across a stenotic pulmonary valve. By convention, flows toward the transducer are above the baseline and flows away from the transducer are below the baseline. Using calipers, we can measure the peak blood flow velocity across a stenotic valve. In the case on the top left facing page, the peak velocity value is 5 m/sec. In addition, information from spectral Doppler flow tracings includes peak flow velocity, mean flow velocity, and velocity time integrals (VTI).

Evaluation of pressure gradients

Normal blood flow is laminar (turbulence free). When blood flows from a high to low pressure zone, blood flow velocities increase causing turbulence. Blood flow acceleration may occur at the stenotic or insufficient valve; across a vessel obstruction or narrowing; across an atrial or ventricular septal defect; or across a patent ductus arteriosus. We use a simplified Bernoulli equation to measure gradients. Formula below:

$$\text{Peak gradient in mm Hg} = (PFV\ m/sec)^2 \times 4$$

➤PFV = the peak flow velocity. The Echo machine's computer can also determine a mean pressure gradient from the tracing of the transvalvular Doppler flow signal.

From the example in the figure on the facing page above left, the pulmonary valve gradient is 100 mm Hg or $(5\ m/sec)^2 \times 4 = 100$.

Pressure gradient applications

- Valvular stenosis or vessel obstruction
- RV systolic pressure from tricuspid regurgitation
- PA systolic pressure from RV systolic pressure values

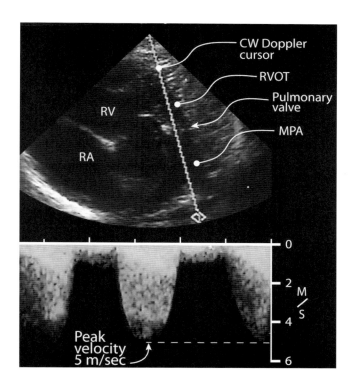

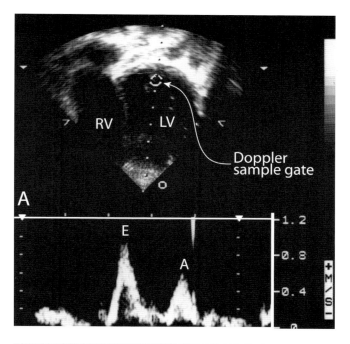

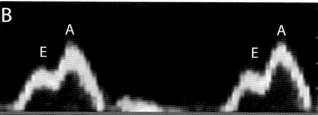

Diastolic function

Evaluation of flow pattern across the mitral or tricuspid valves provides information about diastolic function. As most of the ventricular filling normally occurs in early diastole, the mitral or tricuspid Doppler inflow tracing shows a higher E-wave than A-wave (figure A above on the right). Abnormal relaxation delays ventricular filling until later in diastole, decreasing the flow velocity of early ventricular filling making the E-wave smaller than the A-wave (figure B above on the right). With progression of diastolic dysfunction, the increased filling pressure augments the flow velocity of the E-wave, causing pseudonormalization of the Doppler tracing where the E-wave is again higher than the A-wave. With severe diastolic dysfunction (restrictive phase) the E-wave becomes much higher than the A-wave. Doppler examination of pulmonary vein flow in patients with pseudonormal or restrictive diastolic dysfunction shows abnormally increased retrograde flow during atrial systole.

Estimation of flow

We can calculate a cardiac output by measuring the flow across the aortic valve and measuring the diameter of the aortic valve annulus. The LV stroke volume equation requires the aortic valve cross-sectional area and the VTI of the aortic Doppler flow signal. Cardiac output is stroke volume times heart rate. The formulas for LV stroke volume

22 Echocardiogram

and cardiac output is below:

> **LV stroke volume (SV) in cm³ = cross-sectional area of the aortic valve in cm² × the VTI of the aortic flow tracing**
>
> **Cardiac output in L/min = SV × heart rate in bpm ÷ 1,000**

Myocardial performance index (MPI)

MPI can evaluate systolic and diastolic function. We obtain a pulsed Doppler recording from the inlet and outlet of the left ventricle, displaying transmitral and left ventricular outflow tract flows. With systolic or diastolic dysfunction the isovolumetric systolic or diastolic times increase, rendering an increase in the MPI

Tissue Doppler

Tissue Doppler (figure above right) measures velocity of myocardial motion. We can display tissue Doppler information as a color map (similar to color flow Doppler) or as a spectral signal for quantitative analysis. We usually obtain the sample from the tricuspid and mitral annulus or the myocardium immediately below. Doppler tissue allows measurement of indices of systolic and diastolic motion or function. References provide normative values for peak systolic velocity (S′) and peak diastolic velocities (E′ and A′). Diastolic dysfunction makes the E′-wave smaller than the A′-wave. We can also use tissue Doppler to estimate ventricular end-diastolic pressures and to measure a MPI.

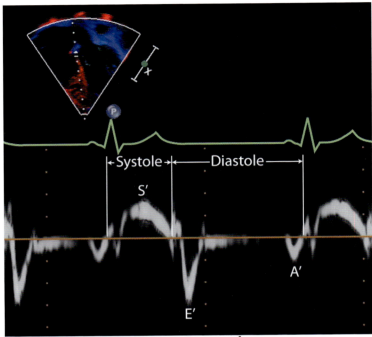

Tissue Doppler

OTHER ECHO METHODS

Transesophageal Echocardiography (TEE)

TEE utilizes a transducer similar to an endoscope. Under sedation or anesthesia, we pass the probe down the esophagus and into the stomach for echocardiographic images. Transthoracic echocardiography (TTE) images the heart from the front, and TEE images the heart from behind. Without lung interference, TEE renders excellent images. Similar to TTE, we can obtain color and spectral Doppler information with TEE. TEE probes with capability of 3-D echo are also available. Contrary to 3-D TTE Echo, we use 3-D TEE routinely in the cardiac catheterization laboratory and operating room.

We obtain TEE images through probe (transducer) manipulation that includes advancing, withdrawing, rotating, and flexing the probe head. Current TEE probes acquire images from a continuum of different planes, within a 180° range (omniplane probe).

Indications
- For poor transthoracic widows
- For pre-op, intra-op, & post-cardiac surgery evaluation
- For guidance during interventional catheterization

Contraindications
- For neonates < 3 kg, standard pediatric probe too large
- Esophageal atresia
- Recent esophageal surgery or constriction.

Complications
- Airway & ventilation compromise
- Hypotension from probe compression
- Lacerations & bleeding
- Rarely, esophageal or gastric perforation

Intravascular Ultrasound (IVUS)

IVUS uses a specialized vascular catheter with an ultrasound transducer fixed to the tip. IVUS is useful for ultrasound evaluation of vessel interiors like the coronary arteries. Intravascular evaluation includes examination of the vessel's endothelium and the location and characterization of intravascular plaques.

Intracardiac Echocardiography (ICE)

ICE uses a specialized intracardiac catheter equipped with an ultrasound transducer. We introduce the ICE catheter-transducer transvascularly into the heart's chambers. The ICE transducer can provide 2-D images, spectral Doppler, and color flow Doppler information. We use ICE for invasive electrophysiology procedures and interventional cardiac catheterization.

REFERENCES

1 WW Lai, Mertens L, Cohen M, Geva T. Echocardiography in Pediatric and Congenital Heart Disease From Fetus to Adult. Hoboken, Wiley-Blackwell, 2009

2 Acierno LJ. Profiles in Cardiology - Inge Edler: father of echocardiography. Clin Cardiol 2002; 25: 197-199

3 Edler I, Hertz CH. Use of ultrasonic reflectoscope for the continuous recording of movements of heart walls. Kungl Fysiogr Sallsk Lund Forh 1954; 24: 40-46

4 Evans WN, Acherman RJ, Mayman GA, Berthoty DP, Rollins RV, Kip K, Restrepo H. Simple echocardiographic evaluation of right ventricular size in children. Congenital Heart Disease 2009; 4: 91-95

5 Christian Doppler http: //en.wikipedia.org/wiki/Christian_doppler

23 Fetal Echocardiogram

Contents

Background	369
Risk Factor Indications	370
Normal Screening Echo	371
Doppler Growth Restricted	379
Fetal Anemia & Heart Failure	382
Fetal Cardiac Arrhythmias	384

23 Fetal Echocardiogram

ruben acherman • william evans • william castillo

BACKGROUND

Most infants born with serious congenital heart disease undergo rapid evaluation and life-saving treatment. Most fetuses with significant cardiovascular malformations, however, are not diagnosed prenatally. Those not diagnosed prenatally cannot receive state-of-the art, fetal-cardiology evaluation and treatment, a situation tantamount to sending a cyanotic newborn home without the benefit of currently available diagnostic and treatment methods.

Cardiovascular malformations are the most frequent anomalies of human development. Cardiovascular defects occur in about 1 in 100 live births. Among congenital abnormalities tabulated in the United States, cardiovascular malformations are the number one cause of death. Even today, 1 out of 10 infants dying from congenital heart disease do so without diagnosis until autopsy, a sobering fact that universal fetal cardiovascular evaluation could alter. Nonetheless, fetal cardiac evaluations are currently limited to those women who are referred because of risk factors for fetal heart disease (see table on the following page). Most pregnant women undergo only a general obstetric ultrasound which, following the joint recommendations by the American Institute of Ultrasound in Medicine, the American College of Radiology, and the American College of Obstetric and Gynecologists, includes a limited evaluation of the 4 chambers of the heart, and if possible, a view of the outflows. Studies, however, show that the majority of newborns with congenital heart disease are born to women without risk factors.

The first reports on the use of ultrasound to evaluate the fetal heart appeared in the 1960s and 1970s. The work by Kleinman and colleagues, first published in 1980, marked the beginning of modern fetal echocardiography and the birth of fetal cardiology as a new super specialty of pediatric cardiology. Thus, prenatal cardiovascular diagnosis has been possible for over 30 years. With today's clinical knowledge and technical advancements, the prenatal diagnosis of serious congenital heart diseases by fetal echocardiogram approaches 100%. Because of limitations placed on the use of fetal cardiovascular evaluation (expertise and financial), these advancements have not improved the general prenatal detection of serious cardiovascular abnormalities. [1-7]

Risk Factors for Fetal Heart Disease and Current Indications for Fetal Echocardiography

Maternal

Advanced maternal age
Alcohol
Autoimmune diseases
Illicit drugs
Infections
Maternal congenital heart disease
Maternal diabetes
Maternal obesity
Medications
Methylene tetrahydrofolate reductase (MTHFR) gene mutations
Phenylketonuria
Pregnancies of assisted reproductive technology
Suspected fetal cardiac anomaly during obstetric ultrasound

Familial

Congenital heart disease
Nonchromosomal syndromes

Fetal

Abnormal first trimester markers
Cardiac arrhythmias
Chromosomal abnormalities
Extracardiac abnormalities
Hydrops fetalis
Increased nuchal transluscency thickness
Multiple pregnancy
Single umbilical artery

NORMAL SCREENING FETAL ECHOCARDIOGRAM

In our opinion, a screening fetal echocardiogram, as proposed by Yagel and colleagues, should replace the current 4-chamber view strategy [3, 8]. The screening evaluation includes 5 axial slices of the fetal abdomen and chest obtained by sliding the transducer cephalad beginning from the upper abdominal view. We reserve a detailed fetal echocardiogram for patients with risk factors (see table on previous page), and those with clear or suspected abnormalities noted in screening fetal echocardiograms. Experienced specialists should perform the detailed fetal echocardiographic studies.

Upper Abdominal View

The upper abdominal slice (figure A on the right and figures B and C below) evaluates abdominal situs. In usual situs solitus, the stomach (St) is on the left side of the abdomen, the descending aorta (Ao) is to the left of the spine (S), the inferior vena cava (IVC) is anterior and to the right of the aorta, and the umbilical vein (UV) turns towards the right (dashed arrows) into the portal sinus.

When visible, the gallbladder (G) is to right of the umbilical vein.

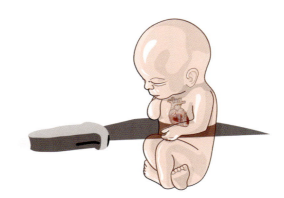

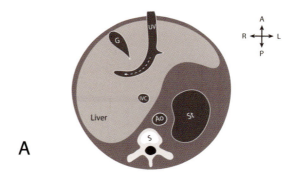

A

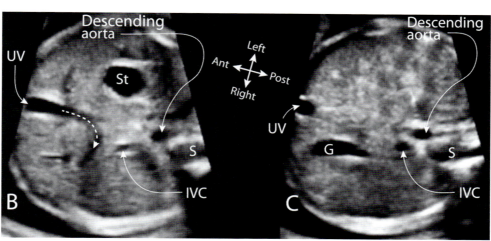

4-Chamber View

The 4-chamber view (figure A below) is obtained from a transverse slice of the fetal chest slightly above the upper abdominal view. Before concentrating on the cardiac chambers, the examiner should pay attention to the position of the heart within the chest, the cardiac axis, cardiac size, and the structures surrounding the heart. For all figures: right atrium (RA); left atrium (LA); right ventricle (RV); left ventricle (LV); descending aorta (Ao); spine (S).

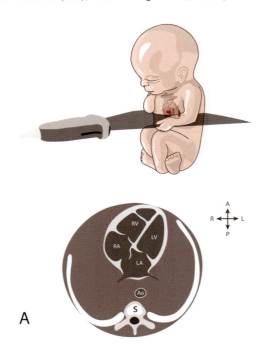

Cardiac position

The heart is normally positioned towards the left chest, and in the 4-chamber view the left lung usually appears slightly smaller than the right (figure A above and figure B on the right). The right ventricular free wall is in contact with the anterior chest wall (arrowheads in figure B). Mass effect on either side of the chest, from diaphragmatic hernias, tumors, or pleural effusions may deviate the heart towards the contralateral chest side. Figure C below shows the heart pushed against the right chest wall (arrows) by abdominal content (AC) herniating into the chest via a diaphragmatic hernia. The descending aorta is deviated to the right of the spine and the stomach (St) is positioned in the right chest and behind the heart. Mass impingement on cardiovascular structures may significantly affect hemodynamics and cause hydrops.

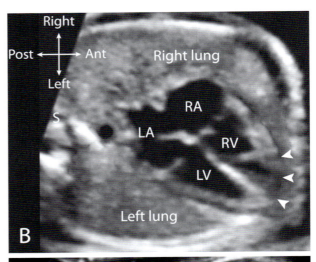

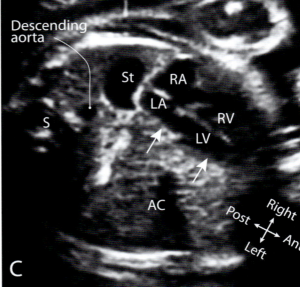

Cardiac axis

Figure A below shows that the normal angle between the ventricular septum (dashed arrows) and the midline of the chest (arrows) is about 45°. Extreme levocardia with angles above 50° (figure B below), and dextrocardia, are associated with increased incidence of congenital heart disease. For example, the fetus in figure B has a complete atrioventricular septal defect.

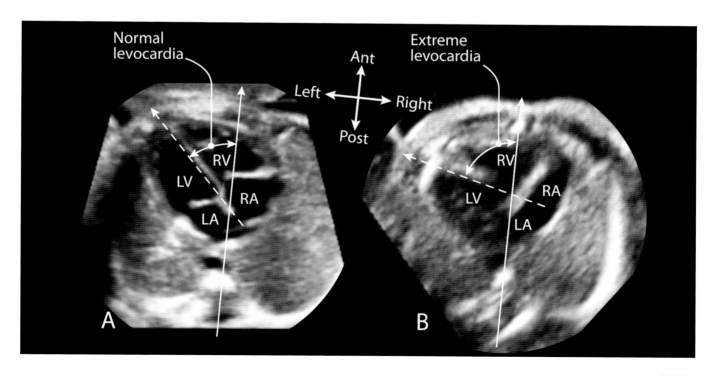

23 Fetal Echocardiogram

Cardiac size

The normal cardiac area is about 1/3 of the chest area. Modern ultrasound equipment software facilitates measurements of cardiac and chest areas that are needed to calculate the cardiac/thoracic (C/T) ratio. Figure A on the right and figures B and C below demonstrate the method of calculating a C/T ratio. A C/T ratio of > 35% indicates cardiomegaly.

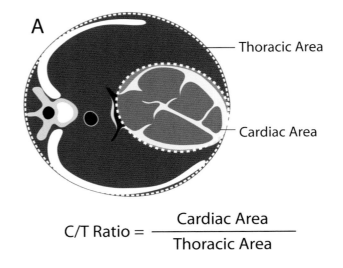

$$C/T\ Ratio = \frac{Cardiac\ Area}{Thoracic\ Area}$$

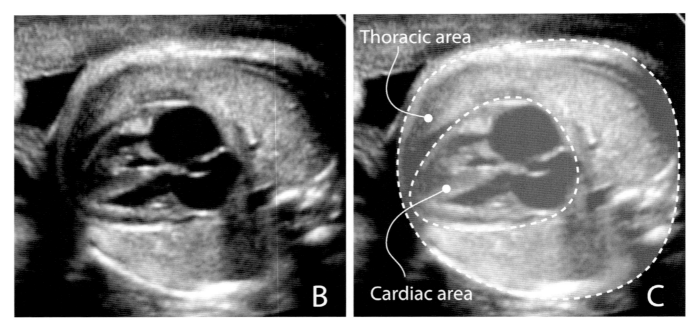

Structures surrounding the heart

As seen in figure A on the right, the descending aorta (DAo) is anterior and to the left of the spine (S), and the left atrium (LA) is anterior to the descending aorta. The echogenicity of the lungs is more or less homogeneous. Areas of significant increased or decreased echogenicity may represent masses. Areas of absent echogenicity suggest the presence within the chest of abdominal viscera, cysts, or effusions.

Cardiac chambers

The 4-chamber view, illustrated in figures A, B, and C, shows the 2 atria (LA, RA), 2 ventricles (LV, RV), the tricuspid (TV) and mitral (MV) valves, and the atrial and ventricular septa. Both atria are about the same size. The atrial septum contains the foramen ovale. The foramen ovale flap normally opens towards the left atrium; the foramen ovale excursion is normally 50% of the left atrial width or less. Exaggerated foramen ovale flap excursion, also known as atrial septal aneurysm or foramen ovale aneurysm, is associated with fetal arrhythmias, congenital

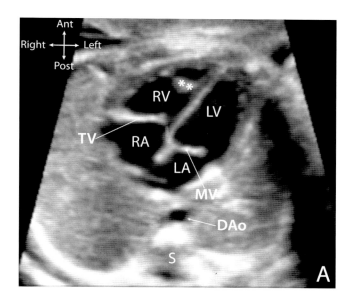

heart diseases, and increased incidence of postnatal atrial septal defects. Both ventricles are about the same size. The right ventricle contains the moderator band (asterisks in figure A above and labeled in figure B below). The normal TV is slightly closer to the apex than the MV. Large ventricular septal defects are seen with 2D imaging, smaller defects are visualized only with the help of color flow Doppler.

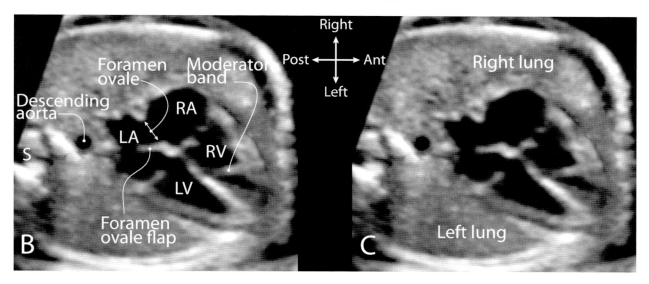

23 Fetal Echocardiogram

Left-Outflow View

Angling cephalad from the 4-chamber view, the aorta appears exiting the left ventricle (LV) (figure A below and figure B on the right). The anterior wall of the aorta is in continuity with the interventricular septum (arrowheads in figure B). The aortic valve is seen opening and closing between the left ventricle and the ascending aorta.

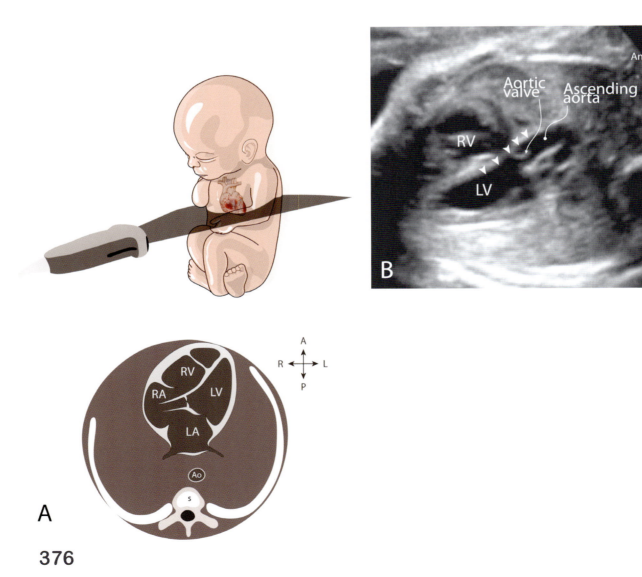

Right-Outflow View

The right ventricular outflow lies immediately cephalad to the left outflow (figure A below and figure B on the right). Usually seen together with the ascending aorta (AAo) and the superior vena cava (SVC) or the upper right atrium (RA). The ascending aorta is immediately to the right of the right outflow and the superior vena cava is just to the right of the ascending aorta. Increased distance between the ascending aorta and the superior vena cava in the 3-vessel view may indicate the presence of a right diaphragmatic hernia [9].

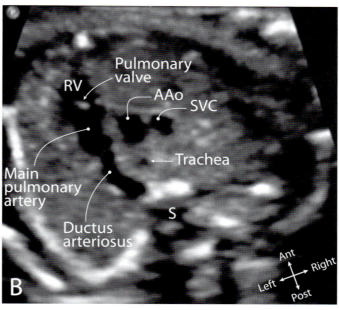

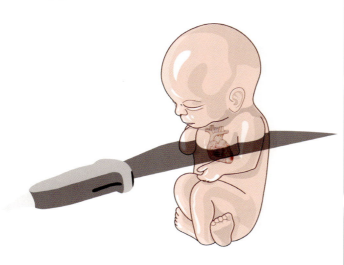

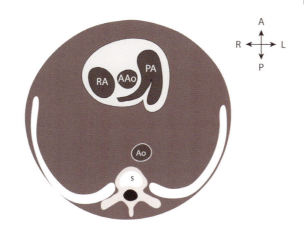

3-Vessel & Trachea View

Slightly cephalad from the right outflow view, we find the 3-vessel and trachea view (figure A below and figure B on the right). This view is ideal to evaluate the size and position of the aortic arch, between the superior vena cava (SVC) and the descending aorta. In cases of right aortic arch, the trachea is to the left of the aortic arch. If there is a vascular ring, then the trachea is between the aortic and ductal arches.

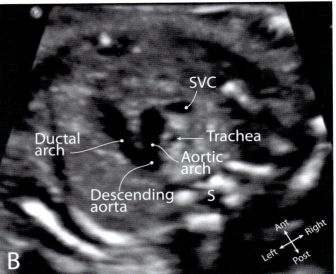

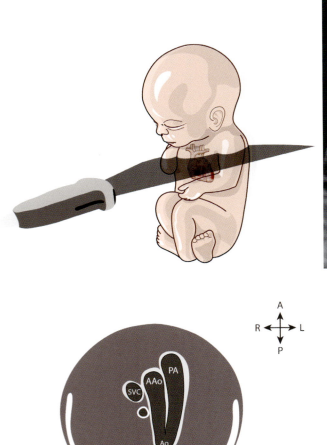

DOPPLER IN THE GROWTH RESTRICTED FETUS

Diagnosis and management of fetal-growth restriction decreases fetal and neonatal morbidity and mortality. Fetal Doppler helps to differentiate a healthy, small for gestational age fetus from a growth-restricted fetus [10]. Umbilical artery, middle cerebral artery, umbilical vein, inferior vena cava, and ductus venosus flow Doppler are useful for monitoring growth-restricted fetuses [11]. In growth-restricted fetuses, arterial Doppler changes occur before those in the venous channels, and venous Doppler changes precede abnormalities on cardiotocography (fetal heart monitoring). In addition, recent studies report fetal aortic isthmus flow changes, fetal cardiac diastolic dysfunction, and elevated fetal B-type natriuretic peptide are associated with poor perinatal outcome in intrauterine growth restriction; however, these latter methods are still under evaluation [12, 13].

Umbilical Artery flow

Figure A below shows normal, forward umbilical arterial flow throughout systole (S) and diastole (arrow heads). The systolic-diastolic ratio (S/D) is normally < 3 in the 3rd trimester. With placental insufficiency and increasing placental resistance, there is decreased, absent, or reversed end diastolic flow in the umbilical arteries, resulting in an

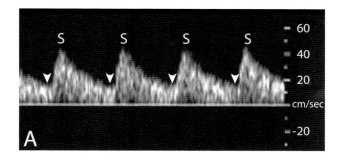

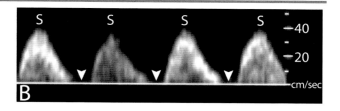

elevated S/D ratio. In figure B above, absent or reversed end diastolic flow is associated with poor perinatal outcome (arrow heads show absent diastolic flow).

Middle Cerebral Artery Flow

Growth restricted fetuses have limited oxygen and nutrient supply, leading the fetal cardiovascular physiology to redistribute flow to vital organs. Doppler evaluation of the middle cerebral artery may detect increased diastolic velocities that indicate decreased cerebral vascular resistance, so-called brain sparing effect. Figures C and D below depict Doppler flow in the middle cerebral arteries; in C, arrowheads show normal diastolic flow. In D, arrowheads indicate abnormally increased diastolic flow. In more severe cases, there is a pseudonormalization of the

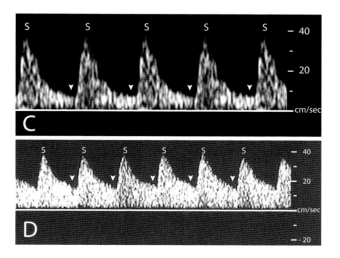

middle cerebral artery Doppler where the diastolic velocity decreases, resembling normal flow. This pseudonormalization occurs because there is inadequate fetal-cardiovascular reserve to maintain favorable redistribution of flow to the brain.

Inferior Vena Cava & Hepatic Veins Flow

The normal inferior vena cava and the hepatic vein Doppler waveforms (figure A below) consist of an initial forward wave during ventricular systole (S), a 2nd forward wave during early diastole (D) that is less prominent that than the forward wave during systole, and a 3rd retrograde wave during atrial contraction (a). Systemic venous Doppler abnormalities may be consequences of deteriorating systemic or placental resistance and increased right atrial pressure. With increased right atrial pressure, there is an increase in the velocity and duration of the retrograde inferior vena cava and hepatic venous flows during atrial contraction (a) (figure B below left)

Ductus Venosus Flow

In figure C below, the normal Doppler profile of the ductus venosus flow consists of 2 peaks of forward flow, the 1st during systole (S), and the 2nd during early diastole (D). A nadir of flow occurs during atrial contraction (a). With increasing venous pressure, the ductus venosus flow velocity, during "a", progressively decreases and even may reverse during more adverse conditions. Figure D below shows the retrograde flow during atrial contraction (a).

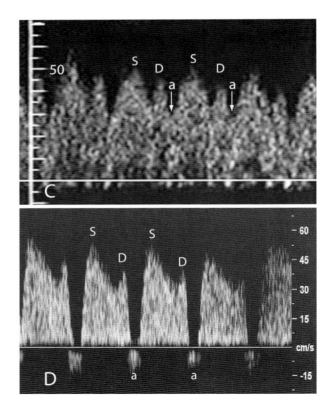

Umbilical Vein Flow

The normal umbilical vein flow is continuous (figure A below). In figure B below, venous pulsations (arrows) in the umbilical vein flow may result from increased venous pressure and from tricuspid valve regurgitation secondary to right ventricular dilatation.

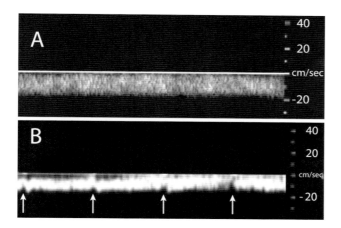

FETAL ANEMIA & HEART FAILURE

Fetal Anemia

Fetal anemia causes increased cardiac output without redistribution of blood flow. The increased cardiac output generates increased venous and arterial flow velocities and cardiomegaly, also leading to pleural effusions (E in the figure below) and thickened chest wall (C in the figure below). Doppler studies show a relationship between flow velocities and fetal hematocrit. The Doppler flow velocities in the fetal aorta and middle cerebral arteries are helpful monitors in the anemic fetus. Monitoring these Doppler flows helps determine when the fetal hemoglobin should be checked by cordocentesis and when to perform intrauterine transfusion. In fetal anemias, serial Doppler evaluations of the middle cerebral artery have led to a > 70% reduction in the number of invasive tests [14, 15].

Fetal Heart Failure

Fetal heart failure may result in fetal hydrops. Figures A and B on the facing page show severe skin edema (asterisks), ascites, and pleural effusion in a hydropic fetus. Hydrops may result in fetal demise. The fetus with effusions and suspected cardiomegaly need, at a minimum, evaluation of the cardiothoracic ratio, color Doppler of the cardiac valves, and spectral Doppler of the umbilical vein, ductus venosus, and umbilical artery. A fetal cardiothoracic ratio ≥ 0.35 constitutes cardiomegaly. Refer to the "Doppler in the Growth Restricted Fetus" section for the normal venous and arterial flow profiles and changes associated with increased resistance and increased venous pressure.

As in postnatal life, fetal heart failure has numerous etiologies including cardiac malformations, anemia, arrhythmia, valvular regurgitation, primary myocardial disease, absence of the ductus venous, and others. Prognosis depends on the cause, response to therapy, and timing of delivery. Valvular regurgitation is easily detected by color Doppler. Figure C on the facing page shows a 4-chamber view; the yellow-green color indicates a tricuspid valve regurgitation jet (TR). Arteriovenous malformations are rare but should be suspected in the fetus with cardiomegaly and effusions of unclear etiology. Color Doppler interrogation of the brain, liver, umbilical vein and placenta helps identify ateriovenous malformations. Figure

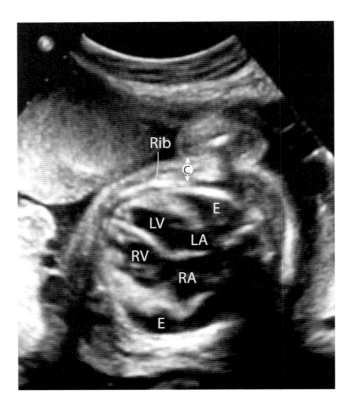

D below shows the fetal head with a vein of Galen malformation (large blue venous lake). Primary myocardial disease, particularly with decreased systolic function, may cause fetal heart failure. Fetal heart failure may also be due to myocarditis or dilated cardiomyopathy. The absence of the ductus venosus may lead to congestive heart failure from volume overload; the overload may be the result of an abnormal direct, unrestricted connection between the umbilical vein and the systemic venous system or the right atrium. However, areas of stenosis within the umbilical venous pathway may mitigate volume overload [16, 17].

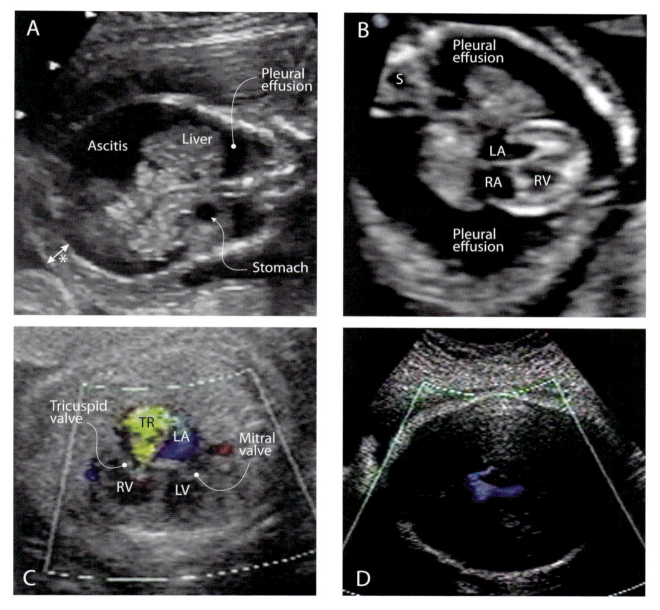

FETAL CARDIAC ARRHYTHMIAS

The evaluation of fetal cardiac rhythm requires all echocardiographic modalities including M-mode, Doppler, and 2-dimensional imaging. Refer to other references for fetal electrocardiography and magnetocardiography, as these techniques are not usually available in most clinical settings.

2-Dimensional Imaging

2-dimensional imaging permits evaluation of the heart size (see cardiothoracic ratio above), systolic function, effusions, cardiac structure, myocardial appearance, and abdominal situs. All these characteristics may affect, or be affected by, cardiac rhythm abnormalities. Examples include bradycardia related to left atrial isomerism [18], cardiac arrhythmias, and long QT syndrome associated with myocardial noncompaction [19, 20], and the association of premature atrial contractions and supraventricular tachycardia with atrial septal aneurysms [21]. The figure below shows the ultrasound guided introduction of a transuterine needle placed into a fetal thigh to deliver digoxin.

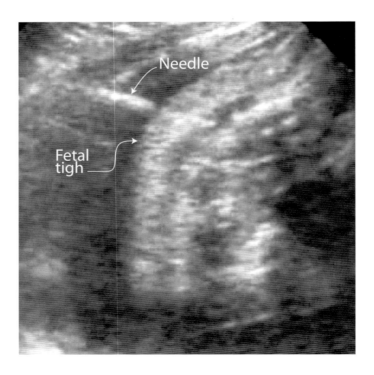

M-Mode Echocardiography

M-mode echocardiography is useful for evaluating cardiac systolic function and for diagnosing an arrhythmia mechanism. The M-mode cursor is placed across the atrial and ventricular walls to display the movement of both chambers. The figure below shows how chamber movements are used to time atrial (a) and ventricular (v) systole. The atrial appendages and lateral ventricular walls are typically areas of maximal wall motion. In the normal example below, the rhythm is regular and the atrial contractions always precede the ventricular contractions at regular intervals.

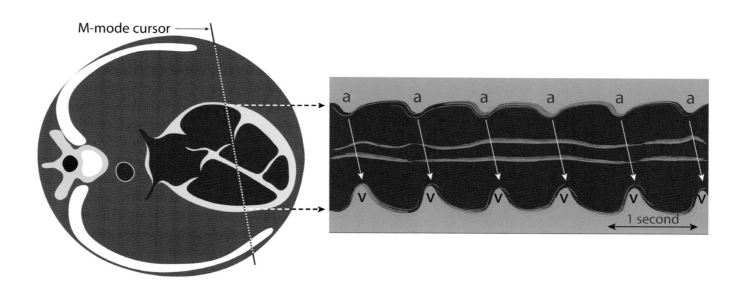

Pulsed Doppler

There are several techniques for recording atrial (a) and ventricular (v) events simultaneously. In the 5-chamber view (figure A on the right), the cursor is placed between the mitral valve (MV) inflow and the left ventricular outflow (indicated by Ao). The MV inflow consists of two waves (E and A). In normal 1:1 atrioventricular conduction, systolic antegrade flow (v) through the subaortic area follows each atrial (a) contraction.

Alternatively, in figure B below, the cursor can be placed to simultaneously record the superior vena cava (SVC) and the ascending aorta Ao; inferior vena cava and abdominal aorta (not shown); or the pulmonary artery branch and pulmonary vein (not shown); or in the pulmonary artery branch and the pulmonary vein (also not shown). The pulsed Doppler sample-volume gate size is adjusted to include both targeted flows.

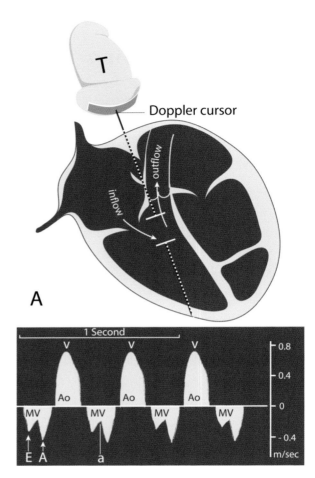

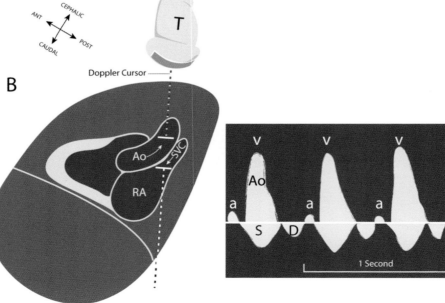

References

1 Stümpflen I, Stümpflen A, Wimmer M, Bernasheck G. Effect of detailed fetal echocardiography as part of routine prenatal ultrasonographic screening on detection of congenital heart disease. Lancet 1996; 348: 854-857

2 Kleinman CS, Hobbins JC, Jaffe CC, Lynch DC, Talner NS. Echocardiographics studies of the human fetus: prenatal diagnosis of congenital heart disease and cardiac dysrhythmias. Pediatrics 1980; 65: 1059-1067

3 Acherman RJ, Evans WN, Luna CF, Rollins R, Kip KT, Collazos JC, Restrepo H, Adasheck J, Iriye BK, Roberts D, Sacks AJ. Prenatal detection of congenital heart disease in Southern Nevada: the need for universal fetal cardiac evaluation. J Ultrasound Med. 2007; 26: 1715-1719

4 American Institute of Ultrasound in Medicine. AIUM Practice Guideline for the Performance of Obstetric Ultrasound Examinations. Laurel, MD; American Institute of Ultrasound in Medicine; 2007. Available at: http://www.aium.org/publications/guidelines/obstetric.pdf

5 Friedberg MK, Silverman NH, Moon-Grady AJ, Tong E, Nourse J, Sorenson B, Lee J, Hornberger LK. Prenatal detection of congenital heart disease. J Pediatr. 2009; 155: 26-31

6 Hollier LM, Leveno KJ, Kelly MA, MCIntire DD, Cunningham FG. Maternal age and malformations in singleton births. Obstet Gynecol 2000; 96: 701-706

7 Reefhuis J, Honein MA. Maternal age and non-chromosomal birth defects, Atlanta--1968-2000: teenager or thirty-something, who is at risk? Birth Defects Res A Clin Mol Teratol 2004: 70: 572-579

8 Yagel S, Cohen SM, Achiron R. Examination of the fetal heart by five short-axis views: a proposed screening method for comprehensive cardiac evaluation. Ultrasound Obstet Gynecol. 2001; 17: 367-369

9 Luna CF, Acherman RJ, Rollins RC, Castillo WJ, Berthoty DP, Evans WN. Laterally displaced superior vena cava on the fetal 3-vessel view from a diaphragmatic hernia. J Ultrasound Med 2011; 30: 1161-1162

10 Soothill PW, Bobrow CS, Holmes R. Small for gestational age is not a diagnosis.Ultrasound Obstet Gynecol 1999; 13: 225-228

11 Craigo SD, Beach ML, Harvey-Wilkes KB, D'Alton ME. Ultrasound predictors of neonatal outcome in intrauterine growth restriction. Am J Perinatol 1996; 13: 465-471

12 Cruz-Martínez R, Figueras F, Benavides-Serralde A, Crispi F, Hernandez-Andrade E, Gratacós E. Sequence of changes in myocardial performance index in relation with aortic isthmus and ductus venosus Doppler in fetuses with early-onset intrauterine growth restriction. Ultrasound Obstet Gynecol 2011; 38: 179-184

13 Crispi F, Comas M, Hernández-Andrade E, Eixarch E, Gómez O, Figueras F. Gratacós E. Does pre-eclampsia influence fetal cardiovascular function in early-onset intrauterine growth restriction? Ultrasound Obstet Gynecol 2009; 34: 660-665

14 Delle Chiaie L, Buck G, Grab D, Terinde R. Prediction of fetal anemia with Doppler measurement of the middle cerebral artery peak systolic velocity in pregnancies complicated by maternal blood group alloimmunization or parvovirus B19 infection. Ultrasound Obstet Gynecol 2001; 18: 232-236

15 Mari G. Middle cerebral artery peak systolic velocity for the diagnosis of fetal anemia: the untold story. Ultrasound Obstet Gynecol 2005; 25: 323-330

16 Acherman RJ, Evans WN, Galindo A, Collazos JC, Rothman A, Mayman GA, Luna CF, Rollins R, Kip KT, Berthoty DP, Restrepo H. Diagnosis of absent ductus venosus in a population referred for fetal echocardiography: association with a persistent portosystemic shunt requiring postnatal device occlusion. J Ultrasound Med. 2007; 26: 1077-1082

17 Acherman RJ, Rollins RC, Castillo WJ, Evans WN. Stenosis of alternative umbilical venous pathways in absence of the ductus venosus. J Ultrasound Med. 2010; 29: 1227-1231

18 Acherman RJ, Evans WN, Luna CF, Castillo W, Rollins R, Kip

K, Law IH, Collazos JC, Restrepo H. Fetal bradycardia. A practical approach. Fetal Matern Med Rev 2007; 18: 225-255

19 Acherman RJ, Evans WN, Schwartz JK, Dombrowski M, Rollins RC, Castillo W, Haltore S, Berthoty DP. Right ventricular noncompaction associated with long QT in a fetus with right ventricular hypertrophy and cardiac arrhythmias. Prenat Diagn. 2008; 28: 551-553

20 Drago F, Stefano Silvetti M, Annichiarico M, Michielon G, Brancaccio G, Zanoni S, Valsecchi S. Biventricular pacing in an infant with noncompaction of the ventricular myocardium, congenital AV block, and prolonged QT interval. J Interv Card Electrophysiol. 2010; 28: 67-70

21 Papa M, Fragasso G, Camesasca C, Di Turi RP, Spagnolo D, Valsecchi L, Calori G, Margonato A. Prevalence and prognosis of atrial septal aneurysm in high-risk fetuses without structural heart defects. Ital Heart J 2002; 3: 318-321

24 Magnetic Resonance Imaging & Computed Tomography

Contents

Background	391
MRI versus CT	392
Example Studies	393

24 Magnetic Resonance Imaging & Computed Tomography

dean berthoty

BACKGROUND

Imaging is key for cardiovascular malformation evaluation and treatment. Echocardiography (Echo) is the most common noninvasive imaging modality. However, Echo has limitations for viewing branch pulmonary arteries; aspects of the aorta and aortic arch; coronary arteries; systemic and pulmonary veins; postoperative structures including systemic-to-pulmonary artery shunts; and other extracardiac structures. Additional imaging methods include angiography (which we address in the next chapter), magnetic resonance imaging (MRI), and computed tomography (CT). However, MRI and CT are safer than catheter based angiography. Also, MRI and CT use less iodine-laden contrast—lower volumes for CT and none for MRI.

MRI and CT provide detailed 2- and 3-dimensional intra- and extracardiac structure imaging. Additionally, MRI can provide information on flows and pressure gradients, similar to Doppler Echo. Contrary to Echo, which various professionals perform with mobile units in many settings, those needing MRI or CT scans must go to imaging facilities or radiology departments. Also, MRI and CT require patients to remain motionless for protracted periods. This usually requires anesthesia in uncooperative infants and young children.

MRI and CT fundamentally differ. MRI uses strong magnetic fields and radio waves that alter the energy states of hydrogen-atom protons and causes photon discharges that the scanner uses to create images. MRI may create some tissue heat from radio waves, but studies show no long-term side effects. CT, however, uses ionizing radiation (X-ray), which causes long-term health problems. [1-4]

CT versus MRI

Radiation Dose Comparisons

The table below lists the radiation doses from testing procedures. Natural and artificial environmental sources emit the annual background radiation. We express radiation doses in milli-sievert (mSv) units.

Radiation Dose Comparison	
Exposure	Radiation in mSv
MRI	0.00
Chest X-ray	0.05
Dental X-rays	0.09
Annual background	1.80 - 4.00
CT	0.5 - 25 (10 - 500 CXRs)
Cardiac catheterization	10 (minimum)

CT Advantages

- Faster & less anesthesia
- Extracardiac anatomy better imaged
- Less complicated to perform than MRI
- Use with pacemakers & other metal structures
- CT is more available than MRI

MRI Advantages

- No radiation
- Contrast is not mandatory like CT
- Usually better imaging of intracardiac structures
- Provides better pericardium characterization
- Super tissue characterization of masses
- Cardiac function
- Pressure gradients
- Chamber volumes
- Valve regurgitation
- Valve motion
- Calculate Qp:Qs ratios

Examples

CT

Figure 1 on the facing page is a CT scan of a newborn that demonstrates a coarctation of the aorta, transverse aortic arch hypoplasia, and a patent ductus arteriosus. Figure 2 is a CT scan of an infant showing a vascular ring (from behind) that encircles the trachea.

MRI

Figure 3 on the facing page is an MRI of a child showing a small apical muscular ventricular septal defect (VSD). Figure 4 is an MRI of a child that demonstrates a secundum atrial septal defect (ASD).

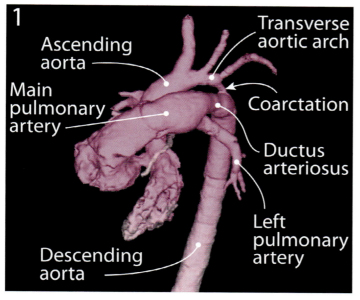

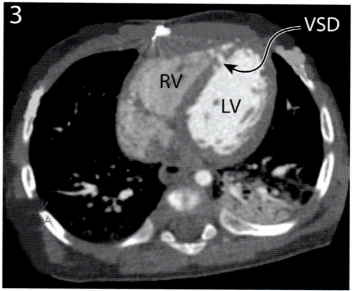

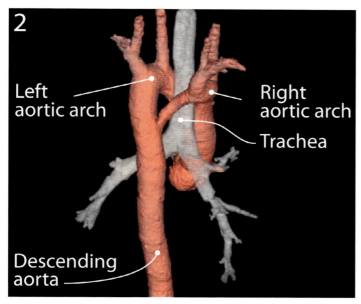

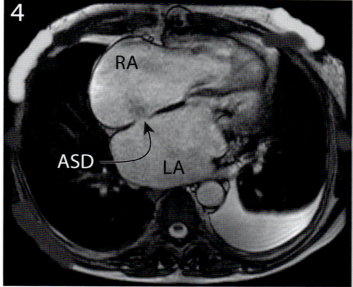

REFERENCES

1 Cook SC, Raman SV. Multidetector computed tomography in the adolescent and young adult with congenital heart disease. J Cardiovasc Comput Tomogr 2008; 2: 36-49

2 Krishnamurthy R. The role of MRI and CT in congenital heart disease. Pediatr Radiol 2009; 39 Suppl 2: S196-204

3 Marcotte F, Poirier N, Pressacco J, Paquet E, Mercier LA, Dore A, Ibrahim R, Khairy P. Evaluation of adult congenital heart disease by cardiac magnetic resonance imaging. Congenit Heart Dis 2009; 4: 216-230

4 Krishnamurthy R. Neonatal cardiac imaging. Pediatr Radiol 2010; 40: 518-527

25 Cardiac Catheterization & Intervention

Contents

Background	397
Diagnostic Cath Indications	398
Patient prep & Safety	398
Procedure	399
Calculations	402
Angiography	404
Interventional Cath	405
Opening Structures	406
Closing Structures	410
Other Procedures	412

396

25 Cardiac Catheterization & Intervention

alvaro galindo • abraham rothman

BACKGROUND

In 1870, German physiologist Adolph Fick theorized that cardiac output (CO) is proportional to the body's oxygen consumption [2]. Fick's theory resulted from intellectual intuition rather than from experimental data. Although late-19th century researchers confirmed Fick's theory by calculating cardiac outputs in animals, 60 more years passed before clinicians confirmed Fick's theory in humans. In 1930, Prague physician Otto Klein was the first to calculate a Fick CO from human cardiac-catheterization data. In the 1930s and early 1940s, André Cournand and Dickinson Richards, at Columbia's Bellevue Hospital, and others also obtained catheterization data that supported Fick's equation. In 1935, Cuban physician Agustín Castellanos was the first to employ angiography in children with congenital heart disease. Then in the late 1940s, physicians in Boston and Johns Hopkins combined intracardiac pressure measurements, Fick CO, and angiography for cardiovascular malformations. In the 1950s, cineangiography became the standard method for imaging cardiovascular defects.

During the later 20th century, clinicians began performing interventional procedures along with the acquisition of physiological data and cineangiography. In the early 21st century, cardiac catheterization-based intervention has now become about equal in importance to surgery as a treatment method for children with cardiovascular malformations. The earliest descriptions of interventional procedures include pulmonary valvotomy by Víctor Rubio-Alvarez, Rodolfo Limón, and Jorge Soní in 1953, balloon atrial septostomy for transposition of the great arteries by Rashkind and Miller in 1966, and static pulmonary valve balloon dilation by Kan and colleagues in 1982. Subsequently, interventionalists have devised multiple procedures to treat many cardiovascular malformations.

For many cardiovascular malformations, we prefer interventional cardiac catheterization. The success rates are high and complication rates are low. Interventional catheterization procedures are possible for patients from premature infants weighing < 1,000 grams to adults with congenital or acquired structural heart disease. Fetal intervention is currently under development.

Despite the advent of other diagnostic modalities including echocardiography (Echo), MRI, and CT scans, cardiac catheterization remains an important tool for assessing the anatomy and physiology of cardiovascular malformations. [1-4]

DIAGNOSTIC CARDIAC CATHETERIZATION

Information from Catheterization

- Oxygen saturations from chambers & vessels
- Pressures from chambers & vessels
- Anatomy from angiography
- Ventricular function from angiography
- Calculations of shunts & vascular resistance
- Calculation of ventricular function
- Calculation of vessel size & valve areas

Indications

Determine shunts & vascular resistances

- Confirm echocardiographic findings
- Check conflicting Echo findings

Cardiac function evaluation

- Correlate findings with Echo
- Evaluation for transplant

Anatomy not resolved by Echo

MRI and CT scan can also provide this information.

- Coronary artery anatomy
- Aortic arch
- Pulmonary arteries & pulmonary veins
- Systemic veins
- RV-dependent coronary arteries in pulmonary atresia with intact ventricular septum (see also Chapter 19)

Preoperative assessment

- For pre-Glenn or pre-Fontan procedures
- Other conditions needing invasive pre-op evaluation

Pulmonary hypertension evaluation

- **Unrestricted pulmonary blood flow**

As is large ventricular septal defect (VSD), a large patient ductus arteriosus (PDA), or a heart with 1-functional ventricle without PS.

- **Living at high altitude**

Especially those with large left-to-right atrial shunts including large atrial septal defects (ASD) or anomalies of pulmonary venous return.

- **Elevated pulmonary venous pressure**

In pulmonary vein stenosis, obstructed left atrial outflow, or elevated left ventricular end-diastolic pressures.

- **Primary pulmonary hypertension**

Complex evaluation to obtain pulmonary arterial pressures, pulmonary vascular resistance, pulmonary vasodilator challenges, and ruling in or out causes of pulmonary hypertension

Patient Preparation & Safety

- Avoid hypothermia, especially infants
- Monitor vital signs
- EKG monitoring
- Oximetry & end-tidal CO_2 monitoring
- A pediatric anesthesiologist to manage the airway
- Limit radiation exposure
- Minimize risk of brachial plexus injury
- Minimize embolism with anticoagulants
- Use CO_2 in balloon catheters & air filters for IV lines
- Blood available
- Snares, pericardiocentesis, & pleurocentesis trays

- Beware of potential latex allergy
- Availability of surgical backup & ECMO if needed
- Low ionic contrast to minimize renal side effects

➤Consider N-acetylcysteine (mucolytic agent) and sodium bicarbonate in renal dysfunction before catheterization to minimize further risk of worsening renal dysfunction.

Catheterization Procedure

Sedation
- Conscious sedation
- General anesthesia

Vascular access

Peripheral veins & arteries
- Femoral vein & femoral artery

➤This approach remains the preferred route for most diagnostic and interventional procedures, particularly for device closure of atrial septal defects and atrial transseptal puncture.

Internal jugular & subclavian veins
- Favored for device closure of muscular VSDs
- Endomyocardial biopsies
- Pulmonary artery angioplasty & stent placement
- Poor for atrial septal interventions

Radial artery
- May provide access to the aorta & the coronaries
- We rarely use in pediatrics

Carotid artery cutdown
- Cardiovascular surgeon

An experienced cardiovascular surgeon should perform the procedure, especially on an infant.

- Intervention

Provides a controlled access for interventional procedures in small children including aortic balloon valvuloplasty, stent placement in the ductus arteriosus, and stent placement in pulmonary arteries via Blalock-Taussig shunts

Transhepatic venous access
- When no other venous vascular access possible
- Access to a hepatic vein & right atrium
- Heart access similar to femoral venous approach

Direct surgical access via midline sternotomy or thoracotomy

A cardiac surgeon provides direct access to a vascular structure such as the pulmonary artery or a cardiac chamber, allowing interventionalists to place a pulmonary artery stent or a ventricular septal closure device.

Data

On the following page, the heart diagram figure displays normal oxygen saturation and pressure data.

Oxygen saturation

We obtain small blood samples from each cardiac chamber. Without left-to-right or right-to-left shunts, the oxygen saturations vary < 4% throughout the right heart.
- A step-up > 4% suggests a left-to-right shunt
- Low mixed venous values suggest low cardiac output

Pressure data

The ideal catheter for pressure measurements is short, stiff, with a large lumen, filled with a low-density fluid, and connected to a pressure transducer by few stopcocks.
- Record at end-expiration when breathing spontaneously
- Extra care for recording pressures in ventilated patients

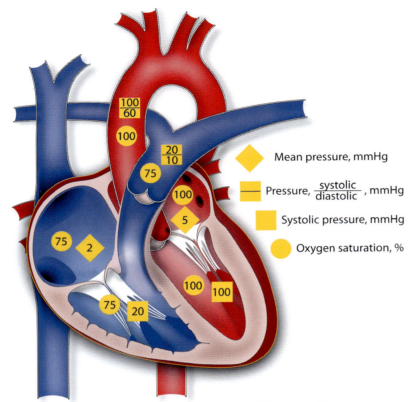

Normal Oxygen Saturation and Pressure Data

Atrial pressures

On the facing page, we display a right atrial pressure tracing in figure 1 and a left atrial tracing in figure 2.

a-wave

Atrial contraction (EKG p-wave) generates the a-wave.

- The RA a-wave is normally < 9 mm Hg
- The LA a-wave is normally about 6-9 mm Hg

➤ High ventricular end-diastolic pressure, tricuspid or mitral stenosis or atresia, and arrhythmias with atrial ventricular dissociation all increase the a-wave. The a-wave is absent in junctional rhythm (no atrial contractions).

v-wave

The v-wave results from continued venous return and resultant rising pressure in the atrium during ventricular systole before opening of the atrioventricular valves.

- The RA v-wave is normally 2-3 mm Hg < the RA a-wave
- The LA v-wave is normally slightly > the LA a-wave

➤ The v-wave increases with tricuspid or mitral insufficiency. The right atrial v-wave elevation can also be from a left ventricle to right atrial shunt. Increased pulmonary venous return, as in atrial or ventricular septal defects or patent ductus arteriosus, increases the left atrial v-wave.

Ventricular pressures

On the facing page, we display right ventricular (RV) pressure in figure 3 and left ventricular (LV) pressure in figure 4. Values are in mm Hg. Ventricular pressure tracings have a rapid upstroke during isovolumic contraction followed by a plateau during ejection and a drop to near 0 mm Hg during isovolumic relaxation. During isovolumic contraction and relaxation, the atrioventricular and semilunar valves close. In diastole, a slow rise in pressure to end-diastolic pressure occurs. The end-diastolic pressure is equal to the atrial a-wave.

- Elevated RV systolic pressures

RV systolic pressure is high with pulmonic stenosis, pulmonary hypertension, a large VSD, a large PDA, and a volume-loaded right ventricle.

- Elevated LV systolic pressures

LV systolic pressure is high with obstruction of the left ventricular outflow tract, coarctation of the aorta, and systemic hypertension.

- Elevated diastolic pressures

Ventricular end-diastolic pressures (LVEDP and RVEDP) are high in conditions that cause ventricular dysfunction for various reasons including restrictive cardiomyopathy.

25 Cardiac Catheterization & Intervention

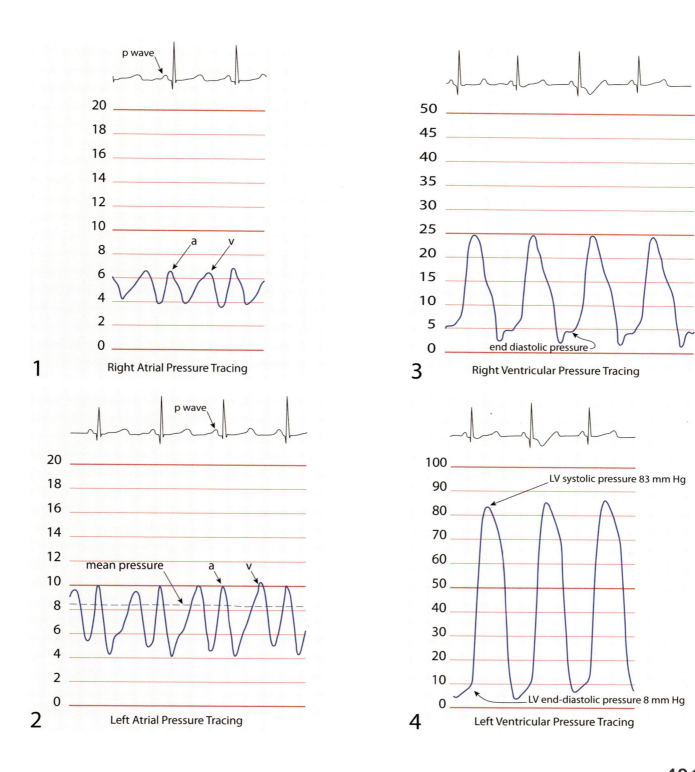

Arterial pressure

Figure 1 on the right displays pulmonary arterial pressure, and figure 2 displays aortic pressure. Values are in mm of Hg. The arterial pressure rises abruptly at the end of isovolumic contraction upon opening of the semilunar valve. The pressure tracing is identical to the ventricle until the onset of isovolumic relaxation. The closure of the semilunar valve inscribes a dicrotic notch on the pulse tracing. Arterial pressure then falls from continued flow into the vascular bed, until arterial pressure rises again with the next ventricular contraction. Arterial pressure tracing findings include the following:
- No dicrotic notch suggests semilunar valve regurgitation
- A low dicrotic notch suggests a PDA or anemia

Systolic & diastolic gradients

By measuring pressure differences across structures, we can determine pressure gradients. Pressure gradients can be systolic or diastolic.
- Systolic across semilunar valves, VSDs, & coarctation of the aorta (CoA)
- Diastolic across atrioventricular (AV) valves or ASDs

Calculations from saturation & pressure data

Fick Principle

The Fick principle uses oxygen in the blood as an indicator. Oxygen chiefly binds to hemoglobin with a small fraction dissolved in serum. When calculating a Fick cardiac output in room air, we ignore the dissolved oxygen. When we make measurements in high-inspired concentrations of oxygen, we include the dissolved oxygen content. Data necessary for calculating a Fick cardiac output (for both the systemic flow and the pulmonary flow) include the oxygen

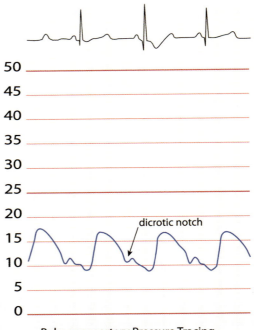

1 Pulmonary artery Pressure Tracing

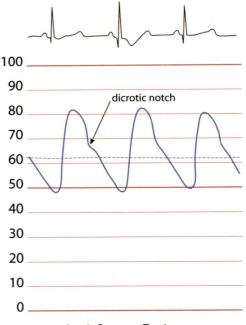

2 Aortic Pressure Tracing

consumption (VO_2 in mL O_2/min); the hemoglobin; and oxygen saturation data from the aorta, the superior vena cava (mixed venous saturation), pulmonary artery, and pulmonary veins. Usually, we assume VO_2 in mL O_2/min from a table of values rather than from measurement (a difficult procedure). Also, as we note in Chapter 7, an oximeter measures the percentage of hemoglobin bound to oxygen, but we commonly refer to this percentage as "oxygen saturation." Normally systemic flow (Qs) equals pulmonary flow (QP), and the Qp:Qs ratio is 1:1. With a left-to-right shunt, the pulmonary blood flow is greater than the systemic blood flow and the Qp:Qs ratio is > 1. However, with a right-to-left shunt, the Qp:Qs ratio is < 1. The formulas for Qs, Qp, and Qp:Qs ratio follow below:

- Systemic flow (Qs)

> *Qs (L/min) = VO_2 (oxygen consumption) ÷ [Hgb g/dL × 1.36 × 10 (aortic oxygen saturation – mixed venous oxygen saturation)]*

- Pulmonary flow (Qp)

> *Qp (L/min) = VO_2 (oxygen consumption) ÷ [Hgb g/dL × 1.36 × 10 (pulmonary venous oxygen saturation – pulmonary artery oxygen saturation)]*

- Qp:Qs ratio

> *Result of Qp ÷ result of Qs*

Quick Qp:Qs ratio calculation

We can obtain a quick Qp to Qs ratio estimate by using just the oxygen saturation data from the formula below:

> *Qp:QS = (aortic oxygen saturation – mixed venous oxygen saturation) ÷ (pulmonary venous oxygen saturation – pulmonary artery oxygen saturation)*

Thermodilution

Without significant tricuspid or pulmonary regurgitation, we can measure cardiac output by using cold saline as an indicator. Using a Swan-Ganz type catheter, we inject cold saline in or near the right atrium. The cold saline mixes completely with systemic venous blood in the right ventricle. We monitor blood temperature continuously using a thermistor tipped catheter in the pulmonary artery. The blood temperature drops briefly then returns to baseline. The equipment electronically inscribes a curve, and the area under the curve equates to the cardiac output.

Vascular resistance

We also discuss pulmonary and systemic vascular resistances (PVR and SVR) in Chapter 19. The formulas to calculate pulmonary and systemic arteriolar vascular resistance from catheterization pressure data follow below:

> *PVR = (pulmonary artery mean pressure – left atrial mean pressure) ÷ Qp*
>
> *SVR = (aortic mean pressure – right atrial mean pressure) ÷ QS*

Values

We record values in Wood units.
- Normal PVR is 1-3 Wood units, high if > 4 wood units
- Normal SVR is < 20 Wood units, high if > 20 wood units

Valve area

We can calculate valve area by using the Gorlin-Gorlin formula. The formula for aortic valve area (AVA) follows below:

> AVA (cm²) = [CO ÷ (SEP × HR)] ÷ [44.5 × (the square root of the LVSM − ASM)]

CO - cardiac output in mL/min
SEP - systolic ejection period in sec
HR - heart rate
LVSM - left ventricular systolic mean pressure in mmHg
ASM - aortic systolic mean in mmHg

Values

For pediatric valvular aortic stenosis, aortic valve areas are indexed as cm²/m².

Mild AS	0.80 – 2.0 cm²/m²
Moderate AS	0.50 – 0.8 cm²/m²
Severe AS	< 0.50 cm²/m²

Angiography

Angiography of congenital heart defects requires biplane X-ray equipment. Because of the complex 3-dimensional nature of the heart, we need multiple X-ray projections to highlight the cardiac anatomy.

Calculations from angiography

Ejection fraction

We can calculate a LV ejection fraction from frozen angiographic images of the LV in systole and diastole.

The Nakata Index & the McGoon ratio for pulmonary artery sizes

The sizes of the pulmonary arteries underlie the success of operative repairs in tetralogy of Fallot and other defects where the pulmonary arteries (PAs) may be hypoplastic. The 2 methodologies of quantitatively assessing the size of PAs are the McGoon ratio and the Nakata index. For each angiographic assessment, we make measurements of the PAs in mm at the hilum (proximal to the main left and right PAs branch points). The formulas for the McGoon ratio and the Nakata index follow below:

> McGoon ratio = RPA (right pulmonary artery) diameter + LPA (left pulmonary artery) diameter ÷ DAo (descending aorta) diameter at the diaphragm

Values

McGoon ratios are unitless.
- Normal is > 2.0
- Significantly hypoplastic PAs < 0.8

> Nakata Index = RPA cross-sectional area (mm²) + LPA cross-sectional area (mm²) ÷ BSA (body surface area) in m²

Values

The Nakata index units are mm²/m².
- Normal 330 ± 30 mm²/m²
- Significantly hypoplastic PAs < 150 mm²/m²

CATHETER INTERVENTION

INTRODUCTION

Types

• **Opening or enlarging structures**

Including opening atrial septums, enlarging narrowed valves, arteries, veins or surgically placed conduits.

• **Closing structures**

Including atrial septal defects, a ventricular septal defects, a patent ductus arteriosus, extra vascular connections, and surgically-placed conduits.

• **Other procedures**

Including hybrid procedures that combine surgery with catheter intervention, endomyocardial biopsy, or retrieving stray catheters or devices.

Possible Complications

- Vascular injury
- Hemorrhage
- Thrombosis
- Vessel aneurysm formation
- Vessel arteriovenous fistula
- Infection
- Arrhythmias
- Seizures or stroke
- Allergic reactions to contrast
- Renal failure
- Rupture of arteries, veins, or cardiac structures
- Balloon rupture & device malfunction
- Embolization of stents or devices
- Death

OPENING OR ENLARGING STRUCTURES

Atrial Septostomy & Septectomy

Newborns with transposition of the great arteries atrial usually require balloon atrial septostomy (BAS) to improve mixing of atrial blood. BAS can open an obstructed atrial communication, which may be present in tricuspid atresia or hypoplastic left heart syndrome. Beyond the newborn, thicker atrial septums need extensive interventional procedures

- Thin newborn atrial septums

We pass a balloon into the left atrium and, after inflating, pull the balloon back vigorously into the right atrium, tearing the atrial septum and creating an atrial septal defect.

- Thicker atrial septums

May need balloon dilation, a transcatheter blade septostomy, or stent placement.

- Intact atrial septums

For intact atrial septums, we advance a long Brockenbrough needle through a long femoral venous sheath to the right atrial side of the septum and then push the needle through to create a septal puncture. Following this procedure, we can open the atrial septum by the procedures we describe above.

Valvular Pulmonic Stenosis

We recommend balloon valvuloplasty of the pulmonary valve (PV) when the peak gradient is > 40 mm Hg by invasive measurement. We may use a lower gradient in the face of right ventricular dysfunction or the presence of a PDA. The figures on the facing page illustrate pulmonary valvuloplasty: figure A is an RV angiogram, figure B illustrates the inflation and opening a stenotic doming valve, figure C and D show the fluoroscopic images of an actual balloon valvuloplasty. We cross the valve with a catheter or a wire. We advance a balloon catheter over the wire. We use a balloon 20-40% larger than the PV annulus.

- Highly successful for typical valvular PS
- Less successful for dysplastic PV as in Noonan syndrome
- Complications are rare
- Long-term results are excellent

Pulmonary Atresia & Intact Ventricular Septum

When the pulmonary valve is atretic and membrane-like, we can perforate the membrane by placing a catheter right up to the atretic valve and using radiofrequency energy or a stiff guidewire to cross the membrane. Once we create a hole, we dilate in the same manner as for valvular pulmonic stenosis.

Branch Pulmonary Artery Stenosis

Indications for pulmonary artery dilation include a significant right ventricular systolic pressure, marked asymmetry in pulmonary blood flow, or hypertension in unaffected pulmonary arteries. We use a balloon measuring 3 to 4 times larger than the diameter of the stenosis for dilation. In cases of long-segment stenoses or failed balloon dilation, we perform a stent implantation. Complications are rare but may include pulmonary artery rupture, aneurysm formation, and stent embolization. [9, 10]

- Stenting's long-term success is good
- Redilation of stents with growth usually successful

25 Cardiac Catheterization & Intervention

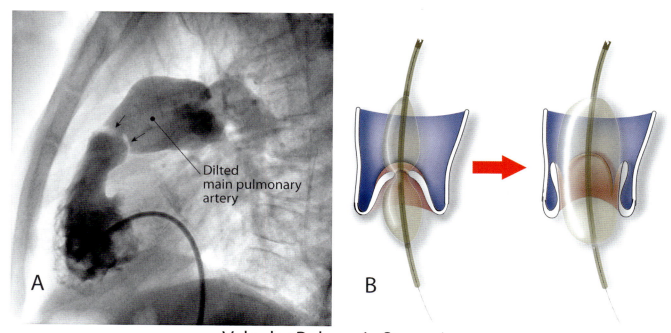

Valvular Pulmonic Stenosis
A, Lateral view, the arrows show the doming pulmonary valve. B, schematic of pulmonary balloon valvuloplasty

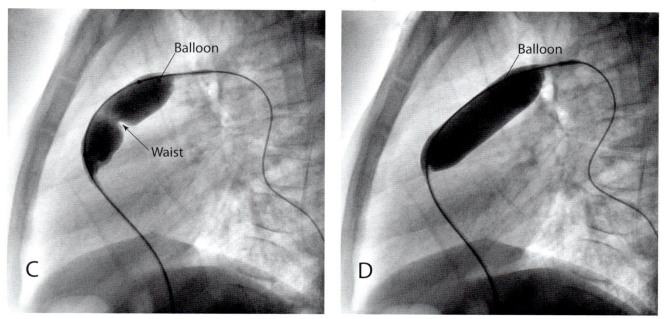

Balloon Dilatation of Valvular Pulmonic Stenosis
C, partial inflation of the balloon. D, fully inflated balloon with disappearance of the waist

Systemic & Pulmonary Vein Stenosis

Indications for intervention of stenotic veins include a significant pressure gradient, venous stasis such as swelling of the head and upper extremities (superior vena cava syndrome), or pulmonary hypertension with multiple stenotic pulmonary veins. Stent implantation has a significantly higher success rate acutely than balloon dilatation, but restenosis is common. We expand the stent up to the diameter of the adjacent normal vein. Because of neointimal growth within the stent, we need to redilate the stent frequently to keep up with the child's growth.

Right Ventricular to Pulmonary Artery Conduit Stenosis

Surgically-placed conduits, which create or enlarge the outflow from right ventricle to main pulmonary artery, often develop stenosis. Stenosis mechanisms include tissue ingrowth, kinking, and calcification. Balloon dilation may be partially or transiently successful, but the procedure can aid in postponing surgery for a few years. Stent placement achieves better, acute, and long-term gradient reduction, but stents may cause pulmonary regurgitation. Percutaneously delivered valves are currently available, and these valves are useful for significant pulmonary regurgitation. Patients need close followup for possible restenosis, pulmonary regurgitation, and stent fracture.

Valvular aortic Stenosis

We recommend balloon valvuloplasty of the aortic valve for a peak gradient > 50 mm Hg by invasive measurement, or lower gradients with left ventricular dysfunction. Figures A and B above on the facing page illustrates an aortic valvuloplasty. Pacing the heart stabilizes the balloon catheter, allowing for an effective valvuloplasty. We cross the valve from the aorta or from the left ventricle, and we use a balloon with a diameter about 90-100% of the aortic valve annulus.

- The success rate is high
- Mild aortic valve regurgitation occurs commonly
- Mild aortic regurgitation can worsen over time
- Moderate or severe AR is rare
- Re-intervention common after catheter or surgery

Coarctation of the Aorta

Pediatric cardiologists accept balloon dilation of postoperative-recurrent coarctation more so than for balloon dilation of unoperated-native coarctations, especially in newborns. Figures C and D below on the facing age show the placement of a stent to relieve coarctation. We perform intervention for gradients > 20 mm Hg. Gradient reduction is better with stenting versus balloon dilation, but disadvantages include a larger sheath size for stent delivery and the need for stent redilation with somatic growth. [5-8]

- Successful acute gradient reduction is common
- Restenosis may occur, especially in small patients
- Long-term aneurysm formation exists in 3-5%
- In larger patients, stents may be preferable

Blalock-Taussig Shunt Stenosis or Occlusion

A stenotic or occluded Blalock-Taussig shunt is often life-threatening. We cross the stenotic shunt with a soft guidewire. We then implant a stent with a diameter the same size as the shunt. We give post-procedure anti-platelet agents to prevent recurrent thrombosis.

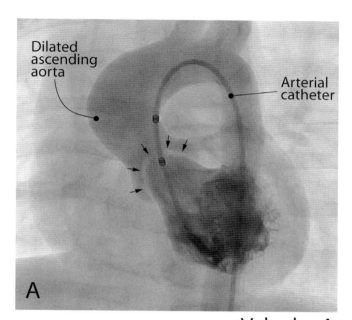
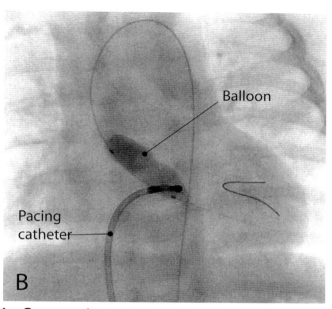

Valvular Aortic Stenosis
A, the short arrows show the doming aortic valve
B, balloon inflation with right ventricular pacing

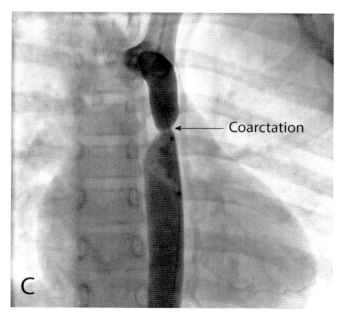
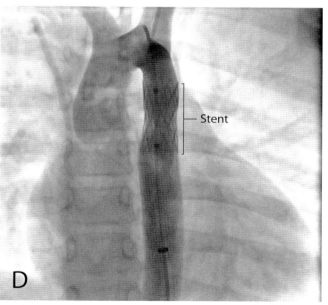

Coarctation of Aorta
C, before dilatation. D, after stent placement

CLOSING CARDIAC STRUCTURES
Patent Ductus Arteriosus

Figures A and B on the facing page demonstrate device closure of a PDA. We close most PDAs with catheter intervention rather than surgery. The exceptions include large PDAs in newborns, when surgery is best. Acute success and long-term results are excellent. Complications are rare, but occasionally coils or devices may embolize.

- PDAs <2 mm in diameter

Small PDAs are amenable to closure with coil, spring-like devices covered with thrombogenic material, which causes thrombosis and subsequent endothelialization. We use coils to also close aortopulmonary collaterals that may produce similar hemodynamic consequences, as a PDA, in preterm infants with chronic lung disease and oxygen dependence. [11-13]

- PDAs >2 mm in diameter

PDAs larger than 2 mm usually require larger occluder devices.

Atrial Septal Defect

Indications for percutaneous ASD closure include a significant volume load to the right ventricle and adequate defect edges to secure the device. Most devices have double discs or umbrellas, which occlude the defect from both sides of the atrial septum. We size the defect with a compliant balloon, which we inflate gently across the defect. We cross the defect with a long sheath. We then advance the collapsed device through the sheath. As we sequentially display in the lower figure on the facing page, we deliver a distal disc in the left atrium and then pull the distal disc back on to the atrial septum. We open the proximal disc or umbrella on the right atrial side of the defect. When transesophageal echocardiography confirms a good position, we release the device and close the ASD. Approximately 10% of defects are too large or have deficient edges precluding device closure.

- Acute & long-term results are excellent
- Complications are rare, but devices may embolize

Ventricular Septal Defect

Currently, we chiefly limit device closure of VSDs to muscular defects. Early experience with device closure of membranous VSDs reported a significant risk of complete heart block. Inlet and outlet VSDs are not currently amenable to device closure. For muscular VSDs, we initially cross the VSD with a soft guidewire from left to the right ventricle. We snare the guidewire in the right ventricle, right atrium, or pulmonary artery, and then we exteriorize the wire through the venous sheath, creating an arteriovenous loop. We advance a long venous sheath into the left ventricle. We then deliver the distal disc or umbrella in the left ventricle and the proximal disc or umbrella in the right ventricle. In small patients, we may have a surgeon perform a limited sternotomy, through which we advance a short sheath directly through the anterior wall of the right ventricle and through the VSD into the left ventricle, all under transesophageal guidance. We then load the device and deliver it in standard fashion. [14]

- Complications higher than for PDA or ASD closure
- Complications include transient arrhythmias, device embolization, & residual leaks
- Long-term results are excellent

Fontan Procedure Fenestrations

Surgeons may create a small (4-5 mm) fenestration in the

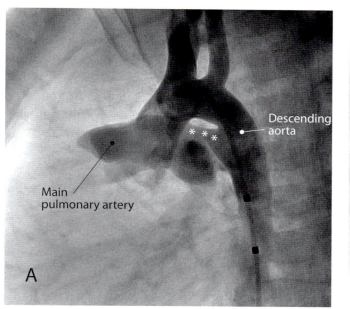 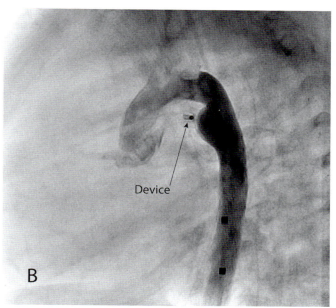

Patent Ductus Arteriosus
A, before occlusion, the asterisks show the patent ductus. B, after device occlusion

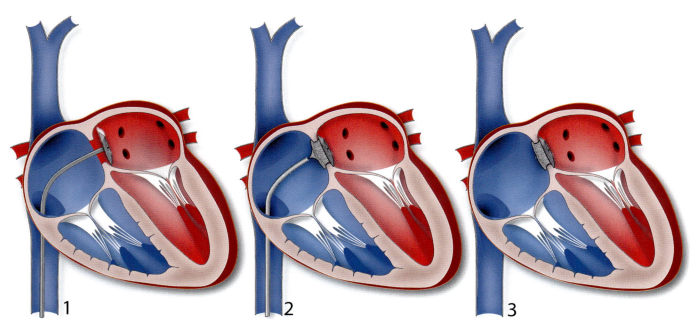

ASD device closure

Fontan conduit that communicates with the pulmonary venous atrium. The fenestration may be beneficial in the early postoperative period possibly leading to quicker recovery and earlier discharge than those undergoing a Fontan procedure without a fenestration. We can subsequently close the defect with a variety of small devices and techniques similar to those we described for ASD device closure above. Fontan fenestration closures sometimes need unique procedures [15].

Aortopulmonary Collaterals & Obsolete Shunts

Aortopulmonary collaterals and obsolete aorto-pulmonary shunts provide an unwanted volume load to a systemic ventricle. We close them with coils, vascular plugs, and double disc or double umbrella devices.
- Complications are rare
- Short & long-term results are excellent

OTHER PROCEDURES

Miscellaneous Procedures

Endomyocardial biopsy

For biopsy, we advance a sheath into the right ventricle from a jugular or femoral venous approach, and advance the bioptome catheter through the sheath to the right ventricle. We use endomyocardial biopsy for heart transplantation surveillance or to diagnose cardiac rejection. The procedure is also useful in myocarditis and some cardiomyopathies.
- Success rate is high
- Complications are rare

Retrieval of broken or stray catheters & devices

Using loop snares, basket catheters, hook-like snares, and bioptomes we trap stray objects and exteriorize them through the access sheath [16].
- Success rate is high
- Complications are rare

Hybrid Procedures

Hybrid procedures use interventional cardiac catheterization procedures and surgery together or close in time to treat or palliate cardiovascular malformations. Hybrid procedures can avoid cardiopulmonary bypass (CPB) in low birth weight neonates or infants in poor hemodynamic states. Avoiding CPB may improve outcome. The preliminary results from hybrid procedures in newborns with HLHS or severe aortic arch abnormalities are favorable. Also see Chapter 27 for surgical procedures.

Hypoplasia of left-sided cardiac structures

25 Cardiac Catheterization & Intervention

- **1st stage**

For HLHS or variants (severe aortic arch obstruction) we place surgical bands on both branch pulmonary arteries, and we place a stent in the PDA to maintain its patency long term. When placing the PDA stent, we may also perform a balloon atrial septostomy for a restrictive atrial septum, minimizing the obstruction to pulmonary venous return. Occasionally, a thick atrial septum requires a stent in the foramen ovale to maintain an unobstructed communication to the right atrium. Figure 1 below left illustrates HLHS prior to intervention, and figure 2 below right is post hybrid intervention with bilateral pulmonary artery bands, a PDA stent, and a stent across the atrial septum.

- **2nd stage palliation for HLHS or variants**

A few months after the 1st stage for HLHS or variants, the surgeon performs a 2nd stage, consisting of aortic arch repair and a Glenn procedure.

- **2nd stage repair for 2-ventricle hearts**

Complete surgical repair that includes VSD closure and arch augmentation weeks or months, following a hybrid procedure for interrupted aortic arch or severe arch hypoplasia and VSD.

- **3rd stage palliation for HLHS or variants**

A Fontan procedure for hearts with 1-functional ventricle at 2 to 3 years old, similar to standard staged palliation for 1-functional ventricles that uses exclusively surgical procedures

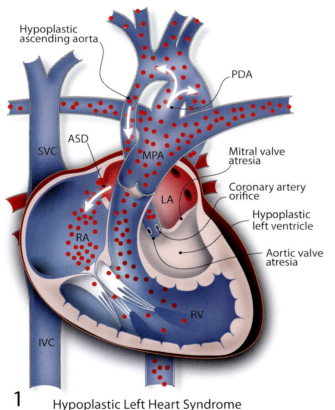

1 Hypoplastic Left Heart Syndrome

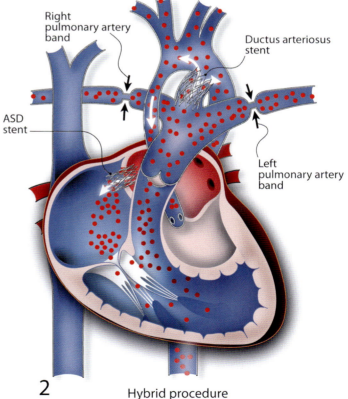

2 Hybrid procedure

REFERENCES

1 Mullins CE. History of pediatric interventional catheterization: Pediatric therapeutic cardiac catheterizations. Pediatr Cardiol 1998; 19: 3-7

2 Rubio-Alvarez V, Limon R, Soni J. [Intracardiac valvulotomy by means of a catheter]. Arch Inst Cardiol Mex 1953; 23: 183-192

3 Kan JS, White RI Jr, Mitchell SE, Gardner TJ. Percutaneous balloon valvuloplasty: a new method for treating congenital pulmonary-valve stenosis. N Engl J Med 1982; 307: 540-542

4 Rothman A, Lock JE. Percutaneous balloon valvotomy in pediatric congenital and acquired heart disease. Cardiac Surgery: State of the Art Reviews 1991; 5: 197-219

5 Rothman A. Coarctation of the aorta: an update. Curr Probl Pediatr 1998; 28: 33-60

6 Sohn S, Rothman A, Shiota T, Luk G, Tong A, Swenson R, Shan DJ. Acute and follow-up intravascular ultrasound findings after balloon dilation of coarctation of the aorta. Circulation 1994; 90: 340-347

7 Rothman A, Galindo A, Evans WN, Collazos JC, Restrepo H. Effectiveness and safety of balloon dilation of native coarctation in premature neonates weighing < or = 2,500 grams. Am J Cardiol 2010; 105: 1176-1180

8 Park Y, Lucas VW, Sklansky MS, Kashani IA, Rothman A. Balloon angioplasty of native aortic coarctation in infants 3 months of age and younger. Am Heart J 1997; 134: 917-923

9 Rothman A, Perry SB, Keane JF, Lock JE. Early results and follow-up of balloon angioplasty for branch pulmonary artery stenosis. J Am Coll Cardiol 1990; 15: 1109-1117

10 Movahhedian H, Lucas VW, Moore JW, Kashani IA, Sklansky MS, Luk G, Rothman A. Comparison of results of stent implantation in small (< 2 kg) children vs larger children with pulmonary artery stenoses. Am J Cardiol 1996; 78: 1180-1183

11 Rothman A, Lucas VW, Sklansky MS, Cocalis MW, Kashani IA. Percutaneous coil occlusion of patent ductus arteriosus. J Pediatr 1997; 130: 447-454

12 Acherman RJ, Siassi B, Pratti-Madrid G, Luna C, Lewis AB, Ebrahimi M, Castillo W, Kamat P, Ramanathan R. Systemic to pulmonary collaterals in very low birth weight infants: color doppler detection of systemic to pulmonary connections during neonatal and early infancy period. Pediatrics 2000; 105: 528-532

13 Evans WN, Acherman RJ, Collazos JC, Restrepo H, Mayman GA, Rothman A. Expedited oxygen wean after coil embolization of systemic-to-pulmonary collaterals in a premature infant with bronchopulmonary dysplasia. J Ultrasound Med 2007; 26: 695-697

14 Lim DS, Forbes TJ, Rothman A, Lock JE, Landzberg MJ. Transcatheter closure of high-risk muscular ventricular septal defects with the CardioSEAL occluder: initial report from the CardioSEAL VSD Registry. Catheter Cardiovasc Interv. 2007; 70: 704-744

15 Rothman A, Evans WN, Mayman GA. Percutaneous fenestration closure with problematic residual native atrial septum. Catheter Cardiovas Interv 2005; 66: 286-290

16 Rothman A, Kung FH. Percutaneous retrieval of an embolized Mediport catheter in a patient receiving therapy for Hodgkins lymphoma. Pediatr Hematol Oncol 1993; 10: 179-82

26 Electrophysiology Pacemakers & ICDs

Contents

Background EP	417
EP Procedure	418
Catheter Ablation	420
Background Pacers & ICDs	421
Pacer & ICD Indications	423
Pacer & ICD Follow-Up	424

26 Electrophysiology Pacemakers & ICDs

ian law • nicholas von bergen • vincent thomas

BACKGROUND ELECTROPHYSIOLOGY

William His Jr discovered the "His" bundle in 1893. In 1930, Werner Forssmann, who was the first to place an invasive catheter in the heart (his own), casually suggested the possible future use of intracardiac catheters for obtaining electrocardiograms. The first intracardiac recordings in humans began in the 1970s. The first pediatric therapeutic applications of radiofrequency occurred in the late 1980s, making this method of invasive cardiovascular therapy historically the newest.

Intracardiac electrophysiology (EP) procedures and therapies are now the basis for definitive pediatric arrhythmia treatment. The procedures carry some risk, but the risk is minimal compared to the therapeutic benefit. Besides pathway ablations, current intracardiac EP procedures can help define an arrhythmia's mechanism, evaluate response to drug therapy, and guide pacemaker and implantable cardioverter defibrillator (ICD) placements.

We can also use a transesophageal EP procedure for arrhythmia diagnosis. We place the probe in the esophagus behind the left atrium, allowing atrial pacing and recording. We can perform this abbreviated EP procedure with minimal sedation. Nevertheless, this method has limitations. Other than the location of the pacing and recording catheter within the esophagus, performing an esophageal study is similar to an invasive EP procedure. We can also use the transesophageal method to convert supraventricular tachycardia with overdrive pacing. [1-4]

TECHNIQUE

We perform EP procedures in the cardiac catheterization laboratory under moderate sedation or anesthesia. However, sedation can cause arrhythmia suppression. We place catheters via the percutaneous technique, similar to a typical cardiac catheterization. We place the EP catheters in strategic, intracardiac locations to map the normal conduction system, abnormal pathways, and areas of abnormal electrical activity or automaticity (figure below). We frequently administer pharmacological agents to elicit normal and abnormal electrophysiological responses.

Typical Intracardiac Evaluations

- Sinus node recovery time

A prolonged recovery time occurs in sinus node dysfunction, but we do not commonly perform this measurement in children unless they have a history of extensive atrial surgery, resulting in sick sinus syndrome.

- Atrioventricular (AV) nodal function

We can measure values both on and off medications and

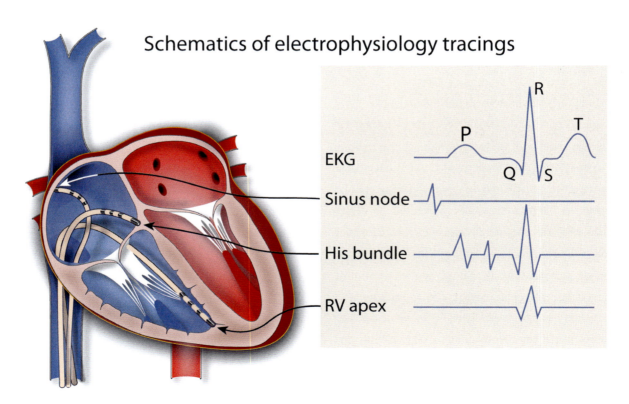

Schematics of electrophysiology tracings

assess atrioventricular node properties including conduction and refractory periods.

- **Refractory period**

A prolonged refractory period of atrial, atrioventricular node, or ventricular tissue may mean diseased myocardium or conduction tissue.

- **Arrhythmia risk**

We can assess the ease of inducing an arrhythmia.

- **Arrhythmia mechanism**

We can determine the location and mechanism of arrhythmias.

Programmed Pacing

Programmed pacing helps evaluate the intrinsic electrophysiological properties of the conduction system. Pacing maneuvers are also useful in inducing arrhythmias. Programmed pacing includes fixed pacing, pacing at successively faster heart rates, and extra-stimulus pacing. Each pacing protocol evaluates different electrophysiological properties.

Mapping Arrhythmia Substrate

Once we map the arrhythmia mechanism and substrate, we target the abnormal tissue for ablation. We use 3 standard methods to map the location of arrhythmia substrates:

Fluoroscopy

- Traditional anatomical method
- Shows catheters in 2 X-ray planes
- Major disadvantage is radiation exposure

Electrical mapping with intracardiac signals

- Identification and location of reentrant circuits
- Identification and location of automatic foci

3-Dimensional mapping

- 3-dimensional geometry of the heart
- Tracks the catheters within the heart
- Catheter positions accurate to within millimeters
- Allows reliable catheter repositioning

CATHETER ABLATION

The success of pediatric catheter ablation approaches 95% (figure below), with recurrence rates around 5%. Serious complications are rare but may include vessel injury, cardiac perforation, valve injury, inadvertent heart block, stroke, myocardial infarction, and death. Given this high success rate and relative low risk, catheter ablation for treating pediatric arrhythmias is now routine. Ablation methods include radiofrequency (RF) and cryothermal (Cryo) energy applications. [5-9]

Radiofrequency

Most children with typical SVT undergo RF ablation with a catheter tip heated to temperatures between 50° and 70° Celsius.

• Advantages

Advantages include a rapid tissue injury and a wide variety of catheters that industry has designed for children.

• Disadvantages

Disadvantages include relative instability of the catheter tip, possible damage to the AV node when ablating accessory pathway near the AV node, lesion extension, and clot formation.

Cryothermal

SVT from abnormal electrical pathways near the AV node likely need Cryo ablation, which is much less likely to cause permanent damage to the AV node. The equipment cools the catheter tip to a temperature of about minus 70° Celsius.

• Advantages

Advantages include stable catheter tip adherence during energy application, minimizing possible tip dislodgment, and the reversibility of tissue injury.

• Disadvantages

Disadvantages include less pliable catheters, longer energy application periods, and incompatibility of the catheters with some of the 3-dimensional mapping technology.

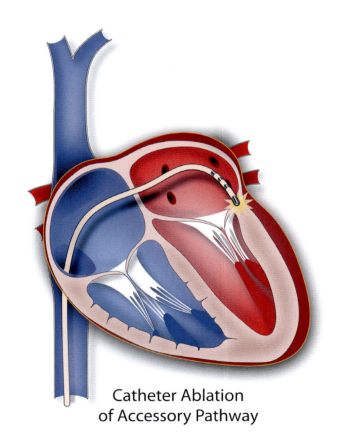

Catheter Ablation of Accessory Pathway

BACKGROUND PACEMAKERS & ICDs

A pacemaker is simply an implantable battery-operated computer with electrodes connected to the heart. The electrodes function as 2-way streets. The electrodes can both sense intrinsic cardiac electrical activity and relay electrical impulses from the generator back to the heart. In the young, we implant pacemakers in the abdomen. In older children, we place pacemakers beneath the clavicle. Surgeons attach pacemaker leads to the outside of the heart (epicardial leads), or electrophysiologists place leads inside the heart (transvenous leads). Lead placements depend on the child's size, with epicardial systems usually in younger children and transvenous systems more often in older children.

As seen in the figure below, implantable cardioverter defibrillators (ICDs) have all pacemaker functions, with the additional capability to treat arrhythmias like ventricular tachycardia. ICDs can pace, sense, and shock (defibrillate). We can program ICDs to pace the heart quickly in an

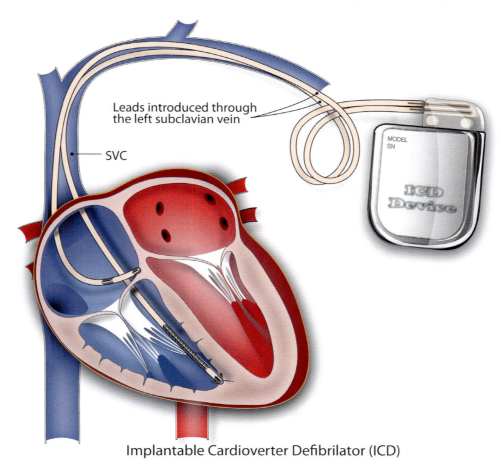

Implantable Cardioverter Defibrilator (ICD)

attempt to terminate an arrhythmia before the device delivers a shock. Pacemakers or ICDs may be single chamber with electrodes to 1 cardiac chamber for sensing and pacing, or dual chamber with electrodes to an atrium and a ventricle. We abbreviate pacemaker nomenclature, for example, DDD or VVI. The 1st letter in the abbreviation represents the chamber paced, the 2nd letter the chamber sensed, and the 3rd letter signifies the pacemaker's response to intrinsic cardiac electrical activity. For DDD pacing (**D**ual pacing, **D**ual sensing, **D**ual inhibiting or triggering), the device paces the atrium and the ventricle, senses the atrium and the ventricle for intrinsic cardiac electrical activity, which inhibits the device (when not needed) or triggers the device (when needed). For VVI pacing (**V**entricle paced, **V**entricle sensed, and sensing **I**nhibits the pacemaker), the device only paces the ventricle, only senses the ventricle, and the ventricle's intrinsic electrical activity inhibits the device (when not needed). More letters for pacemaker nomenclature may appear. For simplicity, however, we limit the description to the first 3 letters. [10-13]

INDICATIONS

Pacemaker Placement

The recommendations for pacemaker placement are in published guidelines from the American College of Cardiology, the American Heart Association, and the Heart Rhythm Society. Controversy exists for some relative pacing indications. For simplicity, we list the undisputed Class I indications for implantation. These indications include the following:

- **Advanced 2nd- or 3rd-degree AV block (AVB)**

Particularly, advanced AV block with symptomatic bradycardia, ventricular dysfunction, or low cardiac output.

- **Sinus node dysfunction**

Especially with symptoms during age-inappropriate bradycardia (low heart rate varies by age).

- **Postoperative advanced 2nd- or 3rd-degree AVB**

Particularly AV block persisting for at least 7 days postoperatively.

- **Congenital 3rd-degree AVB**

Block with a wide-QRS escape rhythm, complex ventricular ectopy, ventricular dysfunction, infants with ventricular rates < 50 to 55 bpm, or infants with congenital heart disease and ventricular rates < 70 bpm.

- **Sustained pause-dependent VT**

Ventricular tachycardia, with or without long QT syndrome, with documented pacing efficacy.

- **Cardiac resynchronization therapy**

For patients with all of the following: (1) Poor heart function, (2) QRS duration > 120 ms, (3) Sinus rhythm, and (4) New York Heart Association class IV heart failure on optimal medical therapy.

ICD Placement

The following indications are the recommendation of the American College of Cardiology, the American Heart Association, and the Heart Rhythm Society:

- **Survivors of cardiac arrest**

Cardiac arrest from ventricular fibrillation (VF) or hemodynamically unstable sustained ventricular tachycardia following an evaluation to define the event and to exclude any reversible causes.

- **Structural heart disease**

Structural heart disease with spontaneous sustained VT, whether hemodynamically stable or not.

- **Syncope**

Syncope of undetermined origin with clinically relevant, hemodynamically significant sustained VT or VF induced during an EP procedure.

FOLLOW-UP

Pacemakers & ICDs

Pacemakers and ICDs need close followup with regularly scheduled device evaluations that pediatric cardiologists or pediatric electrophysiologists supervise. We list the common problems and concerns below:

- Acute wound infections that can track back to the heart
- Lead dislodgment
- Lead fracture
- Battery depletion
- Avoidance of magnets like MRI scanners
- Avoidance of high-energy electrical fields including chain saws, arc welders, & radio transmitters
- Avoid contact sports
- Other sports at discretion of a pediatric cardiologist
- Hold cell phones & small electronic devices 6" from pacemaker
- Microwave ovens & X-rays are safe
- Airport metal detectors ok but patients should carry pacemaker ID cards

REFERENCES

1 Dick M. Clinical Cardiac Electrophysiology in the Young. Boston, Springer Science Business Media, 2006

2 Gillette PC, Reitman MJ, Gutgesell HP, Vargo TA, Mullins CE, McNamara DG. Intracardiac electrography in children and young adults. Am Heart J 1975: 89: 36-44

3 Forssman W. Experiments on Myself: Memoirs of a Surgeon in Germany. New York, St. Martin's Press, 1972

4 Dick M 2nd, Law IH, Dorostkar PC, Armstrong B, Reppert C. Use of the His/RVA electrode catheter in children. J Electrocardiol 1996; 29 Suppl: 227-233

5 Law IH, Fischbach PS, LeRoy S, Lloyd TR, Rocchini AP, Dick M. Access to the left atrium for delivery of radiofrequency ablation in young patients: retrograde aortic vs transseptal approach. Cardiol 2001; 22: 204-209

6 Makhoul M, Von Bergen NH, Rabi F, Gingerich J, Evans WN, Law IH. Successful transcatheter cryoablation in infants with drug-resistant supraventricular tachycardia: a case series. Interv Card Electrophysiol 2010; 29: 209-215

7 Von Bergen NH, Abu Rasheed H, Law IH. Transcatheter cryoablation with 3-D mapping of an atrial ectopic tachycardia in a pediatric patient with tachycardia induced heart failure. J Interv Card Electrophysiol 2007; 18: 273-279

8 Law IH, Von Bergen NH, Gingerich JC, Saarel EV, Fischbach PS, Dick M 2nd. Transcatheter cryothermal ablation of junctional ectopic tachycardia in the normal heart. Rhythm 2006; 3: 903-907

9 Thomas V, Lawrence D, Kogon B, Frias P. Epicardial ablation of ventricular tachycardia in a child on venoarterial extracorporeal membrane oxygenation. Pediatr Cardiol 2010; 31: 901-904

10 Lawrence D, Von Bergen N, Law IH, Bradley DJ, Dick M 2nd, Frias PA, Streiper MJ, Fischbach PS. Inappropriate ICD discharges in single-chamber versus dual-chamber devices in the pediatric and young adult population. J Cardiovasc Electrophysiol 2009; 20: 287-29

11 Atkins DL, Scott WA, Blaufox AD, Law IH, Dick M 2nd, Geheb F, Sobh J, Brewer JE. Sensitivity and specificity of an automated external defibrillator algorithm designed for pediatric patients. Resuscitation 2008; 76: 168-174

12 Epstein AE, DiMarco JP, Ellenbogen KA, et al. ACC/AHA/HRS 2008 Guidelines for Device-Based Therapy of Cardiac Rhythm Abnormalities: a report of the American College of Cardiology/American Heart Association Task Force on Practice Guidelines (Writing Committee to Revise the ACC/AHA/NASPE 2002 Guideline Update for Implantation of Cardiac Pacemakers and Antiarrhythmia Devices) developed in collaboration with the American Association for Thoracic Surgery and Society of Thoracic Surgeons. J Am Coll Cardiol 2008; 51: e1-e 62.

13 Von Bergen NH, Atkins DL, Dick M 2nd, Bradley DJ, Etheridge SP, Saarel EV, Fischbach PS, Balaji S, Sreeram N, Evans WN, Law IH. Multicenter study of the effectiveness of implantable cardioverter defibrillators in children and young adults with heart disease. Pediatr Cardiol 2011; 32: 399-405

26 Electrophysiology Pacemakers & ICDs

27 Cardiovascular Surgery

Contents

Background	429
Procedure Descriptions	432
Operative Terms	446
Postoperative Care	449

27 Cardiovascular Surgery

michael ciccolo • gary mayman

BACKGROUND

In 1896, the prominent London surgeon Stephen Paget wrote, "Surgery of the heart has probably reached the limits set by nature; no new method and no new discovery can overcome the natural difficulties that attend a wound of the heart." Nonetheless, in a 1902 Lancet article, the London physician Lauder Brunton described his experiments on dead animals where he detailed a credible surgical method for manually dilating stenotic mitral valves. In another set of live-animal experiments, Brunton noted the heart's surprising resiliency during open-chest handling. He recommended further investigations. The Lancet sharply criticized Brunton's visionary ideas by writing, "Sir Lauder Brunton would have been better advised to have himself completed his experiments, even at considerable inconvenience, rather than incite others to pursue a path into the unknown which must be beset with very grave difficulties and responsibility."

Similar to Brunton's animal experiments, surgeons performed the first intracardiac operations in humans by passing their finger or a dilating instrument into the beating heart to force open a stenotic valve. In July of 1912, Paris surgeon Théodore Tuffier undertook the world's first such surgery. Tuffier opened the chest and used his finger to dilate a stenotic aortic valve. Miraculously, the patient survived. A few months after Tuffier's first successful surgery, Eugène Louis Doyen, again in France, attempted surgery on a 27-year-old patient thought to have valvular pulmonic stenosis. The patient died within hours. An autopsy revealed anatomy consistent with tetralogy of Fallot, rather than simple valvular pulmonic stenosis, explaining the poor outcome. Following World War I, Elliot Cutler in Boston, Evarts Graham in St. Louis, and Henry Souttar in London also performed a handful of valve dilation procedures.

Before 1938, surgery for children with cardiovascular malformations did not exist. Nonetheless, visionaries dreamed of possible corrective procedures. In 1907, Boston surgeon John Munro proposed a patent ductus arteriosus ligation. Robert Gross, at Boston Children's Hospital, finally carried out the first successful patent ductus arteriosus ligation 3 decades later in August of 1938. Six years later at Johns Hopkins in November of 1944, Alfred Blalock, assisted by Vivien Thomas and inspired by Helen Taussig, performed the first systemic-to-pulmonary artery shunt for tetralogy of Fallot. Other surgeries followed such as repairs for coarctation of the aorta and vascular rings. A decade and a half later, following the end of World War II and rapid technological advances, surgeons commenced open-heart surgery, first for congenital defects and later for coronary artery disease.

Advances in surgery for cardiovascular malformations have continued into the 21st century. The current era demonstrates an evolving collaboration between cardiac surgeons and interventional cardiologists. Together, surgeons and cardiologists can accomplish treatment with hybrid procedures. Hybrid procedures combine surgical palliation with interventional catheterization. Newborn hybrid procedures' major benefit is avoiding cardiopulmonary bypass (CPB) in small, ill infants. The hybrid procedure reduces risk by postponing surgical procedures that require CPB until infants are beyond the newborn period.

Ultimately, treatment depends on whether the heart has 2-functional ventricles, 1 to pump blood to the lungs and 1 to the body, or 1-functional ventricle that provides the force to circulate blood through the lungs and the body. We use the term, "functional ventricle," as some hearts have additional hypoplastic ventricular chambers too small to function as a pumping chamber for the body or the lungs. The successful treatment of hearts with 1-functional ventricle or 2 ventricles also relies on the anatomy of the pulmonary circulation, pulmonary veins, systemic veins, systemic circulation, and other cardiovascular malformations.

The short- and long-term treatment goals include using the best methods, with the least risk, to achieve an optimum result. With 2 ventricles, the surgical approach is either an effective primary repair or an approach including 1 or more staged procedures that leads to an effective repair. Nonetheless, some hearts with 2 ventricles have complicated malformations rendering an initial complete repair difficult to achieve. Further, patients having undergone an initial successful 2-ventricle repair may require future procedures such as conduit replacements or artificial valves. In contrast, all hearts with 1-functional ventricle require a series of staged palliative procedures, as no current method for initial complete anatomic repair is available.

Despite the best surgical correction or palliation, some patients may go on to develop end-stage heart failure, sometimes leading to cardiac transplantation. Also, primary cardiac transplantation continues to play a role for extraordinarily complex heart disease, where an attempt at surgical correction or palliation would be ineffective or pose an unacceptably high operative risk. [1-6]

Treatment Approaches

The most common conditions include those with 2 ventricles that lend themselves to complete correction such as a patent ductus arteriosus (PDA), most ventricular septal defects (VSD), atrial septal defects (ASD), valvular regurgitation, pulmonic or aortic stenosis, and coarctation of the aorta (CoA) with or without a VSD. A PDA requires surgical ligation or division or device closure. For VSDs, most require surgical patch closure; although, device closure is available for some VSDs. Many secundum ASDs are closable with a device; whereas, most large secundum ASDs and ASDs in other locations usually need surgery. Valvular regurgitation may be amenable to valve repair; nonetheless, some require replacement with a tissue or mechanical valve. Typical valvular pulmonic and aortic stenosis can usually be ballooned; however, surgery plays a role for some valvular stenosis and most supra- and subvalvular stenosis. Some CoAs can undergo catheter intervention; nevertheless, certain types of CoAs and CoA with VSD need surgical resection, plus or minus VSD patch closure. As all these procedures are straightforward, we do not illustrate them in the following figures.

Some complex conditions with 2 ventricles are also amenable to primary repair that may require septal patch closures, sometimes additional primary arterial or venous vessel surgery, and occasionally repair or replacement of cardiac valves. Such conditions include some interrupted aortic arch with VSDs, some tetralogy of Fallots, most forms of total anomalous pulmonary venous return, some double outlet right ventricles, some Ebstein anomalies, pulmonary arteriovenous malformations, and vascular rings. As these procedures are also usually straightforward, we do not illustrate them.

Except for conditions like D-transposition of the great arteries (with or without a VSD), complex congenital heart disease often requires a staged treatment approach. Staging implies > 1 procedure usually performed over a defined period of time. Staged procedures may be combinations of surgical and cardiac interventional procedures. Frequently, staged procedures require the placement of artificial material beyond standard septal defect patches. Such artificial material may include additional patch placements, conduits, artificial valves, and devices placed by cardiac intervention.

Illustrations

The following figures illustrate procedures primarily used in staged treatment approaches and initial primary repairs of complex malformations. In order, the illustrations include palliative systemic-to-pulmonary artery shunts; palliative pulmonary artery bands; procedures for repairing tetralogy of Fallot; the arterial switch operation for D-transposition of the great arteries; the Rastelli procedure for truncus arteriosus and some forms of double outlet right ventricle; staged palliation of 1-functional ventricle hearts with normal systemic flow; and staged palliation of 1-functional ventricle hearts with abnormal systemic flow.

PROCEDURE DESCRIPTIONS & ILLUSTRATIONS

Shunts & Pulmonary Artery Bands

Systemic-to-pulmonary artery shunts and pulmonary artery bands play central roles in palliating complex congenital heart disease through the control of pulmonary blood flow, whether the malformation is associated with restricted or excessive pulmonary flow.

In most patients with tetralogy of Fallot and in those with other conditions that have obstruction to pulmonary blood flow, an alternative source of blood flow to the lungs may be needed, particularly if a complete repair is either not possible or high risk. Figure A on the facing page illustrates a "classic" Blalock-Taussig (BT) shunt, accomplished by connecting the right subclavian artery to the right pulmonary artery. However, a classic BT shunt disrupts the subclavian artery and renders the affected arm pulseless. Currently, as in figure B on the facing page, surgeons usually create systemic-to-pulmonary artery shunts using Gore-Tex® graft tubes that they anastomose between a systemic artery and a pulmonary artery, creating a "modified" BT shunt. A Gore-Tex® shunt does not interrupt the subclavian artery. Alternatively, an interventional cardiologist could place a stent in the ductus arteriosus to create a systemic-to-pulmonary artery shunt without surgery. Also, rather than a systemic artery, a systemic vein (the superior vena cava) can also be anastomosed to the right pulmonary artery (Glenn procedure) to deliver more blood flow to the lungs in the face of obstructed flow. We illustrate and discuss Glenn procedures in the next section.

In contrast to conditions that have obstructed flow to the lungs, some malformations may have excessive pulmonary blood flow (figure C on the facing page), which leads to pulmonary overcirculation and congestive heart failure. Also, excessive pulmonary blood flow is often accompanied by elevated pulmonary arterial pressure, which if left unregulated often leads to irreversible pulmonary hypertension. Thus, banding the pulmonary artery (figure D on the facing page) regulates pulmonary blood by reducing excessive flow and reducing elevated pressure, until a more definitive procedure can be performed.

27 Cardiovascular Surgery

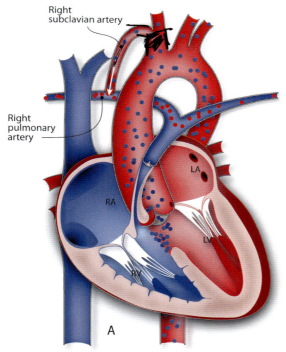

A
Tetralogy of Fallot
Classic Blalock-Taussig Shunt

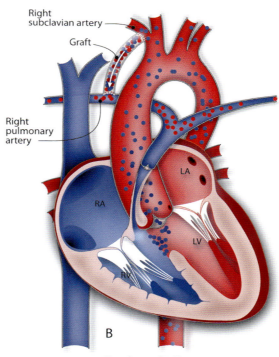

B
Tetralogy of Fallot
Modified Blalock-Taussig Shunt

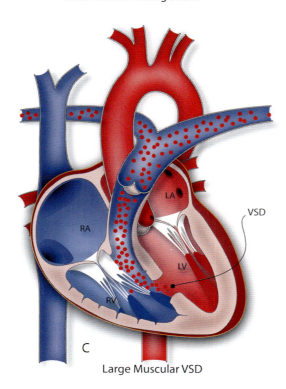

C
Large Muscular VSD

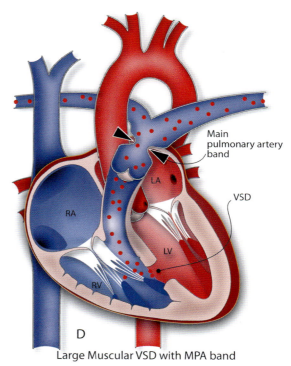

D
Large Muscular VSD with MPA band

Repair of Tetralogy of Fallot

Tetralogy of Fallot (ToF) is a common complex cardiac malformation with a wide spectrum of severity (figure on the right). When pulmonic stenosis is mild, repair is straightforward and includes a patch VSD closure and surgical relief of mild pulmonic stenosis without the need for additional pulmonary artery patching or use of artificial materials like right ventricle-to-pulmonary artery (RV-to-PA) conduits. However, some forms of ToF have severe pulmonic stenosis that may extend from the subvalvular to the supravalvular location and even include diminutive branch pulmonary arteries.

Patients with severe ToF usually need a staged approach that includes an initial modified BT shunt or a newborn patent ductus arteriosus stent, placed by an interventional cardiologist, to provide an additional stable source of pulmonary blood flow. Later, a second surgery may include a VSD patch closure, extensive resection of areas of pulmonic stenosis and patching of the right ventricular outflow tract (figure A on the facing page). Further, some forms of ToF require an RV-to-PA conduit when the pulmonary artery is too small to use in an effective repair (figure B on the facing page). After a second procedure, a third procedure may be needed to replace the RV-to-PA conduit with a larger one to keep up with somatic growth. Currently, patients with failing RV-to-PA conduits may also be candidates for the placements of artificial pulmonary valves through interventional cardiac catheterization procedures.

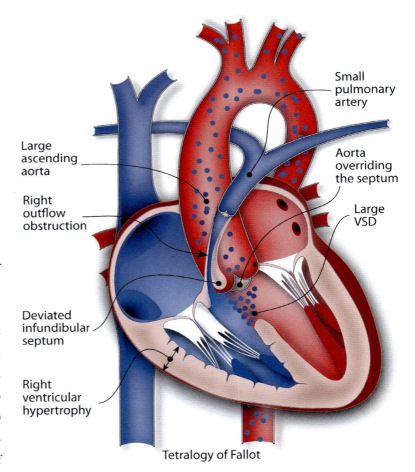

Tetralogy of Fallot

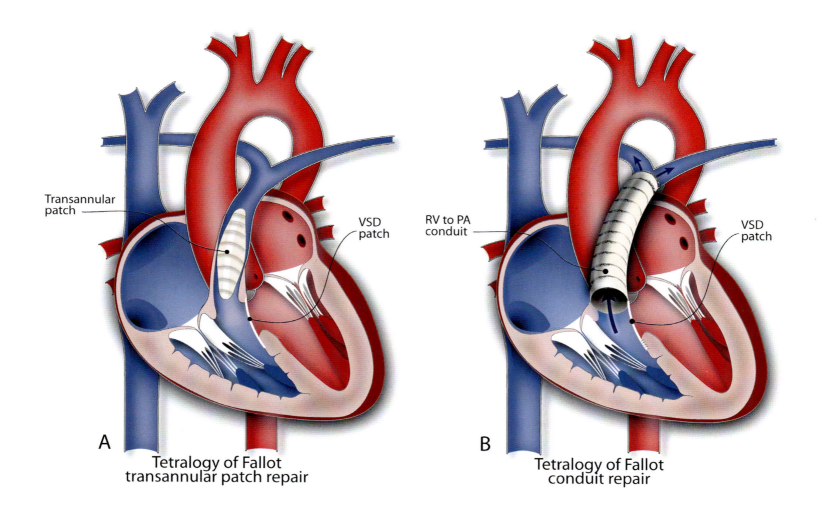

Repair of D-Transposition of the Great Arteries

D-transposition of the great arteries (D-TGA) with an intact ventricular septum (figure below) is a complex cardiac malformation that is amenable to a complete anatomic repair in the newborn period. Prior to successful arterial switch operations, "correction" was accomplished by switching the direction of the systemic and pulmonary venous returns.

Prior to the late 1970s and early 1908s, surgeons used the Senning or Mustard procedure (figures A and B on the facing page) to reroute desaturated systemic venous return to the left ventricle (1 and 2 in figure A), which pumps to the lungs, and reroute saturated pulmonary venous blood to the right ventricle (3 in figure A), which pumps to the body. The basic problem with the "venous switch" procedure was that the patient was left with an anatomic right ventricle to pump blood to the body, and the RV often failed over time. Currently, there is a significant population of adults in their 30s and older who underwent venous switch operations and require longterm follow-up, as such patients often have ongoing cardiac problems.

The "arterial switch," or Jatene procedure, allows for the the morphological left ventricle to become the correct, life-long systemic ventricle, by surgically switching the great arteries to their appropriate ventricles (figures C and D on the facing page). Patients undergoing an arterial switch do not develop systemic ventricular failure like patients with Senning or Mustard procedures. Nonetheless, the fundamental problem that faced early surgeons attempting the arterial switch operation was the delicate nature of transferring the coronary arteries. The coronary arteries embryologically develop from the aorta even when it is transposed to the right ventricle. The coronary arteries must be successfully translocated to the "neoaorta" now arising from the left ventricle. Abnormal coronaries increase surgical risk. Currently, surgical techniques allow for successful arterial switch operations in the vast majority of newborns.

D-TGA can also occur with additional cardiac malformations such as VSDs, pulmonic stenosis, and myriad others. Additional malformations increase the risk and complexity of the repair. Some patients with transposition of the great arteries and associated complex malformations require a staged approach, rather than a primary repair.

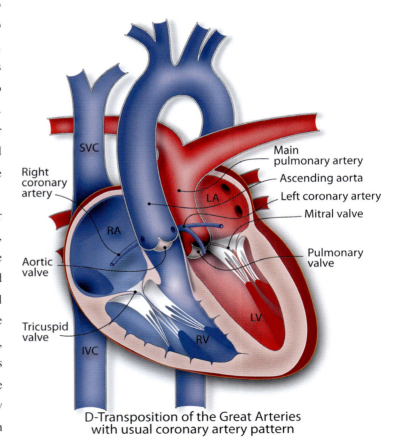

D-Transposition of the Great Arteries with usual coronary artery pattern

27 Cardiovascular Surgery

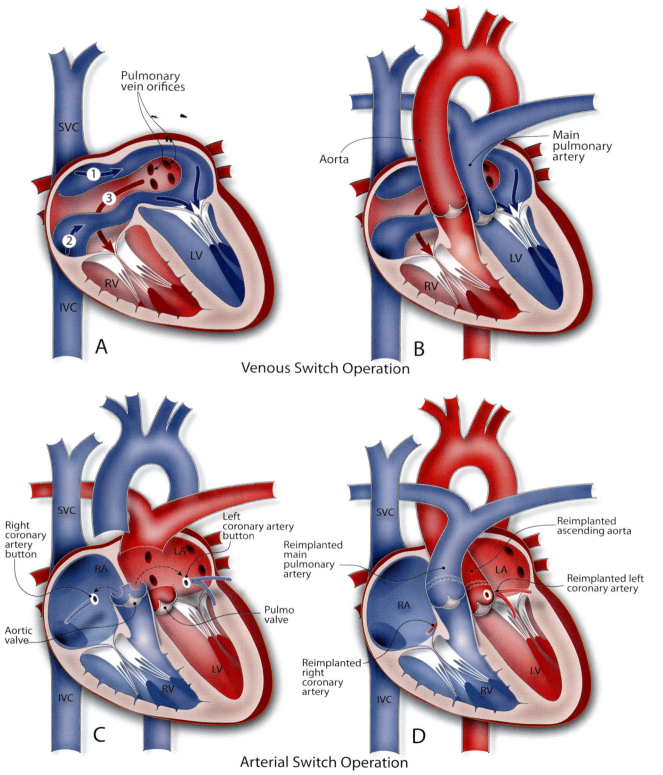

Venous Switch Operation

Arterial Switch Operation

437

Repair of Truncus Arteriosus & Double Outlet Right Ventricle

All forms of truncus arteriosus (figure A on the facing page) and many forms of double outlet right ventricle require a repair that includes a long intracardiac VSD patch, which connects the left ventricle with a somewhat anterior and rightward positioned aorta. In addition, especially in truncus, an RV-to-PA conduit is needed between the right ventricle and the pulmonary arteries. The combination of the long intracardiac patch and an RV-to-PA conduit is called a Rastelli procedure (figures B and C on the facing page).

Over time, depending on the patient's age at the time of the the first procedure, additional conduit replacement surgeries are likely needed to keep up with somatic growth. Also, in some patients, the long outflow from the left ventricle to the aorta occasionally becomes narrowed and further surgery is needed to revise the intracardiac patch. Subsequent RV-to-PA conduits, which fail over time, are often also amenable to placement of stents and valves by cardiac catheterization interventional procedures.

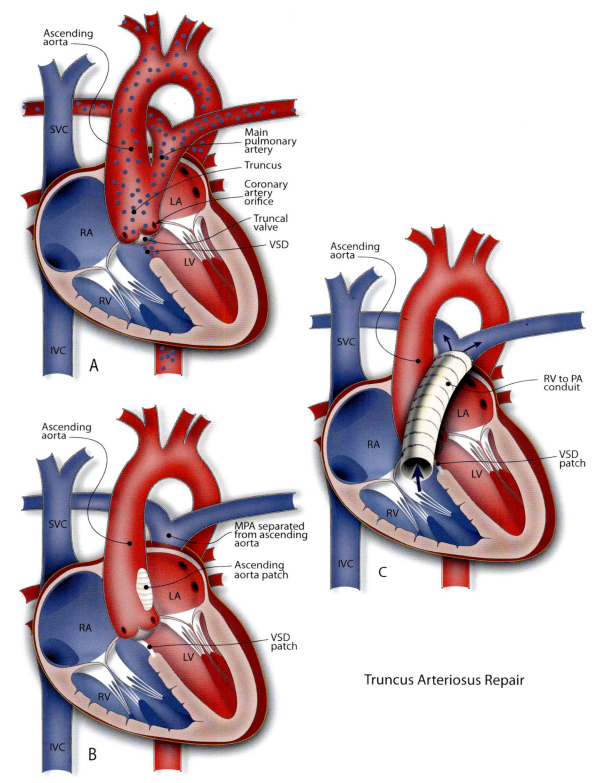

Truncus Arteriosus Repair

Staged Palliation for 1-Functional Ventricles

Hearts with 1-functional ventricle require staged palliation. The goals of staged palliation include protecting the pulmonary circulation, ensuring unobstructed systemic flow, and preserving the 1-functional ventricle as the pump for the body. As there is no effective pump for the pulmonary circulation, staged palliation includes rerouting the systemic venous return via direct connections of the superior and inferior vena cavas to the pulmonary arteries. The lack of a pump to the lungs results in predominately "passive" blood flow through the lungs. Passive flow occurs best when the pulmonary arteries are normal size and the pulmonary artery vascularity is normal. Any pulmonary artery abnormalities impair the ease of blood flow through the lungs.

In addition to passive flow, the ventricle does exert some negative pressure during diastole when the ventricle actually "pulls" or "sucks" blood through the lungs. Good ventricular function, therefore, is also important to the success of effective staged palliation. With ventricular dysfunction, the ventricular end-diastolic pressure is high, which may eliminate the ventricles's ability to pull blood through the lungs.

Conditions usually fall into 2 categories: 1) Malformations associated with normal systemic blood flow but either excessive or restricted pulmonary blood flow, and 2) Conditions with impaired systemic blood flow but usually with unimpaired pulmonary flow. Palliation consists of 3 stages. Stage 1 involves controlling pulmonary blood flow and ensuring good systemic flow. Stage 2 begins the process of connecting the systemic venous return directly to the pulmonary arteries (superior vena cava to the pulmonary arteries or the Glenn procedure). Stage 3 completes the direct connection of the remaining systemic venous return to the lungs (the inferior vena cava to the pulmonary arteries or modified Fontan). We preserve the 1-functional ventricle to pump blood to the body, leaving no chamber to pump blood to the lungs.

1-Functional ventricles with normal systemic flow

Tricuspid atresia (the condition illustrated in the series of figures on the facing page) is an example of a 1-functional ventricle heart with normal systemic flow. In tricuspid atresia, the right ventricle is usually hypoplastic. Because complex congenital heart disease can occur with unusual situs and dextrocardia, "right" ventricles may neither be on the right nor even have the appearance of a normal right ventricle; thus, some prefer the term "pulmonary ventricle." Despite a hypoplastic right (or pulmonary) ventricle, the pulmonary blood flow may be excessive if a large VSD is present, as in figure A on the facing page, or restricted with pulmonic stenosis, as in figure B on the facing page.

Stage 1

For excessive pulmonary blood flow, stage 1 consists of placing a pulmonary artery band, as per figure C on the facing page. For restricted pulmonary flow, stage 1 consists of placing a systemic-to-pulmonary artery shunt (modified B-T shunt), as per figure D on the facing page. Sometimes a pulmonary artery band is combined with a systemic-to-pulmonary artery shunt, when surgical planning calls for a tight band that results in too little pulmonary blood flow without the addition of a shunt. We perform stage 1 procedures in newborns.

27 Cardiovascular Surgery

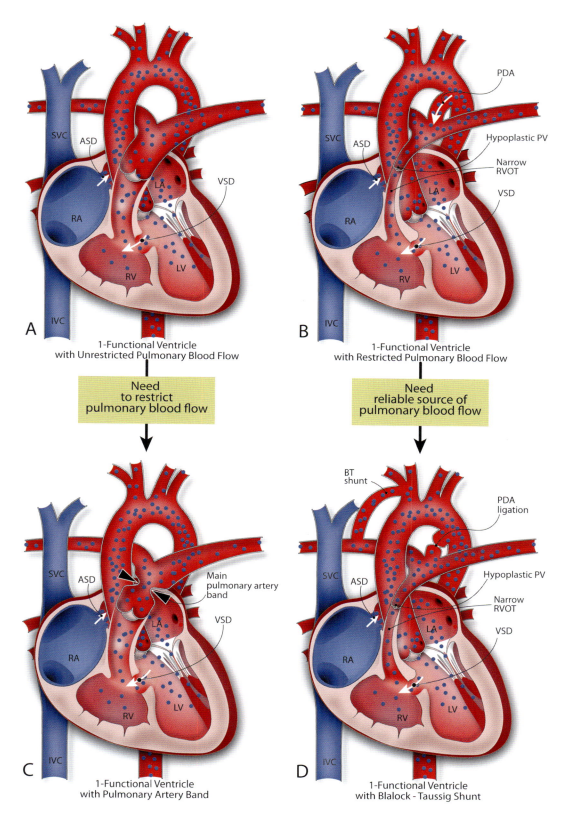

441

Stage 2

Usually, we perform stage 2 palliation at about 6 months old. Sometimes clinical circumstances require an earlier stage 2 procedure. Also, some patients' clinical findings delay this stage beyond 6 months. On occasion, a patient's anatomy and physiology preclude proceeding to stage 2 or stage 3.

• Glenn procedure

For either a banded or shunted patient, a Glenn shunt (facing page figures A and B) is the connection of the systemic venous return from the upper body (the superior vena cava or SVC) directly to the lungs. Usually at the time of the Glenn, we also divide the main pulmonary artery (figures A and B on the facing page) to eliminate any forward flow from the heart, allowing only desaturated blood to enter the pulmonary arteries via the Glenn shunt. Additional saturated blood from the heart, reentering the lungs, is of no benefit.

Also, to function properly, a Glenn shunt requires a low pulmonary arterial pressure and low pulmonary vascular resistance. Pulmonary vascular resistance falls over time from birth. Thus, a Glenn shunt cannot be successfully used for a stage 1 procedure in newborns. Having served its purpose, we take down the systemic-to-pulmonary artery shunt during the stage 2 Glenn procedure.

• Kawashima procedure (not illustrated)

With the presence of an interrupted inferior vena cava connecting to the superior vena cava via an azygos vein, the modified Glenn procedure becomes a Kawashima procedure.

Stage 3

Stage 3 consists of a modified Fontan procedure at about 2 to 3 years old. A modified Fontan (figure C on the facing page) includes connecting the lower body systemic venous return (inferior vena cava) to the lungs. We use the term "modified Fontan" procedure, because the procedures we use now differ substantially from Fontan's original description. Following stage 3, all the systemic venous return enters the lungs and the 1-functional ventricle pumps blood to the body.

27 Cardiovascular Surgery

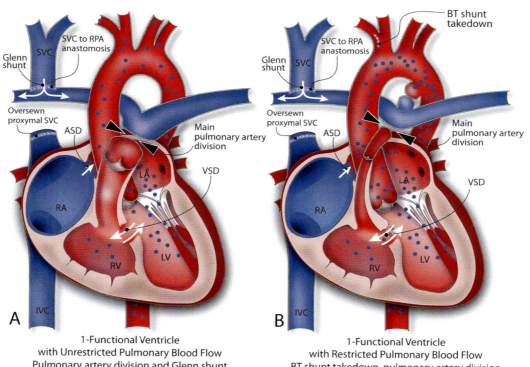

A
1-Functional Ventricle
with Unrestricted Pulmonary Blood Flow
Pulmonary artery division and Glenn shunt

B
1-Functional Ventricle
with Restricted Pulmonary Blood Flow
BT shunt takedown, pulmonary artery division
and Glenn shunt

Completion of Fontan

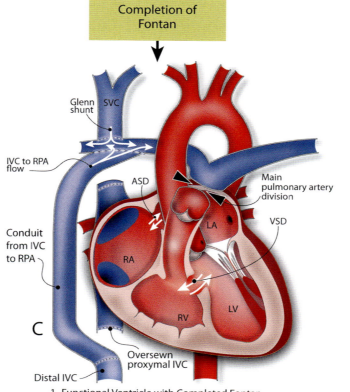

C
1- Functional Ventricle with Completed Fontan

443

27 Cardiovascular Surgery

1-Functional ventricles with abnormal systemic flow

This group of malformations is typified by the hypoplastic left heart syndrome (HLHS), which we illustrate in figure A on the facing page. In the presence of a patent ductus arteriosus (PDA), systemic flow is maintained. When the PDA closes, the patient succumbs quickly.

Stage 1

This anatomical substrate requires a Norwood procedure (figure B on the facing page), a Norwood with the Sano modification (not illustrated), or a hybrid procedure (see Chapter 25) to maintain systemic flow through aortic arch reconstruction in the Norwood or Sano and through a PDA stent in the hybrid procedure. Further, with the Norwood, pulmonary flow is regulated via a modified BT shunt and in a Sano with a right ventricle-to-pulmonary artery shunt. With the hybrid approach, pulmonary flow is regulated by bilateral pulmonary artery banding.

Some patients may not be good candidates for any of the stage 1 procedures. Poor candidates may include those whose hearts have significant risk factors including poor right ventricular function, unrepairable tricuspid regurgitation, and serious coronary artery abnormalities. Patients with these conditions often require heart transplantation.

Stage 2

For those that underwent a Norwood with or without a Sano modification, stage 2 consists of placing a Glenn shunt (SVC to RPA connection in figure C on the facing page). For patients that underwent a previous hybrid procedure for HLHS, as newborns, we perform the Glenn procedure along with aortic arch repair.

Stage 3

Similar to the previous example, a modified Fontan procedure constitutes stage 3 (figure D on the facing page). Following the modified Fontan procedure, all the oxygenated blood is pumped to body (1 in figure D) and all the systemic venous return enters the lungs (2 and 3 in figure D)

27 Cardiovascular Surgery

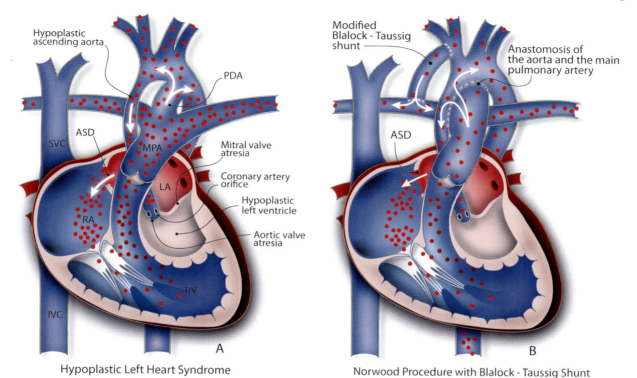

Hypoplastic Left Heart Syndrome

Norwood Procedure with Blalock - Taussig Shunt

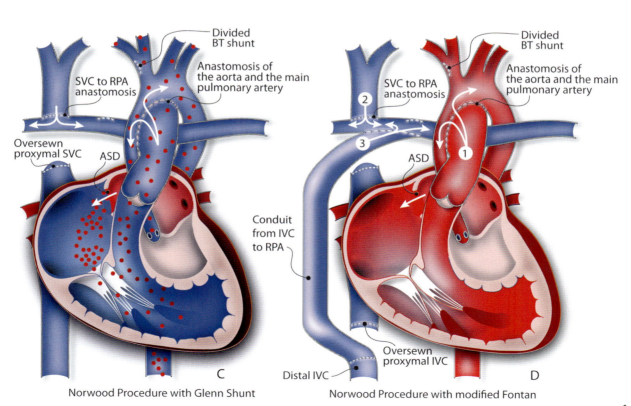

Norwood Procedure with Glenn Shunt

Norwood Procedure with modified Fontan

445

OPERATIVE TERMS

Cardiopulmonary Bypass

Cardiopulmonary bypass (CPB) is an artificial means of cardiopulmonary oxygenation and perfusion via mechanical equipment.

Initiation

- **Vascular cannulation**

We place cannulas in the vena cavas to drain blood from the body and send the blood to a mechanical pump and oxygenator, after which the blood returns to the body via another cannula we place in the aorta (facing page figure).

- **Hemodilution**

We establish hemodilution by priming the pump with a low hematocrit solution. Hemodilution decreases the viscosity of blood and vascular resistance, augmenting capillary perfusion at low flow rates.

- **Anticoagulation**

We use anticoagulation to prevent extravascular coagulation in the bypass circuit, most often with heparin but occasionally with other agents [7].

- **Ventilation**

Once we establish CPB, ventilation is no longer necessary.

- **Aortic cross-clamp**

Prevents back flow of blood into the left ventricle.

- **Cardioplegia & myocardial protection**

We provide for myocardial protection from ischemia by injecting cold (4° C) cardioplegia into the aortic root or coronary arteries. The cardioplegia solution includes a high potassium concentration solution that arrests the heart and decreases myocardial oxygen consumption.

- **Venting**

Venting prevents chamber distention and myocardial damage arising when the heart cannot handle blood return such as during cooling, ventricular fibrillation, aortic cross-clamping, and administration of cardioplegia. Venting also prevents cardiac ejection of air and facilitates surgical exposure.

Weaning

- **Ultrafiltration**

We may perform ultrafiltration (UF) at the end of CPB. UF removes excessive plasma water and removes some low molecular weight solutes like inflammatory factors.

- **Mechanical actions**

We de-air the heart and remove the aortic cross-clamp.

- **Normalize physiology**

We rewarm, normalize electrolytes, ionized calcium, and arterial blood gases. Then we progressively reduce bypass flows, and we administer protamine to counter heparin once off bypass.

- **Evaluate results**

We check the heart's function and the repair's status with transesophageal echocardiography.

Hypothermia & Circulatory Arrest

Hypothermia

Preserves organ function by decreasing metabolic demands during low circulatory flow with CPB, and provides an

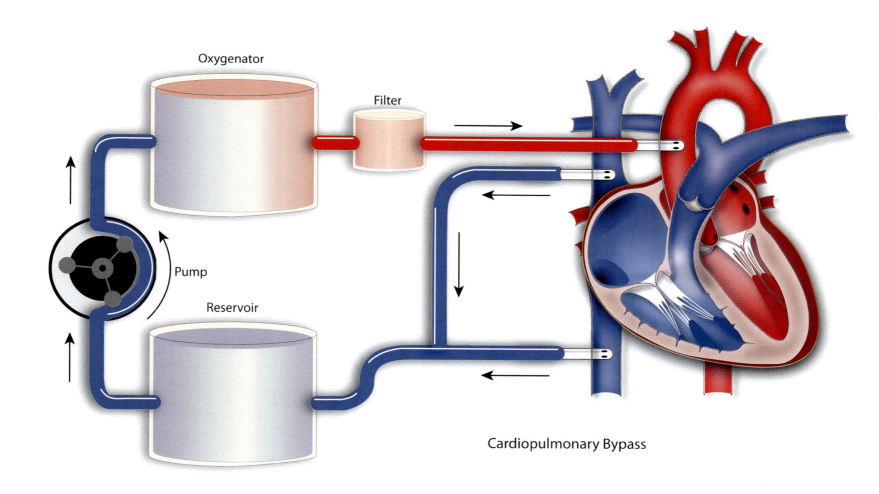

environment for myocardial protection during myocardial ischemia.
- Moderate hypothermia at 20 to 25° C
- Deep hypothermia at 18 to 20° C

Circulatory arrest

Cessation of CPB can occur with hypothermia. Cessation of CPB allows removal of intracardiac cannulas, creating an unobstructed operative field.
- Up to 60 minutes at temperatures ≤ 20° C
- May increase myocardial & CNS complications

POSTOPERATIVE CARE

Whether a surgical procedure is closed-heart or open-heart, postoperative evaluation is similar; although, monitoring devices and pharmacological agents vary. Cardiac surgery frequently results in a temporary impairment in the heart's ability to pump blood effectively, negatively impacting cardiac output (CO). Therefore, most postoperative patients frequently require inotropic support. Nevertheless, the expected outcome is improving cardiac function. If monitoring suggests a declining cardiac output, then the patient needs quick attention and therapeutic intervention. Prompt attention improves outcome.

Exam

Initial postoperative and ongoing physical exam findings:
- Temperature, pulse, respiratory rate, & blood pressure
- Note the skin as pink, cyanotic, or pale
- Extremities for warmth & good perfusion
- Pulses palpable, increased, or decreased
- Breath sounds, wheezes, or rales
- Precordial activity, murmurs, or rubs
- Presence of hepatomegaly

Patient Support

Monitoring equipment, lines, & tubes
- EKG monitor
- Pulse oximeter
- Nasogastric tube for stomach decompression
- Arterial line for blood pressure & blood samples
- Central venous pressure monitoring
- Pulmonary artery line if pulmonary hypertension
- Temporary epicardial pacemaker wires
- Foley catheter
- Chest tubes & mediastinal tubes

Ventilation

We may extubate stable patients in the operating room. However, some postoperative patients require ventilation with relative respiratory acidosis to keep pulmonary vascular resistance high, while others require a relative respiratory alkalosis to keep the pulmonary vascular resistance low. Important ventilation points include the following:
- Endotracheal tube size & proper placement
- Ventilation for stable, physiological blood gases
- Wean from ventilation & extubate quickly

Enhancing inotropy & cardiac output

Use inotropes judiciously, as excessive inotropic dosing can cause excessive myocardial oxygen utilization and subendocardial ischemia that worsens myocardial function. We include medication doses in Appendix C.

- **Dopamine**

Besides inotropic action, low dose dopamine can improve renal blood flow.

- **Dobutamine**

This agent does not improve renal flow like low dose dopamine.

- **Milrinone**

Milrinone is a weak inotrope, but the medication also produces salutary vasodilation and afterload reduction.

27 Cardiovascular Surgery

- Calcium

Low ionized calcium causes myocardial systolic dysfunction; excessive calcium may cause diastolic dysfunction.

- Epinephrine

Powerful inotrope and chronotrope (affect heart rate), especially for low CO and bradycardia. However, may cause excessive tachycardia that then may impair cardiac output.

- Norepinephrine

For increasing systemic vascular resistance (SVR) in patients with hypotension from significant vasodilation.

- Systemic vasodilators

Agents such as nitroprusside and nitroglycerin may decrease afterload improving cardiac output but can also cause significant hypotension.

Fluid balance

Capillary leak causes pulmonary edema, peripheral edema, gastrointestinal edema, and myocardial edema. Tissue edema increases postoperative morbidity and lengthens intensive care stay. Thus, the importance of early fluid restriction and diuresis with an IV furosemide infusion.

Fluid balance includes all fluid in "I" and all fluid out "O." "I" includes IV maintenance, IV fluid from medication drips, volume expanders, blood products, and oral intake if any. "O" includes urine, bleeding, chest tube drainage, insensible loss, and nasogastric tube loss if any.

Keep urine output at > 1 cc/kg/hour. Low urine output can herald low cardiac output or renal insufficiency. Quickly investigate possible causes of low urine output. Renal insufficiency may require peritoneal dialysis. Bleeding from chest tubes is significant when the flow exceeds > 10 cc/kg/hour, a bleeding rate that may indicate a coagulopathy or a persistent surgical bleeding site.

- I & O need frequent assessments
- Aim for net negative I & Os, if not hypotensive
- A net positive I & O promotes capillary leak

Pain management

Apart from obvious need for pain relief, unregulated immediate post operative pain can cause tachycardia and hypertension that can negatively impact cardiac output. Medications, among others, may include:

- Fentanyl

Immediate post operative IV drip.

- Morphine

Occasionally used, but watch for respiratory depression if not ventilated.

- Hydrocodone/acetaminophen

After immediate post-operative period for oral analgesia.

- Codeine/acetaminophen

After immediate post-operative period for oral analgesia, but less effective than hydrocodone/acetaminophen.

Diagnostic & Monitoring Studies

Echocardiogram

Either by a transesophageal (TEE) or a transthoracic approach, we preform echocardiography after most cardiac surgeries, especially intraoperatively to evaluate the immediate postoperative results. Intraoperative TEE can help the surgeon decide if additional procedures are necessary prior to transfer to the critical unit. Further, we strongly consider an Echo to evaluate any clinical change in the critical or noncritical care units. Also, all patients need an Echo before discharge to check for residual

pathology and to rule out a developing pericardial effusion from early post-pericardiotomy syndrome. Echo is excellent for the following:
- Measure cardiac function & diastolic filling
- Residual defects
- Detect pericardial effusions

EKG
- Arrhythmias
- Ischemic changes
- Metabolic changes
- Bundle branch block

Chest X-ray
- Pneumothorax & pleural effusions
- Central venous line placement
- Intracardiac lines
- Endotracheal tube placement
- Chest tube placement
- Pacing wires
- Heart size
- Pulmonary vascular markings
- Pulmonary parenchyma
- Mediastinal evaluation

Laboratory values
- Desirable lactate < 2, if rising then low CO
- CBC
- Electrolytes sodium, potassium, chloride
- Arterial blood gas
- PT, PTT, ACT, platelets
- Glucose
- Calcium & magnesium
- BUN & creatinine
- Liver function tests

Early Complications

Bleeding
Correct the known coagulopathies present after cardiopulmonary bypass including dilution of coagulation factors, platelet destruction, denaturation of coagulation factors, heparinization, and production of vasoactive peptides.

℞ options for bleeding
- Protamine to correct heparinization
- Platelets, fresh frozen plasma, or cryoprecipitate
- Consider aminocaproic acid (Amicar)
- Return to the OR, if bleeding persists

Low cardiac output
Cause of low cardiac output can be single or multifactorial. Major categories include inadequate ventilation, myocardial dysfunction, cardiac tamponade, arrhythmias, residual defects, pulmonary hypertension, and systemic hypertension.

Inadequate ventilation
- Endotracheal tube (ET) too small
- ET tube plug or displacement
- Pleural effusions, & pneumothorax
- Capillary leak & pulmonary edema
- Diaphragmatic paralysis

℞ options for inadequate ventilation
- Change ET tube if too small or plugged
- Decompress pleural effusions or pneumothorax
- Diuresis for pulmonary edema

➤Although a paralyzed diaphragm or a persistent chylothorax rarely causes immediate postoperative low cardiac output, these conditions may require treatment as a paralyzed diaphragm or persistent chylothorax may prolong assisted ventilation. A paralyzed diaphragm may need surgical plication, and a persistent chylothorax may need, drainage, nonfat nutrition, and IV octreotide.

Myocardial dysfunction
- Ischemia from CPB or surgical technique
- Hypocalcemia, especially post CPB
- Hypocalcemia with chromosome 22q11 deletion
- Hypomagnesemia
- Thromboembolic event or air embolism

℞ options for myocardial dysfunction
- Adjust inotropic support
- Decrease afterload
- Correct electrolyte abnormalities, especially calcium
- May need ECMO or ventricular assist devices

Cardiac tamponade
Surgeons may initially leave the chest open in many complex surgeries in newborns and young infants to avoid early post-operative tamponade. With a closed chest, a minimal pericardial fluid collection can cause tamponade, especially when surgery compromises cardiac function.

Signs of tamponade
- Increased central venous pressure
- Pulsus paradoxus of > 20 mm Hg on arterial line tracing or cuff blood pressure monitoring

℞ options for tamponade
- Open the chest to relieve tamponade
- Immediate pericardiocentesis

Arrhythmias
Electrolyte abnormalities, hypoxia, hypercapnea, acidosis, surgical trauma, and medications can cause or exacerbate arrhythmias. Sinus tachycardia is the most frequent post-op rhythm arising from pain, fever, hypovolemia, and excess catecholamines both endogenous and exogenous. Pathological arrhythmias can occur as fast, slow, or irregular rhythms.

Fast
- Junctional ectopic tachycardia
- Supraventricular tachycardia
- Ventricular tachycardia

Slow
- Sinus node dysfunction
- Atrioventricular block

Irregular
- Ectopics
- Frequently from indwelling lines
- No antiarrhythmics if hemodynamically insignificant

℞ options for arrhythmias
For more on arrhythmia causes and treatment, see Chapter 4.

Residual defects
- Left-to-right & right-to-left shunts
- Pressure from residual stenotic lesions
- Atrioventricular valve regurgitation
- Semilunar valve regurgitation

℞ options for residual defects
- Pharmacological adjustments
- Return to OR to repair residual defects
- Interventional cardiac catheterization

Pulmonary hypertension
- Especially in Down syndrome

- Especially postoperative large VSD or PDA
- Any condition with preoperative pulmonary HTN

℞ options for pulmonary hypertension

- Hyperventilation
- Sedation
- Nitric oxide
- Other pulmonary vasodilators

Systemic hypertension

- Unusual, as hypotension is more common
- Occasionally following coarctation repair

℞ options for systemic hypertension

- Nitroprusside
- Other IV antihypertensives
- Residual CoA may need return to OR or later balloon angioplasty

Other organ systems complications

- Intracranial hemorrhage, stroke, or air embolism
- Liver dysfunction or shock liver
- Renal failure from ATN
- Gastrointestinal bleeds, perforation, or NEC

℞ options for organ system complications

- Organ specific interventions

Infections

- Sepsis
- Preoperative illness magnified after bypass
- From wound & line infections

℞ options for infections

- Antibiotics
- Debridement & abscess drainage

REFERENCES

1 Paget S. The Surgery of the Chest. London, John Wright and Co, 1896

2 Munro JC. Ligation of the ductus arteriosus. Annals of Surgery 1907; 46: 335-338

3 Johnson SL. The History of Cardiac Surgery, 1896-1955. Baltimore, Johns Hopkins Press, 1970

4 Stark JF, De Leval M, Tsang VT. Surgery for Congenital Heart Defects. Chichester, John Wiley & Sons, 2006

5 Yasui H, Kado H, Masuda M. Cardiovascular Surgery for Congenital Heart Disease. Tokyo, Springer, 2009

6 Bacha EAM, Hijazi ZM. Hybrid procedures in pediatric cardiac surgery. Semin Thorac Cardiovasc Surg Pediatr Card Surg Ann 2005; 8: 78-85

7 Ciccolo ML, Bernstein J, Collazos JC, Acherman RJ, Restrepo H, Winters JM, Krueger J, Evans WN. Argatroban anticoagulation for cardiac surgery with cardiopulmonary bypass in an infant with double outlet right ventricle and a history of heparin-induced thrombocytopenia. Congenit Heart Dis. 2008; 3: 299-302

Appendix

Contents

A - SBE Prophylaxis — 457

B - ADD Meds & Sports Form — 461

C - Formulary — 463

D - Laboratory Values — 489

E - Eponyms — 505

F - Abbreviations — 515

A – Endocarditis Prophylaxis

AMERICAN HEART ASSOCIATION 2007 GUIDELINES*

Conditions that Need Endocarditis Prophylaxis

Congenital heart disease (CHD)

- **Unrepaired cyanotic CHD**

Including those with palliative shunts and conduits.

- **Completely repaired CHD**

For 6 months after placing prosthetic material by surgery or catheter intervention, as 6 months allows prosthetic material to endothelialize.

- **Repaired CHD with residual defects**

Residual defects near prosthetic material, as residual defects can inhibit endothelialization.

Other conditions

- History of previous endocarditis
- Prosthetic cardiac valves
- Cardiac transplantation with valvular disease

*The 2007 publication substantially reduced the number of conditions recommend for endocarditis prophylaxis compared to those contained in 1997 guidelines. Due to this change, the 2007 guidelines introduced an element of controversy regarding the selection of conditions pediatric cardiologists recommend for prophylaxis. At the time of this book's publication, a cross-section of pediatric cardiologists continue to recommend prophylaxis for some conditions removed from the 2007 recommendations such as aortic valve abnormalities and some ventricular septal defects. [2]

Procedures that Need Endocarditis Prophylaxis

- **Dental procedures**

Manipulation of the gingiva, periapical region of the teeth, or perforation of the oral mucosa.

- **Other procedures**

On respiratory tract, infected soft tissues, or infected bone.

Procedures that Do Not Need Endocarditis Prophylaxis

- **Dental procedures**

Routine anesthetic injections through noninfected tissue; dental X-rays; placing removable prosthodontic or orthodontic appliances; adjusting orthodontic appliances; placing orthodontic brackets; shedding deciduous teeth; and bleeding from trauma to the lips or oral mucosa.

- **GI or GU procedures**

Without infection or positive cultures.

A - Endocarditis Prophylaxis

Antibiotic Regimens

The table below lists the recommended oral and parenteral antibiotic regimens for both nonpenicillin sensitive and penicillin allergic individuals.

	Agent	Regimen –Single dose 30-60 minutes before procedure	
		Adults	Children
Oral	Amoxicillin	2 g	50 mg/kg
Unable to take oral medication	Ampicillin	2 g IM or IV*	50 mg/kg IM or IV
	OR		
	Cefazollin or ceftriaxone	1 g IM or IV	50 mg/kg IM or IV
Allergic to Penicillins or Ampicillin – Oral regimen	Cephalexin*†	2 g	50 mg/kg
	OR		
	Clindamycin	500 mg	20 mg/kg
	OR		
	Azithromycin or Clarithromycin	500 mg	15 mg/kg
Allergic to Penicillins or Ampicillin and unable to take oral medication	Cefazollin or ceftriaxone†	1 g IM or IV	50 mg/kg
	OR		
	Clindamycin	500 mg IM or IV	20 mg/kg

IM indicates intramuscular; IV, intravenous.
*Or other first- or second-generation oral cephalosporin in equivalent adult or pediatric dosage.
†Cephalosporins should not be used in an individual with a history of anaphylaxis, angioedema, or urticaria with penicillins or ampicillin

REFERENCES

1 Wilson W, Taubert KA, Gewitz M, et al. Prevention of infective endocarditis: guidelines from the American Heart Association. Circulation 2007; 116: 1736-1754

2 Pharis CS, Conway J, Warren AE, Bullock A, Mackie AS. The impact of 2007 infective endocarditis prophylaxis guidelines on the practice of congenital heart disease specialists. Am Heart J 2011; 161: 123-129

A - Endocarditis Prophylaxis

B – ADD Meds & Sports Clearance

Patient Screening for ADD Medications and Sports Clearance

Patient Name _____ DOB _____

Current Medications (Prescribed and Over the Counter)
_____
_____

CHILD SYMPTOMS
Please Circle "Yes" or "No" to the following:

History of fainting or dizziness with exercise	Yes	No
History of fainting or dizziness without exercise	Yes	No
Seizures	Yes	No
Palpitations (fast heartbeats) or extra heartbeats or skipped beats	Yes	No
High blood pressure	Yes	No
History of heart murmur	Yes	No

A FAMILY MEMBER WITH THE FOLLOWING
Please Circle "Yes" or "No" to the following:

Pacemaker less than 35 years of age	Yes	No
Sudden/unexplained death in family members less than 35 yeras of age	Yes	No
Heart attacks in members less than 35 years of age	Yes	No
Sudden death during exercise	Yes	No
Enlarged heart at less than 35 years of age	Yes	No
Long QT syndrome	Yes	No
Wolff-Parkinson-White syndrome or supraventricular tachycardia	Yes	No
An event requiring CPR in a person less than 35 years of age	Yes	No
Marfan syndrome	Yes	No
Seizures or blacking-out episodes at less than 35 years of age	Yes	No
Family member who drowned at less than 35 years of age	Yes	No

○ Normal EKG

○ No EKG, patient history or family history contraindication to using ADD / ADHD medications

○ Abnormal EKG or positive patient or family history, needs further evaluation

B - ADD Meds & Sports Clearance

C - Formulary

INTRODUCTION

This short formulary provides abbreviated descriptions of pharmacological mechanisms and a limited discussion of side effects. We organize medications alphabetically by generic name. Please refer to comprehensive works for lengthier descriptions. Start medications at lower dosing ranges and carefully titrate to higher levels, monitoring positive and negative side effects. Slowly wean medications, rather than abruptly stopping them. Also, check package inserts for drug interactions. Avoid grapefruit juice, as it impairs the cytochrome P_{450} system, which metabolizes many medications.

We checked dosages and content for accuracy. Because of incomplete data on pediatric dosing, many drug dosages may require modification after this book's publication. We recommend the reader check product information and published literature for changes in dosing, especially for new or seldom used medications. [1-5]

C - Formulary

Trade	Generic	Trade	Generic
Adenocard	adenosine	Florinef	fludrocortisone
Aldactone	spironolactone	Glucophage	metformin
Amicar	aminocaproic acid	Haldol	haloperidol
Apresoline	hydralazine	Hydrodiuril	hydrochlorothiazide
Benadryl	diphenhydramine	Inderal	propranolol
Benicar	olmesartan	Indocin	indomethacin
Betapace	sotalol	Intropin	dopamine
Brevibloc	esmolol	Isuprel	isoproterenol
Capoten	captopril	K-Dur	potassium chloride
Cardene	nicardipine	Lanoxin	digoxin
Cardizem	diltiazem	Lasix	furosemide
Carnitor	carnitine	Levophed	norepinephrine
Cordarone	amiodarone	Lipitor	atorvastatin
Coreg	carvedilol	Lopid	gemfibrozil
Corgard	nadolol	Lopressor	metoprolol
Coumadin	warfarin	Lortab	hydrocodone + acetaminophen
Cozaar	losartan		
Decadron	dexamethasone	Lovenox	enoxaparin
DIGIBIND	digoxin immune Fab	Monopril	fosinopril
DigiFab	digoxin immune Fab	Motrin	ibuprofen
Diovan	valsartan	Naprosyn	naproxen
Diuril	chlorothiazide	Natrecor	nesiritide
Dobutrex	dobutamine	NeoProfen	ibuprofen lysine
Fer-In-Sol	ferrous sulfate	Neosynephrine	phenylephrine

Trade	Generic	Trade	Generic
Niaspan	niacin	Trandate	labetolol
Nipride	nitroprusside	Valium	diazepam
Norpace	disopyramide	Vasotec	enalapril
Norvasc	amlodipine	Ventolin	albuterol
Persantine	dipyridamole	Versed	midazolam
Precedex	dexmedetomidine	Viagra	sildenafil
Prelone	prednisolone	Xopenex	levalbuterol
Primacor	milrinone	Xylocaine	lidocaine
ProAmatine	midodrine	Zantac	ranitidine
Procardia	nifedipine	Zebeta	bisoprolol
Prostin	prostaglandin E1	Zestril	lisinopril
Proventyl	albuterol	Zetia	ezetimibe
PTU	propylthiouracil	Zoloft	sertraline
Questran	cholestyramine resin		
Remicade	infliximab		
Revatio	sildenafil		
Sandostatin	octreotide		
Solu-Cortef	hydrocortisone		
Solu-Medrol	methylprednisolone		
SSKI	potassium iodide		
Synagis	palivizumab		
Tapazole	methimazole		
Tambocor	flecainide acetate		
Tenormin	atenolol		

— A —

Adenosine (Adenocard)

Mechanism

Slows AV nodal conduction

IV for SVT conversion

0.1 mg (100 μg)/kg IV fast push, if no effect then increase

0.2 mg (200 μg)/kg IV fast push, if no effect then increase

0.3 mg (300 μg)/kg IV fast push

Side effects

Flushing, bradycardia, apnea, asystole, bronchospasm

➤ IV fast push + immediate IV saline flush fast push into a venous line as close to the heart as possible. Have cardiac monitoring and a crash cart available. Give doses about 1 to 2 minutes apart. Exercise caution if the patient is also on digoxin, as digoxin can accentuate AV nodal block.

Albuterol (Ventolin, Proventyl)

Mechanism for use in hyperkalemia

Increases cellular uptake of potassium, lowering serum potassium

Nebulized inhalation for hyperkalemia

Age	Albuterol dose in 3 ml of normal saline
0 - 1 year	0.05 - 0.15 mg/kg/dose
1 - 2 years	1.0 - 2.5 mg/dose
> 12 years	2.3 - 5.0 mg/dose

Side effects

Tachycardia

Aminocaproic acid (Amicar)

Mechanism

Acts as an inhibitor of fibrinolysis, promoting clotting

IV Load

100 mg/kg IV slow push

IV Infusion

25 - 30 mg/kg/hr IV infusion

Side effects

Nausea, vomiting, fever, hyperkalemia, hypotension

Amiodarone (Cordarone)

Mechanism

Multiple effects on the cardiac action potential

IV Load

5.0 mg/kg IV slow push over 30 min and repeat × 2 as needed

IV Infusion

5.0 - 10 mg/kg/24 hrs IV infusion

Oral load

10 - 15 mg/kg/day PO QD for 7 days

Oral maintenance

5.0 - 10 mg/kg/day PO QD

Oral dosage forms

Tabs 100, 200, or 400 mg; suspension 5.0 mg/mL

Side effects

Bradycardia, increased QTc, myocardial depression, hypo or hyperthyroidism, pulmonary fibrosis, central and peripheral nervous system abnormalities, rashes, corneal deposits, hepatic toxicity

Amlodipine (Norvasc)

Mechanism
Calcium-channel blocker
Oral
0.1 - 0.6 mg/kg/day PO QD or divided BID
Oral dosage forms
Tabs 2.5, 5.0, or 10 mg; suspension 1.0 mg/mL
Side effects
Hypotension, tachycardia, edema, flushing

Aspirin
Mechanism
Anti-inflammatory
Oral anti-inflammatory high dose
80 - 100 mg/kg/day PO divided QID, or divided as frequently as 5 - 6 times/day
Oral anti-platelet low dose
3.0 - 5.0 mg/kg/day PO QD
Oral dosage forms (OTC)
Baby tabs 81 mg; adult tabs 325 mg; suppositories 120, 200, 300, & 600 mg; enteric coated 81, 165, 325, 500, or 600 mg
Side effects
Gastrointestinal bleeding, tinnitus
➤Hold if influenza or varicella (Reye syndrome risk). If using high dose, then consider ASA levels to avoid toxicity.

Atenolol (Tenormin)
Mechanism
β_1-adrenergic antagonist
Oral
0.5 - 2.0 mg/kg/day PO QD or divided BID
Oral dosage forms
Tabs 25, 50, or 100 mg; suspension 2.0 mg/mL
Side effects
Hypotension, hypoglycemia, bronchospasm, bradycardia

Atorvastatin (Lipitor)
Mechanism
Inhibits hydroxy-methyl-glutaryl-CoA reductase, which acts on the metabolic pathway producing cholesterol
Oral
10 - 20 mg/dose PO QD to start
Oral dosage forms
Tabs 10, 20, 40, or 80 mg
Side effects
Rhabdomyolysis, increased liver enzymes
➤Reserve statin use to post-pubescent children. Obtain liver function tests and CPK before starting, at 3 months, and then at 6-month intervals PRN. Also avoid grapefruit juice. Contraindicated in pregnancy.

Atropine
Mechanism
Blocks acetylcholine action
IV or by endotracheal tube
0.01 - 0.02 mg/kg/dose IV Q 3 -5 minutes × 2 - 3 doses or as needed
Side effects
Tachycardia, anticholinergic effects, fever

— B —

Bisoprolol (Zebeta)
Mechanism
β_1 adrenergic antagonist
Oral adolescents and older

2.5 - 10 mg QD

Oral dosage forms

Tabs 5.0 or 10 mg (tablets scored)

Side effects

Diarrhea, dizziness, drowsiness, fatigue, headache, lightheadedness, nausea, sleeplessness, unusual tiredness, weakness

– C –

Calcium chloride

Mechanism for use in hyperkalemia

Does not lower potassium but decreases myocardial excitability

IV bolus for hyperkalemia

10 - 20 mg/kg IV slow push over 5 - 10 minutes

IV infusion for hypocalcemia

10 - 50 mg/kg/hr IV infusion

Side effects

Bradycardia, extravasations may cause tissue necrosis

Captopril (Capoten)

Mechanism

Angiotensin-converting enzyme inhibitor

Oral neonates

0.1 - 0.3 mg/kg/day PO divided BID or TID (maximum dose 1.5 mg/kg/day)

Oral infants and children

1.0 - 2.0 mg/kg/day PO divided BID or TID (maximum dose 6.0 mg/kg/day)

Oral dosage forms

Tabs 12.5, 25, 50, or 100 mg; suspensions 0.75 mg/mL or 1.0 mg/mL

Side effects

Cough, hyperkalemia, renal dysfunction

Carnitine or L - carnitine (Carnitor)

Mechanism

Transports fatty acids from the cytosol into the mitochondria

Oral

50 - 100 mg/kg/day PO divided BID or TID

Oral dosage forms

Tabs 330 or 500 mg; caps 250 or 300 mg; solution 100 mg/mL

Side effects

Nausea, diarrhea, occasionally hypertension

Carvedilol (Coreg)

Mechanism

Nonselective β-adrenergic antagonist and α_1-adrenergic antagonist

Oral

0.05 - 1.0 mg/kg/day PO divided BID

Oral dosage forms

Tabs 3.125, 6.25, 12.5, or 25 mg; solutions 0.1 mg/mL or 1.67 mg/mL

Side effects

Bronchospasm, bradycardia, hypotension, hyperglycemia
➤Initial dose 0.05 - 0.10 mg/kg/day, then increase slowly with each dosing change no more frequent than Q 1 - 2 week intervals (maximum dose of 1.0 mg/kg/day).

Chlorothiazide (Diuril)

Mechanism

Inhibits sodium chloride transport in the distal tubule

Oral

C - Formulary

< 6 months 20-40 mg/kg/day divided BID, > 6 months 20 mg/kg/day divided BID

Oral dosage forms

Tabs 250, 500 mg; suspension 250mg/5.0 mL

Side effects

Hyponatremia, hypokalemia, hypochloremia, metabolic acidosis, hyperuricemia, hyperglycemia, increased LDL-cholesterol, increased triglycerides, ototoxicity

Cholestyramine resin (Questran)

Mechanism

Bile acid sequestrants that bind bile in the gastrointestinal tract, reducing reabsorption

Oral

4.0 - 8.0 g/day PO QD or divided BID (maximum dose 24 g/day)

Oral dosage forms

4.0 g anhydrous resin in 9.0 g powder

Side effects

Constipation, tooth discoloration, impairs the absorption of fat-soluble vitamins, numerous food interactions

Codeine + acetaminophen (Tylenol # 1-4)

Mechanism

Analgesic

Oral

Child 3 - 6 years 5.0 mL TID or QID, 7 - 12 years 10 mL TID or QID, > 12 years 15 mL TID or QID (codeine dose 0.5 - 1.0 mg/kg/dose)

Adult 1 - 2 tablets TID or QID

Oral dosing forms

Tabs

#1- acetaminophen 300 mg + codeine 7.5 mg

#2 - acetaminophen 300 mg + codeine 15 mg

#3 - acetaminophen 300 mg + codeine 30 mg

#4 - acetaminophen 300 mg + codeine 60 mg

Liquid

no # - acetaminophen 120 mg + codeine 12 mg/5.0 mL

Side effects

Hypotension, bradycardia, sedation, nausea, vomiting, constipation, respiratory depression, hepatotoxicity

— D —

Dexamethasone (Decadron)

Mechanism

Anti-inflammatory through suppressing neutrophil migration, decreases pro-inflammatory mediators, decreases capillary permeability

Oral children

0.02 - 0.3 mg/kg/day divided TID or QID

Oral adults

0.75 - 9.0 mg QD, 4.0 mg QD to mother for maternal antibody SSA/SSB related fetal heart block

IV or IM for airway edema

0.5 - 2.0 mg/kg/24 hrs Q 4 - 6 hrs IV bolus or IM

Oral dosage forms

Tabs 0.25, 0.5, 0.75, 1.0, 1.5, 2.0, 4.0, 6.0 mg; elixir 0.5 mg/5.0 mL; solution 0.5 mg/5.0 mL or 1.0 mg/mL

Side effects

Hypertension, gastrointestinal bleeding, hyperglycemia, pseudotumor cerebri

Dexmedetomidine (Precedex)

Mechanism

For sedation in junctional and atrial ectopic tachycardia

an α₂ - adrenergic agonist in the brain causes sedation

IV Load

0.6 - 1.6 µg/kg IV slow push over 30 minutes

IV Infusion

0.3 - 1.2 µg/kg/hr IV infusion

Side effects

Hypotension, bradycardia

Dextrose with insulin

Mechanism for use in hyperkalemia

Causes a shift of potassium ions into cells, from increased activity of sodium-potassium ATPase

IV

Dextrose @ 0.5 g/kg IV with insulin @ 0.1 U/kg IV over 30 minutes

Side effects

Hypo and hyperglycemia, hypokalemia

Diazepam (Valium)

Mechanism

A benzodiazepine, which enhances the effect of the neurotransmitter gamma-amino-butyric acid (GABA)

IV

0.05 - 0.2 mg/kg/dose Q 2 - 4 hours (sedation)

Oral

0.12 - 0.80 mg/kg/day PO divided TID or QID

Oral dosage forms

Tabs 2.0, 5.0, or 10 mg; solutions 1.0 mg/mL or 5.0 mg/mL

Side effects

Respiratory depression, hypotension, bradycardia

Digoxin (lanoxin)

Mechanism

Inhibits sodium-potassium ATPase, an action that results in increased intracellular calcium, improving ventricular function and slowing the heart rate by effecting the cardiac action potential through increased vagal activity

Digitalizing dose (top table facing page), example

40 µg/kg PO or IV and divide into 3 loading doses:

1. 20 µg/kg IV slow push or PO, followed in 6 - 8 hrs by
2. 10 µg/kg IV slow push or PO, followed in 6 - 8 hrs by
3. 10 µg/kg IV slow push or PO, then follow in 12 - 24 hrs with daily dose divided BID

Oral dosage forms

Tabs 125 µg or 250 µg; elixir 50 µg/mL

Side effects

Arrhythmias, nausea, vomiting, diarrhea, hyperkalemia, CNS changes, and visual changes

➤Obtain EKG with each digitalizing dose to check for arrhythmias and prolongation of the PR interval.

Digoxin immune Fab (DIGIBIND-Glaxo Wellcome or DigiFab-Protherics)

Mechanism

Antidigoxin antibody for digoxin toxicity

IV

Dose from bottom table of the facing page, give IV slow push over 10 - 15 minutes (use 0.22 micron filter)

Side effects

Hypokalemia, decreased cardiac output, rash, edema

➤In the bottom table on the facing page, we provide dosing for the 2 available products in the bottom table on the facing page: DIGIBIND and DigiFab. Using the patient's weight in kg and digoxin level in ng/mL, the table lists DIGIBIND and DigiFab doses. If no dosing range

Digoxin Dosing Chart

Age	Digitalizing dose µg/kg		Daily dose µg/kg/day divided BID	
	PO	IV	PO	IV
Premature	20	15	5	3-4
Full term	30	20	8-10	6-8
< 2 yrs	40-50	30-40	10-12	8-9
2 – 10 yrs	30-40	20-30	8-10	6-8
> 10 yrs	10-15	8-12	3-5	2-3

DIGIBIND & DigiFab Dosing Chart

Patient Weight (kg)	Serum Digoxin Concentration (ng/mL)						
	1	2	4	8	12	16	20
1	0.4* mg	1* mg	1.5* mg	3* mg	5 mg	6-6.5 mg	8 mg
3	1* mg	2-2.5* mg	5 mg	9-10 mg	14 mg	18-19 mg	23-24 mg
5	2* mg	4 mg	8 mg	15-16 mg	23-24 mg	30-32 mg	38-40 mg
10	4 mg	8 mg	15-16 mg	30-32 mg	46-48 mg	61-64 mg	76-80 mg
20	8 mg	15-16 mg	30-32 mg	61-64 mg	91-96 mg	122-128 mg	152-160 mg

* Dilution of reconstituted vial to 1 mg/1 mL may be desirable

If no dose range is given, the doses for either product are identical.
If a dosing range is given, then the lower dose is for DIGIBIND and the higher dose is for DigiFab.

C - Formulary

given, then doses for both products are identical. If dosing range given, then the lower dose is for DIGIBIND and the higher dose is for DigiFab. Avoid if allergic to sheep products.

Diltiazem (Cardizem)

Mechanism

Calcium-channel blocker

IV load

0.25 mg/kg IV over 2 minutes, if no response 0.35 mg/kg IV over 2 minutes 15 minutes after 1st dose

IV infusion

0.05 - 0.15 mg/kg/hr IV infusion

Oral

1.5 - 2.0 mg/kg/day PO divided TID, or QD for sustained release (SR) form (maximum dose 3.5 mg/kg/day)

Oral dosage forms

Tabs 30, 60, 90, 120 mg; SR 120, 180, 240, 300, 360, 420 mg

Side effects

Hypotension, tachycardia

Diphenhydramine (Benadryl)

Mechanism

Antihistamine

IV Bolus

5.0 mg/kg/24 hrs divided Q 6 hrs IV slow push (maximum dose 50 mg)

Oral

5.0 - 10 mg/kg/day PO divided QID

Oral dosage forms

Tabs (OTC) 25, or 50 mg; syrup (OTC) 12.5 mg/5.0 mL

Side effects

Sedation, hypotension, tachycardia, anticholinergic

Dipyridamole (Persantine)

Mechanism

Inhibits thromboxane synthase, antiplatelet agent

Oral

3.0 - 6.0 mg/kg/day PO divided TID

Oral dosage forms

Tabs 25, 50, or 75 mg

Side effects

Bleeding, bruising, rashes

Disopyramide (Norpace)

Mechanism

Sodium-channel blocker

Oral

10 - 20 mg/kg/day PO divided QID

Oral dosage forms

Caps 100 or 150 mg

Side effects

Prolongs QTc, anticholinergic, negative inotrope

Dobutamine (Dobutrex)

Mechanism

β_1-adrenergic agonist

IV Infusion

2.0 - 20 µg/kg/min IV infusion

Side effects

Tachycardia, arrhythmias

Dopamine (Intropin)

Mechanism

Low dose chiefly dopamine agonist, middle dose primarily $β_1$-adrenergic agonist, and higher dose also has $α_1$-adrenergic agonist activity

IV Infusion

2.0 - 20 μg/kg/min IV infusion

Dopamine Dosing Chart	
Dose type	Range
Low	2.0 - 5.0 μg/kg/min
Middle	5.0 - 10 μg/kg/min
High	> 10 μg/kg/min

Side effects

Tachycardia, arrhythmias

— E —

Enalapril (Vasotec)

Mechanism

Angiotensin-converting enzyme inhibitor

IV (enalaprilat) Bolus

5.0 - 20 μg/kg/dose IV over 10 minutes Q 24 hrs up to Q 8 hrs

Oral infants and children

0.1 - 0.5 mg/kg/day PO QD or divided BID (maximum dose 0.6 mg/kg/day

Oral adolescents and adults

2.5 - 5.0 mg/day PO QD (maximum dose 40 mg/day)

Oral dosage forms

Tabs 2.5, 5.0, 10, or 20 mg; suspension 1.0 mg/mL

Side effects

Cough, hyperkalemia, renal dysfunction

Enoxaparin (Lovenox)

Mechanism

Low molecular weight heparin, which binds to antithrombin III and accelerates its activity

SC infants and children up to 17 years

0.5 mg/kg/dose SC BID

Side effects

Bleeding, allergy, fever, thrombocytopenia, increased liver enzymes

Epinephrine

Mechanism

Nonselective α and β-adrenergic agonist

IV Bolus/intraosseous (IO) for CPR (1:10,000 or 0.1 mg/mL)

0.1 mL/kg (0.01 mg/kg) Q 3 - 5 minutes

IV Infusion (1:10,000)

0.05 - 1.0 μg/kg/min IV infusion

Per endotracheal tube for CPR (1:1,000 or 1.0 mg/mL)

0.1 mL/kg (0.10 mg/kg) Q 3 - 5 minutes

IM or SC for anaphylaxis (1:1,000)

0.01 - 0.5 mg/kg/dose IM or SC Q 20 min

Epi-pen Jr (autoinjector) = 0.15 mg for < 30 kg

Epi-pen (autoinjector) = 0.30 mg for > 30 kg

Side effects

Tachycardia, arrhythmias

Esmolol (Brevibloc)

Mechanism

$β_1$-adrenergic antagonist

IV Load

100 - 500 μg/kg IV over 5 minutes

IV Infusion

100 - 1,000 μg/kg/min IV infusion and titrate for effect

Side effects

Hypotension, hypoglycemia, bronchospasm, bradycardia

Ezetimibe (Zetia)

Mechanism

Acts by decreasing cholesterol absorption in the intestine

Oral

10 mg/dose PO QD

Oral dosage forms

Tabs 10 mg

Side effects

Headache, diarrhea, infrequent myalgia or abnormal liver function tests

— F —

Ferrous sulfate (Fer-In-Sol)

Mechanism

Iron replacement

Oral

2.0 - 6.0 mg Fe/kg/day PO QD or divided BID

Oral dosage forms

Tabs 300 mg (60 mg Fe), 325 mg or (65mg Fe); drops 75 mg or (15 mg Fe)/0.60 mL; elixir 220 mg or (44 mg Fe)/5.0 mL;

Side effects

Teeth stain, constipation, dark stools, nausea

Fish oil

Mechanism

Unclear but may inhibit arachidonic acid

Oral

1.0 - 4.0 grams PO QD

Oral dosage forms

Caps (enteric coated) 500 mg;

Side effects

Nausea, fish taste, bloating, diarrhea

Flecainide acetate (Tambocor)

Mechanism

Sodium-channel blocker

Oral

50 - 200 mg/m^2/day PO divided TID, or

1.0 - 4.0 mg/kg/day PO divided TID

Oral dosage forms

Tabs 50, 100, or 150 mg; suspensions 5.0 mg/mL or 20 mg/mL

Side effects

Proarrhythmic, negative inotrope, rash

➤Hospitalize patients to initiate flecainide.

Fludrocortisone acetate (Florinef)

Mechanism

Mineralocorticoid, which augments fluid and salt retention

Oral

0.05 - 0.1 mg/day PO QD

Oral dosage forms

Tabs 0.1 mg

Side effects

Edema, hypertension, hypokalemia

Fosinopril (Monopril)

Mechanism

Angiotensin-converting enzyme inhibitor

Oral

0.10 - 0.60 mg/kg/day PO QD

Oral dosage forms

Tabs 10, 20, 40 mg

Side effects

Cough, hyperkalemia, renal dysfunction

Furosemide (Lasix)

Mechanism

Inhibits sodium chloride transport in the loop of Henle

IV Bolus

0.5 - 2.0 mg/kg/dose IV bolus Q 24 hrs, or may increase to 0.5 - 2.0 mg/kg/dose IV bolus as frequently as Q 6 hrs

IV Infusion

0.05 - 0.4 mg/kg/hr IV infusion

Oral

2.0 - 5.0 mg/kg/day PO divided BID

Oral dosage forms

Tabs 20, 40, or 80 mg; solutions 10 mg/mL or 40 mg/mL

Side effects

Hyponatremia, hypokalemia, hypochloremia, metabolic acidosis, hyperuricemia, hyperglycemia, increased LDL, increase triglycerides, ototoxicity

➤ With a dose > 2.0 mg/kg/day, add spironolactone to spare potassium loss, or IV potassium supplementation with IV dosing along with close monitoring of potassium levels.

Gemfibrozil (Lopid)

Mechanism

Agonists of the peroxisome proliferator-activated receptor α-receptor in muscle, liver, and other tissues that results in decreased hepatic triglyceride section, increased lipoprotein lipase activity, increased HDL, and increased clearance of remnant particles

Oral

600 mg/dose PO BID

Oral dosage forms

Tabs 600 mg

Side effects

Gastrointestinal distress, increased muscle CPK

Haloperidol (Haldol)

Mechanism

Dopamine antagonist

Oral

0.01 - 0.1 mg/kg/day PO divided BID or TID

Oral dosage forms

Tabs 0.5, 1.0, 2.0, 5.0, 10, or 20 mg; solution 2.0 mg/mL

Side effects

Arrhythmias, heart failure, sudden death, dystonia

Heparin

Mechanism

Potentiates antithrombin III, preventing the conversion of fibrinogen to fibrin

IV Bolus

50 - 100 U/kg IV bolus Q 4 hrs

IV Infusion (dosing table top of next page)

C - Formulary

Heparin Dosing Chart	
Age	Dose
< 2 months	28 U/kg/hr IV infusion
2 months - 1 year	25 U/kg/hr IV infusion
> 1 year	18 - 20 U/kg/hr IV infusion

Side effects

Bleeding, allergy, fever, thrombocytopenia, abnormal liver function tests

➤ Maintain PTT > 60 sec < 95 sec. Stop infusion if > 95 sec. Increase infusion dose 10% Q 4 - 6 hrs if < 60 sec, and decrease dose 10% Q 4 - 6 hrs if PTT > 85 sec.

Hydralazine (Apresoline)

Mechanism

Direct peripheral vasodilator

IV Bolus

0.1 - 0.2 mg/kg/dose IV bolus PRN Q 2 - 6 hrs (maximum dose 20 mg/dose)

Oral

0.75 - 1.0 mg/kg/day PO divided BID or QID, may increase dose slowly over 3 - 4 weeks to 5.0 mg/kg/day (maximum dose 25 mg/dose)

Oral dosage forms

Tabs 10, 25, 50, or 100 mg; solutions 1.25 mg/mL, 2.0 mg/mL, or 4.0 mg/mL

Side effects

Lupus-like syndrome, tachycardia, hypotension

➤ As hyperkalemia is not a side effect, hydralazine is useful in renal failure as opposed to ACE inhibitors.

Hydrochlorothiazide (Hydrodiuril)

Mechanism

Inhibits sodium chloride transport in the distal tubule

Oral

1.0 - 2.0 mg/kg/day PO divided BID

Oral dosage forms

Tabs 12.5, 25, 50, or 100 mg; caps 12.5 mg

Side effects

Hyponatremia, hypokalemia, hypochloremia, metabolic acidosis, hyperuricemia, hyperglycemia, increased LDL-cholesterol, increased triglycerides, ototoxicity

Hydrocodone + acetaminophen (Lortab)

Mechanism

Analgesic

Oral (based on hydrocodone dose)

0.6 mg/kg/day divided TID or QID (maximum dose < 2 years old 1.25 mg, 2 to 12 years 5.0 mg, > 12 years 10mg)

Oral dosage forms

Tabs hydrocodone 5.0 mg + acetaminophen 500 mg, hydrocodone 7.5 mg + acetaminophen 500 mg, hydrocodone 10 mg + acetaminophen 500 mg; elixir hydrocodone 10 mg + acetaminophen 500 mg per 15 mL

Side effects

Hypotension, bradycardia, sedation, nausea, constipation, respiratory depression

Hydrocortisone (Solu-Cortef)

Mechanism

Anti-inflammatory through suppressing neutrophil migration, decreases pro-inflammatory mediators, decreases capillary permeability

IV Bolus

1.0 - 5.0 mg/kg/dose IV slow push over 15 minutes Q 24 hrs

Side effects

Hypertension, gastrointestinal bleeding, hyperglycemia, pseudotumor cerebri

— I —

Ibuprofen (Motrin)

Mechanism

Blocks the action of prostaglandin

Oral

10 mg/kg/dose TID or QID

Oral dosage forms

Tabs (OTC) 50, 100, 200 mg; tabs prescription 400, 600, 800 mg; drops (OTC) 40 mg/mL; suspension 100 mg/5.0 mL

Side effects

gastrointestinal distress, GI bleed, rashes, eye problems

Ibuprofen lysine (NeoProfen)

Mechanism

Blocks the action of prostaglandin

IV (3 doses) for PDA in the premature

1. 10 mg/kg IV, followed in 24 hrs by
2. 5.0 mg/kg IV, followed in 24 hrs by
3. 5.0 mg/kg IV

Each dose administered IV slow push over 15 minutes

Side effects

Hyperbilirubinemia; but less renal, bleeding, or enterocolitis than indomethacin

Immune globulin (IVIG)

Mechanism

Probably neutralization of toxins, viruses, and bacteria plus immune modulation

IV Infusion for Kawasaki disease

2.0 g/kg IV infusion over 12 hrs

IV infusion for maternal-autoantibody fetal heart block related to SSA/SSB

1.0 g/kg IV infusion over 12 hrs

Side effects

Fever, hypertension, hypotension, tachycardia, allergic reaction, aseptic meningitis, acute renal failure

Indomethacin (Indocin)

Mechanism

Blocks the action of prostaglandin

IV for PDA in the premature

IV slow push over 20 - 30 minutes Q 24 hrs/dose, or divided Q 12 hrs, and dosing per table below:

Indomethacin Dosing Chart			
Age at 1st dose	1st dose mg/kg	2nd dose mg/kg	3rd dose mg/kg
< 48 hrs	0.2	0.1	0.1
2-7 days	0.2	0.2	0.2
> 7 days	0.2	0.25	0.25

Oral

1.0 - 2.0 mg/kg/day PO divided BID or even QID (maximum dose 4mg/kg/day or 100 - 200 mg/day

C - Formulary

Oral dosage forms

Caps 25, 50 mg; SR 75 mg; suspension 25 mg/5.0 mL

Side effects

Oliguria, renal failure, bleeding, necrotizing enterocolitis (NEC), intestinal perforation in < 1,000-gram premature infants other than NEC, hyponatremia, hyperkalemia

Infliximab (Remicade)

Mechanism

Monoclonal antibody against TNFα (tissue necrosis factor α)

IV Bolus

5.0 mg/kg IV × 1

Side effects

Dyspnea, flushing, headache, rash, pruritis, infections, hepatotoxicty

➤Pretreat with acetaminophen 15 mg/kg PO and diphenhydramine 1.0 mg/kg PO or IV.

Isoproterenol (Isuprel)

Mechanism

Nonselective β-adrenergic agonist

IV Infusion

0.02 - 2.0 µg/kg/min IV infusion

Side effects

Tachycardia, arrhythmias, hypertension

— L —

Labetolol (IV - Trandate)

Mechanism

Nonselective β-adrenergic antagonist and $α_1$-adrenergic antagonist

IV Infusion children

0.25 - 3.0 mg/kg/hr IV infusion

Oral

1.0 - 3.0 mg/kg/day divided BID, to start

10 - 12 mg/kg/day divided BID, maximum

Oral dosage forms

Tabs 100, 200, or 300 mg

Side effects

Bronchospasm, bradycardia, hypotension, hyperglycemia

Levalbuterol (Xopenex)

Mechanism

$β_1$-adrenergic agonist

Nebulized inhalation

6 - 11 years: 0.31 mg in 3 mL Q 8 hr up to Q 6 hr

Aerosol inhaler

> 4 years: 1 - 2 puffs QID up to Q 4 hrs

Dosage forms

Nebulizer solution 0.31 mg in 3 mL, 0.63 mg in 3 mL, 1.25 mg in 3 mL; aerosol inhaler 45 µg/actuation

Side effects

Tachycardia, palpitations, insomnia, headache

Lidocaine (Xylocaine)

Mechanism

Sodium-channel blocker, local anesthetic

IV Load

1.0 - 4.0 mg/kg IV slow push Q 10 - 15 minutes × 2

IV Infusion

20 - 50 µg/kg/min IV infusion (reduce by 50% after 24 hrs)

Side effects

Hypotension, drowsiness, respiratory depression, seizures

➤If left ventricular dysfunction, then use the lowest dose.

C – Formulary

Lisinopril (Zestril)

Mechanism

Angiotensin-converting enzyme inhibitor

Oral children

0.1 mg/kg/day PO QD (titrate up Q 1 - 2 weeks to 0.6 mg/kg/day and maximum dose 5.0 mg/dose)

Oral adolescents and adults

5.0 - 40 mg PO QD

Oral dosage forms

Tabs 2.5, 5.0, 10, 20, 30, or 40 mg; suspensions 1.0 mg/mL or 2.0 mg/mL

Side effects

Cough, hyperkalemia, renal dysfunction

Losartan (Cozaar)

Mechanism

Angiotensin II-receptor blocker

Oral children

0.75 - 1.5 mg/kg/day PO QD (maximum dose 50 mg/day)

Oral adolescents and adults

25 - 100 mg/day PO QD

Oral dosage forms

Tabs 25, 50, or 100 mg; suspension 2.5 mg/mL

Side effects

Headache, dizziness, fatigue, abdominal pain, cough, hyperkalemia, rhabdomyolysis

Magnesium sulfate

Mechanism

Antagonizes calcium entry into smooth muscle cells, promoting vasodilation

IV Load

200 mg/kg IV slow push over 20 min

IV Infusion

20 - 150 mg/kg/hr IV infusion

Side effects

Hypotension, respiratory depression, heart block

Metformin (Glucophage)

Mechanism

Suppresses hepatic gluconeogenesis

Oral (10 - 18 years old)

500 mg/dose PO BID, may increase 250 mg/dose Q weekly to a maximum of 1,000 mg/dose given BID

Oral dosage forms

Tabs 500, 850, or 1,000 mg; suspension 100 mg/mL

Side effects

Diarrhea, cramps, nausea, vomiting, flatulence, occasionally lactic acidosis

Methimazole (Tapazole)

Mechanism

Inhibits the addition of iodine to thyroglobulin, a necessary step for the synthesis of triiodothyronine (T3) and thyroxine (T4)

Oral

0.5 mg - 1.0 mg/kg/day PO divided TID

Oral dosage forms

Tabs 5.0, 10 mg

Side effects

Rash, itching, hair loss

C - Formulary

Methylene blue

Mechanism

Acts to reduce the heme group from methemoglobin to hemoglobin

IV Bolus

1.0 - 2.0 mg/kg of 1.0% solution IV over 5 minutes, may repeat once 1 hr after the 1st dose

Side effects

Nausea, abdominal and precordial pain, dizziness, headache, sweating, mental confusion

Methylprednisolone (Solu-Medrol)

Mechanism

Anti-inflammatory through suppressing neutrophil migration, decreases pro-inflammatory mediators, decreases capillary permeability

IV Bolus (pulse)

30 mg/kg/24 hrs IV slow push over 15 minutes (maximum of 1.0 gram per day for 3 days)

Oral

0.5 - 2.0 mg/kg/day PO divided BID

Oral dosage forms

Tabs 2.0, 4.0, 8.0, 16, 24, 32 mg

Side effects Hypertension, gastrointestinal bleeding, hyperglycemia, pseudotumor cerebri

Metoprolol (Lopressor)

Mechanism

β_1-adrenergic antagonist

Oral

1.0 - 6.0 mg/kg/day PO divided BID, or QD for sustained release (SR)

Oral dosage forms

Tabs 25, 50, or 100 mg; SR 25, 50, 100, or 200 mg; liquid 10 mg/mL

Side effects

Bronchospasm, bradycardia, hyperglycemia

Midazolam (Versed)

Mechanism

A benzodiazepine, which enhances the effect of the neurotransmitter gamma-amino-butyric acid (GABA)

IV Bolus

0.05 - 0.1 mg/kg/dose over 2 - 3 minutes, may repeat PRN for sedation when mechanically ventilated

Nasal

0.2 - 0.3 mg/kg/dose (maximum dose 5.0 mg for < 5 years, 10 mg for > 5 years)

Oral

0.1 - 1.0 mg/kg/dose (maximum dose 5.0 mg for < 5 years, 10 mg for > 5 years)

Oral dosage forms

Syrup 2.0 mg/mL

Side effects

Respiratory depression, hypotension, bradycardia

Midodrine (ProAmatine)

Mechanism

α_1-adrenergic agonist

Oral

2.5 - 10 mg/dose PO TID (AM, midday, and PM 4 - 6 hrs before bed)

Oral dosage forms

Tabs 2.5, 5.0, or 10 mg

Side effects

Hypertension

➤Give the last dose about 4 - 6 hours before bedtime to avoid exaggerated recumbent hypertension.

Milrinone (Primacor)

Mechanism

Inhibits cyclic-AMP phosphodiesterase increasing cyclic-AMP levels for energy production, also acts as vasodilator decreasing afterload

IV Load

50 µg/kg IV slow push load over 20 minutes (no loading in newborns)

IV Infusion

0.1 - 1.0 µg/kg/min IV infusion

Side effects

Hypotension, arrhythmias

Morphine

Mechanism

Binds to opioid receptors, which occur in the central nervous system and the gastrointestinal tract

IM or SC

0.1 - 0.2 mg/kg/dose IM or SC

Side effects

Respiratory depression

— N —

Nadolol (Corgard)

Mechanism

Nonselective β-adrenergic antagonist

Oral

0.50 - 2.5 mg/kg/day PO QD

Oral dosage forms

Tabs 20, 40, 80, 120, 180 mg

Side effects

Bronchospasm, bradycardia, hypotension, hyperglycemia

Naproxen (Naprosyn)

Mechanism

Nonsteroidal anti-inflammatory drug, which is a nonselective inhibitor of cyclooxygenase (COX-1 and COX-2)

Oral

10 mg/kg/day PO divided BID, or QD for sustained release (SR) form (maximum dose 1,250 mg/day)

Oral dosage forms

Tabs 250, 375, or 500 mg; SR 375 or 500 mg; suspension 125 mg/5.0 mL

Side effects

Gastrointestinal bleeding

Nesiritide (Natrecor)

Mechanism

Promotes vasodilation, natriuresis, and diuresis

IV Load

1.0 - 2.0 µg/kg IV bolus over 1 minute

IV Infusion

0.005 - 0.01 µg/kg/min IV infusion

Side effects

Hypotension, arrhythmias, headache

Niacin (Niaspan)

Mechanism

Blocks the breakdown of fat in adipose tissue, which decreases free fatty acids in blood. Niacin also decreases liver secretion of VLDL-cholesterol and increases HDL-cholesterol

Oral

In adolescents start with 250 mg/dose PO QD then increase up to 1,000 mg/dose PO QD (sustained release (SR) tabs)

Oral dosage forms

SR tabs 250, 500, 750, or 1,000 mg

Side effects

Flushing (no-flush niacin caps available OTC), headache, nausea, itching, hypotension, hepatotoxicity

Nicardipine (Cardene)

Mechanism

Calcium-channel blocker

IV infusion

0.50 - 5.0 µg/kg/min IV infusion

Oral

1.0 - 2.0 mg/kg/day divided TID

Oral dosage forms

Caps 20, 30 mg; SR 30, 45, 60 mg

Side effects

Hypotension, tachycardia

Nifedipine (Procardia)

Mechanism

Calcium-channel blocker

Oral

0.25 - 0.9 mg/kg/day PO divided TID, or QD for sustained release (SR) form (maximum dose 10 mg/dose)

Oral dosage forms

Caps 10 mg; SR 30, 60, or 90 mg

Side effects

Hypotension, tachycardia

Nitric oxide or NO

Mechanism

A messenger molecule that induces smooth muscle relaxation

Inhalation

5.0 - 20 ppm

Side effects

Methemoglobinemia

Nitroglycerine

Mechanism

Direct vasodilator

IV Infusion

0.25 - 5.0 µg/kg/min IV infusion

Side effects

Hypotension, tachycardia, flushing, methemoglobinemia

Nitroprusside (Nipride)

Mechanism

Vasodilation by increasing cellular levels of cyclic-GMP

IV Infusion

0.5 - 10.0 µg/kg/min IV infusion

Side effects

Hypotension, cyanide toxicity

➤Monitor thiocyanate levels closely, and the values should remain < 50 mg/L.

Norepinephrine (Levophed)

Mechanism

α₁-adrenergic agonist, predominantly vasoconstriction

IV Infusion

0.05 - 0.1 µg/kg/min IV infusion, may titrate to

2.0 µg/kg/min (maximum dose)

Side effects

Hypertension, local vasoconstriction

— O —

Octreotide (Sandostatin)

Mechanism

An octapeptide that mimics natural somatostatin. The exact mechanism for reduction in a chylothorax is unknown but may be from the multiple effects of octreotide on the gastrointestinal tract and the reduction in splanchnic blood flow to reduce thoracic duct flow and decrease the triglyceride content of chyle

IV Bolus

20 - 70 µg/kg/24 hrs SC divided Q 8 hrs

IV Infusion

1.0 - 4.0 µg/kg/hr IV infusion up to 10 µ/kg/hr

Side effects

Biliary sludge, arrhythmias, diarrhea, abdominal distension, severe epigastric pain, hypoglycemia, hyperglycemia, hypothyroidism

Olmesartan (Benicar)

Mechanism

Calcium-channel blocker

Oral

20 to < 35 kg use 10 mg PO QD (max dose 20 mg/day), > 35 kg use 20 mg PO QD (max dose 40 mg/day)

Oral dosage forms

Tabs 40, 80, 160, 320 mg

Side effects

Headache, dizziness, fatigue, abdominal pain, cough, hyperkalemia, rhabdomyolysis

— P —

Palivizumab (Synagis)

Mechanism

A humanized monoclonal antibody (IgG) directed against an epitope in the "A" antigenic site of the respiratory syncytial virus's (RSV) "F" protein

IM

15 mg/kg IM (divide dose if volume is > 1.0 mL) Q month, commencing during geographically specific RSV season

Side effects

Upper respiratory tract infections, otitis media, fever, rhinitis, rash, diarrhea, cough, vomiting, gastroenteritis wheezing

Phenylephrine (Neosynephrine)

Mechanism

α₁-adrenergic agonist

IV Bolus

5.0 - 20 µg/kg IV Q 10 - 15 minutes PRN

IV Infusion

0.1 - 0.5 µg/kg/min IV infusion

Side effects

Hypertension, arrhythmias

Potassium chloride (K-Dur etc)

Mechanism

483

Potassium replacement

Oral

1.0 - 3.0 mEq/kg/day

Oral dosage forms

SR tabs 8, 10, 15, 20 mEq; SR caps 8, 10 mEq; powder 15, 20, 25 mEq/packet; solution 10% or 20 mEq/15 ml

Side effects

Gastrointestinal disturbance, ulcers

Potassium iodide (SSKI)

Mechanism

Reduces thyroid production of T3 and T4

SSKI (saturated solution of potassium iodide)

Oral

1.0 - 5.0 drops/dose PO TID

Oral dosage forms

1000 mg/mL

Lugol solution

Oral

1.0 drop/dose PO TID

Oral dosage forms

Iodine 50 mg + potassium iodide 100 mg/mL

Side effects

Metallic taste, gastrointestinal distress, rash, headache

Prednisolone (Prelone)

Mechanism

Anti-inflammatory through suppressing neutrophil migration, decreases pro-inflammatory mediators, decreases capillary permeability

Oral

0.5 - 2.0 mg/kg/day PPO QD or divided BID (maximum dose 80 mg per day)

Oral dosage forms

Tabs 10, 15, 30 mg; solutions 5.0 mg/5.0 mL (alcohol free) or 15.0 mg/5.0 mL (2.0% alcohol)

Side effects

Hypertension, gastrointestinal bleeding, hyperglycemia, mood changes, pseudotumor cerebri

➤ If therapy exceeds 5-7 days, then taper the dose over time rather than discontinuing prednisolone abruptly.

Prednisone

Mechanism

Anti-inflammatory through suppressing neutrophil migration, decreases pro-inflammatory mediators, decreases capillary permeability

Oral

0.5 - 2.0 mg/kg/day PO QD or divided BID (maximum dose 80 mg per day)

Oral dosage forms

Tabs 1.0, 2.5, 5.0, 10, 20, 50 mg; solutions 1.0 mg/mL (5.0% alcohol) or 5.0 mg/mL (30% alcohol)

Side effects

Hypertension, gastrointestinal bleeding, hyperglycemia, mood changes, pseudotumor cerebri

➤ If therapy exceeds 5 - 7 days, then taper the dose over time rather than discontinuing prednisone abruptly.

Propranolol (Inderal)

Mechanism

Nonselective β-adrenergic antagonist

IV Bolus for arrhythmias

0.01 - 0.1 mg/kg/dose over 10 minutes PRN Q 8 hrs up to Q 6 hrs

IV Bolus for "Tet" spell

0.15 - 0.25 mg/kg/dose IV slow push may repeat × 1 in 15 min

Oral

1.0 - 4.0 mg/kg/day PO divided TID or QID, or give QD if using sustained release (SR) form

Oral dosage forms

Tabs 10, 20, 40, 60, 80, or 90 mg; SR 60, 80, 120, or 160 mg; solutions 20 mg/5.0 mL, 40 mg/5.0 mL, or 80 mg/mL

Side effects

Bronchospasm, bradycardia, hypotension, hyperglycemia

Propylthiouracil (PTU)

Mechanism

Inhibits the enzyme thyroperoxidase, which impairs thyroglobulin production, a precursor to thyroxine

Oral

5.0 - 10 mg/kg/day PO divided TID

Oral dosage forms

Tabs 50 mg; suspension 5.0 mg/mL

Side effects

Hepatitis, aplastic anemia, drug fever, lupus-like syndrome

Prostaglandin E1 (Prostin)

Mechanism

Maintains ductus arteriosus patency

IV Infusion

0.05 - 0.10 μg/kg/min initial IV infusion, then titrate down to 0.01 μg/kg/min for long term IV infusion if necessary

Side effects

Apnea, vasodilation, fever, seizures

➤Confirm ductal patency with Echo after each dosing change.

Protamine

Mechanism

Coagulant activity from neutralizing heparin through the binding action of a highly cationic peptide, which manufacturers extract from salmon sperm

IV Bolus

1.0 mg IV slow push for every 100 IU of heparin

Side effects

Hypotension or hypertension, bradycardia, pulmonary hypertension, dyspnea, flushing, anaphylaxis

— R —

Ranitidine (Zantac)

Mechanism

Histamaine$_2$ antagonist

Oral

2.0 - 4.0 mg/kg/day PO divided BID or TID

Oral dosage forms

Tabs 75, 150, 300 mg; syrup 15 mg/mL

Side effects

Malaise, insomnia, sedation, arthralgia, hepatotoxicity

— S —

Sertraline (Zoloft)

Mechanism

Selective serotonin reuptake inhibitor (SSRI)

Oral

25 - 100 mg/dose PO QD (maximum dose 200 mg)

Oral dosage forms

Tabs 25, 50, or 100 mg; solution 20 mg/mL

Side effects

Dry mouth, headache, diarrhea, nervousness, and rash

C - Formulary

Sildenafil (Revatio, Viagra)

Mechanism

Inhibits cyclic-GMP phosphodiesterase

IV Load

0.4 mg/kg over 3 hrs

IV Infusion

1.6 mg/kg/24 hrs IV infusion

Oral

1.0 - 2.0 mg/kg/dose PO QID

Oral dosage forms

Revatio tabs 20 mg; Viagra tabs 25, 50, or 100 mg; suspension 2.5 mg/mL

Side effects

Headache, facial flush, upset stomach, and vision changes

Sodium benzoate + sodium phenylacetate (Ammonul)

Mechanism

Provides an alternative pathway for nitrogen disposal in impaired urea cycle and hyperammonemia

IV Load

2.5 mL/kg IV over 90 minutes

IV Infusion

2.5 mL/kg/24 hrs IV infusion

Side effects

Vomiting, hyperglycemia, hypokalemia, seizures

➤Run the IV dose through a central line to avoid local tissue irritation.

Sodium bicarbonate

Mechanism

A base compound, which counteracts metabolic acidosis

IV Bolus per dosing table

| Sodium Bicarbonate Dosing Chart ||
Base Deficit	IV slow push dose
-1 to -5	1.0 mEq/kg/dose
-5 to -10	2.0 mEq/kg/dose
> -10	3.0 mEq/kg/dose

Side effects

Intraventricular hemorrhage in neonates, tetany, local tissue damage with extravasation

Sotalol (Betapace)

Mechanism

Nonselective β-adrenergic antagonist and potassium-channel blocker

Oral

2.0 - 8.0 mg/kg/day or 90 - 200 mg/m^2/day PO divided TID

Oral dosage forms

Tabs 80, 120, 160, or 240 mg

Side effects

Beta-blocker side effects include hypotension, hypoglycemia, bronchospasm, bradycardia, proarrhythmic, and prolongation of QTc

➤Hospitalize patients to initiate sotalol.

Spironolactone (Aldactone)

Mechanism

Aldosterone blocker, preserves potassium

Oral

1.0 - 3.0 mg/kg/day PO QD or divided BID

Oral dosage forms

Tabs 25, 50, or 100 mg; suspensions 1.0 mg/mL, 2.5 mg/mL, 5.0 mg/mL, or 25 mg/mL

Side effects

Hyperkalemia, gastrointestinal distress, gynecomastia, irregular menses

— V —

Valsartan (Diovan)

Mechanism

Angiotensin II-receptor blocker

Oral

0.2 - 5.0 mg/kg/day PO QD

Oral dosage forms

Tabs 40, 80, 160, 320 mg; suspension 4.0 mg/mL

Side effects

Headache, dizziness, fatigue abdominal pain, cough, hyperkalemia, rhabdomyolysis

— W —

Warfarin (Coumadin)

Mechanism

Inhibits synthesis of vitamin K dependent factors (II, VII, IX, X)

Oral

Usually start with 0.2 mg/kg/day PO QD, maximal therapeutic doses are rarely > 5.0 mg QD in patients < 15 years old

Oral dosage forms

Tabs 1.0, 2.0, 2.5, 3.0, 4.0, 5.0, 6.0, 7.5, 10 mg

Side effects

Bleeding

➤ PT/INR monitoring determines a therapeutic dose. For mechanical heart valves, a therapeutic INR is 2.5 - 3.5. Dosing adjustments generally do not always follow predictable patterns. Drug interactions, diet, and illnesses influence dosing.

REFERENCES

1 Zeigler VL, Gillette PC. Practical Management of Pediatric Cardiac Arrhythmias. Armonk, Futura, 2001

2 Webb R, Singer M. Oxford Handbook of Critical Care. New York, Oxford University Press, 2005

3 Taketomo CK, Hodding JH, Kraus DM. Pediatric Dosage Handbook: Including Neonatal Dosing, Drug Administration, & Extemporaneous Preparations. Lexi-Comp's drug reference handbooks. Hudson, Ohio: Lexi-Comp, 2007

4 Saxena A, Juneja R, Ramakrishnan S. Drug therapy of cardiac diseases in children. Indian Pediatr 2009; 46: 310-338

5 Custer JW, Rau RE (eds). The Harriet Lane Handbook. Philadelphia, Elsevier Mosby, 2009

D – Laboratory Values

INTRODUCTION

Normal laboratory values vary by testing facility. We accompany some tests with brief explanations. We note values appropriate by age range, when normal references values vary by age. [1-10] The table below lists the prefixes and related exponents for weights and volumes of laboratory tests:

Prefix	Exponent
m (milli)	10^{-3}
μ (micro)	10^{-6}
n (nano)	10^{-9}
p (pico)	10^{-12}
f (femto)	10^{-15}

Outline of Laboratory Tests

Acute phase reactants
- CRP
- ESR

Antibody tests
- Anti SSA/Ro & anti SSB/La
- Anti-streptococcal

Coagulation
- ACT
- D-dimer
- MTHFR
- Protein C
- PT & INR
- PTT

Genetic testing
- Chromosomal analysis
- Gene analysis

Hematology
- CBC
- HbA1c

Myocardial biomarkers
- B-natriuretic peptide
- CPK-MB
- Troponin

Serum chemistries
- Aldosterone
- Alpha-1 antitrypsin
- Alkaline phosphatase
- Amino acids & organic acids
- Ammonia
- Anion gap
- Blood gases
- BUN & creatinine
- Carnitine
- Catecholamines
- Cortisol
- Electrolytes
- Insulin
- Lactate
- Lipids
- Liver enzymes
- Renin
- Serum proteins
- Thyroid tests

Urine analysis
- Common tests
- Amino acids & organic acids
- Catecholamines

ACUTE PHASE REACTANTS

C-Reactive Protein (CRP)

The liver synthesizes CRP as part of the innate immune system. Macrophages and adipocytes produce an inflammatory byproduct, interleukin-6 (IL-6), which stimulates CRP production. CRP levels rise in response to inflammation.

- All ages

0–1.0 mg/dL

Erythrocyte Sedimentation Rate (ESR)

The ESR measures the rate in mm/hr that a column of red cells settle in a glass tube. The normal ESR is slightly higher in females. With inflammation, the high proportion of fibrinogen causes red blood cells to stick together and form stacks or 'rouleaux.' Stacked red cells settle at a faster rate than nonstacked cells. In contrast, polycythemia, sickle cell anemia, hereditary spherocytosis, and congestive heart failure all decrease the ESR.

- Newborns

0-2 mm/hr

- All others

0-15 mm/hr

ANTIBODY TESTS

Anti-SSA/Ro & Anti-SSB/La

Different laboratories use different methodologies. The 2 most common are ELISA and Luminex. ELISA (enzyme-linked immunosorbent assay) detects an antibody or antigen. ELISA testing results are in EU (ELISA units)/mL The multiplex flow immunoassay (Luminex) method reports results in antibody index (AI) values.

ELISA

- All ages

< 15 U/mL

Luminex

- All ages

< 1.0 AI

Anti-Streptococcal

Streptococci produce several virulence enhancing substances including streptolysin O (lyses red blood cells), hyaluronidase (breaks down hyaluronic acid, a component of connective tissue), and steptodornase (breaks down DNA). The body generates antibodies to these virulence factors, resulting in antistreptolysin O (ASO), anti-hyaluronidase, antideoxyribonuclease-B (anti-DNase B).

ASO

- All ages

≤ 166 Todd units

Anti-hyaluronidase

- All ages

< 250 U/mL

Anti-DNase B

Anti-DNase B	
0 - 5 years	≤ 60 units
5 - 17 years	≤ 70 units

D - Laboratory Values

COAGULATION

Activated Clotting Time (ACT)

The ACT does not correlate with other coagulation tests. ACT demonstrates the inability to coagulate rather than quantifying the ability to clot. Methodology, platelet count and function, hypothermia, hemodilution and certain drugs like aprotinin may affect the results.

- All ages

70–180 seconds

D-Dimer

D-dimer is a fibrin degradation product, a small protein fragment present in blood after fibrinolysis degrades a blood clot. The name derives from its 2 cross-linked D fragments of the fibrinogen protein.

- All ages

< 0.5 µg/mL or < 500 µg/L

Methylenetetrahydrofolate Reductase (MTHFR)

The C677T and A1298C mutations of the MTHFR enzyme cause hyperhomocysteinemia, a risk factor for thrombosis. Signal amplification detects mutations of the MTHFR gene. Homozygotes are at risk for thrombosis but heterozygotes are not.

- All ages

No C677T or A1298C mutations

Protein C

Protein C deficiency predisposes for thrombosis and thromboembolism.

- All ages

700-1400 U/mL

Prothrombin Time (PT), International Normalized Ratio (INR), & Partial Thromboplastin Time (PTT)

The PT evaluates factors I (fibrinogen) II, V, VII, and X. The PTT evaluates factors I (fibrinogen), II, V, VIII, IX, X, XI, XII, as well as prekallikrein (PK) and high molecular weight kininogen (HK). For mechanical heart valves, keep the INR between 2.5 and 3.5 for all ages. PT/INR is also useful for monitoring the effects of liver damage, bleeding disorders, and vitamin K status.

PT - INR - PTT (all ages)	
PT	12 - 15 seconds
INR	0.8 - 1.2
PTT	30 - 45 seconds

GENETIC TESTING

Chromosomal Analysis

Standard analysis
- Trisomies 13, 18, & 21
- XO for Turner syndrome

Fluorescence in situ hybridization (FISH)

FISH identifies chromosomes or chromosomal regions through hybridization (attachment) of fluorescently-labeled DNA probes to denatured chromosomal DNA. An exam with fluorescent lighting detects the hybridized fluorescent signal (presence of chromosome material) or absence of the hybridized fluorescent signal (absence of chromosome material).

- Chromosome 22q11 deletion for DiGeorge syndrome
- Chromosome 7q11 deletion for Williams syndrome

Gene Mutations

Syndromes
- *PTPN11, KRAS, RAF1, & SOS1* genes for Noonan
- *FBN1* genes for Marfan
- *CHD7* gene for CHARGE
- *ELASTIN* gene for SVAS
- *TBX5* gene for Holt-Oram
- *TSC1 & TSC2* genes for tuberous sclerosis
- *JAG1 & NOTCH2* genes for Alagille
- *NF1 & NF2* genes for neurofibromatosis

Hypertrophic cardiomyopathy

In the table above on the right, we list the gene mutations for the common heritable hypertrophic cardiomyopathies.

Ion channelopathies

For individuals with suspected Long QT syndrome (LQTS),

Hypertrophic Cardiomyopathy Genes		
Gene	Protein	Estimated Percentage of HCM Patients
MYH7	β-Myosin heavy chain	20-30%
MYBPC3	Myosin-binding protein C	20-30%
TNNT2	Troponin-T	3-5%
TNNI3	Troponin-I	< 5%
TNNC1	Troponin-C	Rare
TPM1	Tropomyosin-1α	< 5%
MYL2	Regulatory myosin light chain 2	< 5%
MYL3	Essential myosin light chain 3	Rare
ACTC	α-Cardiac actin 1	Rare

the mutation detection rate is approximately 70%; however, the detection rate for Brugada syndrome is < 40%, indicating current limitations in knowledge regarding the array of causative genes in Brugada syndrome. LQTS. Mutations in potassium- and sodium-channel genes lead to LQTS. Mutations in calcium-channel genes lead to catecholaminergic polymorphic ventricular tachycardia (CPVT).

Long QT syndrome

The most common genotypes occur through mutations in the following genes:

Long QT Genes			
Phenotype	Gene	Chromosome location	Percentage of LQTS Patients
LQTS 1	KCNQ1	11p15.5	35 - 45%
LQTS 2	KCNH2	7q35-36	35 - 45%
LQTS 3	SCN5A	3p21-24	5 - 7%

➤In the previous LQTS gene table, KC stands for potassium channel, and SC stands for sodium channel. The *HERG* gene is another name for the *KCNH2* gene, involved in long QT 2. HERG stands for "human ether a-go-go." The *HERG* gene is the human homolog of the *ether-à-go-go* gene found in the Drosophila fruit fly. William Kaplan named the *Ether-à-go-go* gene in the 1960s. Researchers found, when they anesthetized flies with mutations in the *Ether-à-go-go* gene, the flies' legs shook. The shaking looked like the dancing popular then at the Whisky a Go Go nightclub in West Hollywood, California.

Brugada syndrome

Brugada syndrome can also arise from mutations in the *SCN5A* gene, which also underlies LQTS 3.

Catecholaminergic polymorphic ventricular tachycardia (CPVT)

The commonest heritable CPVT (about 50% of cases) is autosomal dominant. Autosomal dominant CPVT results from mutations in RyR2 ryanodine receptor genes. RyR2 ryanodine receptors form a class of intracellular calcium-channel proteins found in muscles and neurons. These receptors are the major cellular mediator of calcium-induced calcium release in animal cells. A rarer CPVT type (about 1% of cases) is autosomal recessive. Autosomal recessive results from mutations in the calsequestrin gene (CASQ2), which codes for proteins related to the RyR2 receptors.

D - Laboratory Values

HEMATOLOGY

CBC

The table lists values by age group.

CBC					
Age	Hb g/dL	Hct %	MCV fL	WBC k/μL	Plts k/μL
Birth	13.5 - 16.5	42 - 54	104 - 108	9 - 30	150 - 350
1 - 2 wks	12.5 - 16	39 - 52	100 - 105	5 - 20	150 - 350
> 2 wks - < 2mon	10 - 14	31 - 43	95 - 100	5 - 20	275 - 615
2 - 6 mon	9 - 11.5	28 - 35	91 - 96	6.8 - 16	275 - 590
0.5 - 2 yrs	11.5 - 12.5	33 - 36	80 - 95	6.2 - 15	220 - 465
> 2 yrs	11.5 - 14	35 - 41	78 - 90	4 - 11	190 - 405

fL: femtoliter; k/μL: 1,000 per microliter

HbA1c

Hyperglycemia causes glycosylated hemoglobin. Elevated levels are risk factors for cardiovascular disease, nephropathy, and retinopathy.

- All ages

< 6.0 % of total hemoglobin

D - Laboratory Values

MYOCARDIAL BIOMARKERS

B-Natriuretic Peptide (BNP)

The cardiac ventricles synthesize and secrete BNP when excess volume or pressure loads the ventricles (including pulmonary hypertension). BNP decreases systemic vascular resistance, decreases central venous pressure, and increases natriuresis.

BNP (values in pg/ml)	
Birth	< 1,000
3 - 4 days old	< 200 - 300
> 1 week old	< 100

CPK-MB & CPK Index

Elevated creatine phosphokinase (CPK) occurs in myocardial infarction, rhabdomyolysis, muscular dystrophy, and acute renal failure. Any CPK-MB value above the 95th percentile may indicate some myocardial necrosis. A CPK index = CPK-MB ÷ Total CPK activity × 100.

- CPK-MB all ages

≤ 3.0 µg/L or ≤ 3.0 ng/mL

- CPK index all ages

≤ 3.0

Troponin

Troponin consists of 3 contractile regulatory proteins, troponin C, T, and I. These proteins control the calcium-mediated interactions between actin and myosin in cardiac and skeletal muscles. Troponin I and T exist in cardiac muscles. Troponin C exists in cardiac and skeletal muscles; thus, troponin C is not an exclusive marker of myocardial damage. Troponin I and T are more specific for myocardial damage than CPK-MB, myoglobin, or LDH isoenzymes. Troponin T levels are slightly less specific for myocardial damage than troponin I.

Troponin I

- All ages

≤ 0.05 ng/mL

Troponin T

- All ages

< 0.01 ng/mL

SERUM CHEMISTRIES

Aldosterone

Mineralocorticoid produced by the adrenal gland.

Aldosterone (values in ng/dL)		
Newborns		< 100
< 1 month		< 175
Infants		< 75
3 - 10 years	Supine	< 20
	Standing	< 45
10 - 18 years	Supine	< 15
	Standing	< 30

Alpha-1 Antitrypsin

Produced in the liver and acts to inhibit the effects of neutrophil elastase, an enzyme that can breakdown connective tissue. 24-hour fecal collection with spot serum measurement:

- All ages

Fecal < 55 mg/dL

Spot serum 80-200 mg/dL

Amino Acids

➤See reference 6 for Quest Diagnostics and Nichols Institute, their website has a list of serum and urine amino acid tests.

Ammonia

High levels occur in inherited urea cycle enzyme defects and in some hemolytic diseases of newborns. In children and adults, elevated ammonia levels may also indicate liver or kidney damage. High ammonia levels are also found in portosystemic shunts that allow portal blood to enter the systemic venous circulation without the filtering effects of the liver.

- Newborns

≤ 150 µg/dL

- Infants and children

≤ 80 µg/dL

Anion Gap

The anion gap increases in lactic acidosis, ketoacidosis, uremia, and poisoning, especially with salicylates. Values are the same for all ages.

Anion Gap (values in mEq/L)	
From $[Na^+] - [Cl^-] + [HCO3^+]$	≤ 12
From ion-selective electrodes	< 11

D – Laboratory Values

Blood Gases

	Blood Gases					
	ABG Normal	VBG Normal	Acute Respiratory Acidosis	Acute Metabolic Acidosis	Acute Respiratory Alkalosis	Chronic Respiratory Acidosis
pH	7.35 - 7.45	7.32 - 7.42	7.25	7.25	7.50	7.35
PaO_2 (mmHg)	80 - 100	28 - 48	60	90	90	75
$PaCO_2$ (mmHg)	35 - 45	38 - 52	50	35	25	70
BE (mEq/L)	-2 to +2	-2 to +2	-1	-10	+1	+15
HCO_3 (mEq/L)	21 - 28	19 - 25	25	15	20	35

Blood Urea Nitrogen (BUN) & Creatinine

BUN
- All ages

≤ 18 mg/dL

Creatinine

Creatinine (values in mg/dl)	
Preterm 1st week	≤ 1.8
Preterm by 4th week	≤ 0.6
Full term 1st week	≤ 1.0
Full term by 4th week	≤ 0.5
3 months - 6 years	≤ 0.6
6 - 15 years	≤ 1.0

Carnitine

Carnitine transports fatty acids from the cytosol into mitochondria where metabolic pathways metabolize fatty acids, releasing energy. L-carnitine is biologically active; thus, the values that follow are for L-carnitine.

Carnitine (values in μmol/L)		
Age	Total	Free
Newborn - < 1 wk	20 - 35	15 - 20
> 1 wk - 1 yr	35 - 70	30 - 50
1 - 17 yrs	30 - 65	20 - 55

Catecholamines

Metanephrine & normetanephrine

The sensitivity of plasma normetanephrine and metanephrine for the detection of tumors is > 95%, and other biochemical tests have sensitivities of < 75%.

Plasma catecholamines (values in pg/ml)			
Sex	Age	Metanephrin	Normetanephrin
Girls	5 - 18 years	< 80	< 80
Boys	5 - 18 years	< 100	< 100

Cortisol

Released by adrenals in response to stress and a low level of blood glucocorticoids. Cortisol's primary functions are to increase blood sugar through gluconeogenesis; suppress the immune system; and aid in fat, protein and carbohydrate metabolism.

Cortisol (values in µg/dL)	
Age	Cortisol
< 1 year	< 10
1 - 2 years	5 - 20
2 - 18 years	AM 10 - 20 PM 5 - 15

Electrolytes

Electrolytes		
Na$^+$	Preterm	128 - 148 mEq/dL
	All other	135 - 145 mEq/dL
K$^+$		3.5 - 5.0 mEq/dL
Cl$^-$		98 - 107 mEq/dL
Ca^{++} (total)		8.8 - 10.8 mg/dL
I Ca^{++} (ionized)		1.1 - 1.3 mmol/L or 4.4 - 5.2 mg/dL
PO$_4$	Newborn	5.0 - 8.0 mg/dL
	All other	4.0 - 6.0 mEq/dL
Mg		1.5 - 2.5 mg/dl

Insulin (fasting)

- All ages

< 17 µIU/mL

D - Laboratory Values

Lactate

Hypoperfusion or hypoxia can cause lactic acidosis. The liver, kidneys, and skeletal muscles clear lactate. In postoperative cardiac patients, a lactate of > 4.5 mmol/L or rising from normal values indicates decreased cardiac output

- All ages

1.0-1.8 mmol/L

Lipids

The following are desirable levels for individuals < 20 years old.

Lipids (values in mg/dL)	
Total cholesterol	≤ 170
LDL-cholesterol	≤ 110
HDL-cholesterol	≥ 45
Triglycerides	≤ 120

Liver enzymes

ALT (alanine transaminase)/SGPT (serum glutamic pyruvic transaminase) exists largely in the liver. AST (aspartate transaminase)/SGOT (serum glutamic oxaloacetic transaminase) is not as liver specific as ALT, because AST also occurs in red cells, cardiac cells, and skeletal muscle cells. Clinically, we measure ALT and AST elevations in multiples of upper limits of normals, such as an ALT of 80 U/L would be 2 × the upper limit of normal (40 U/L).

Liver Enzymes in U/L (units per liter)		
Enzyme	Infants	Older
ALT (SGPT)	5 - 25	5 - 40
AST (SGOT)	5 - 60	10 - 35

Plasma Proteins

Except for gamma globulins, which are synthesized by B lymphocytes (B cells) in lymph nodes and the bone marrow, the liver synthesizes the major plasma proteins. Albumin is the major contributor to plasma osmotic pressure. Albumin also helps transport lipids and steroid hormones. Globulins help transport ions, hormones, and lipids, and participate in the immune system. Of the total globulins about 10% is α 1, 25% α 2, 25% β, and 40% γ.

Proteins (values in g/dL)			
Age	Total protein	Albumin	Total globulins
Preterm		2.0 - 3.6	
< 6 months	4.1 - 6.5	2.6 - 3.6	1.5 - 2.9
6 - 12 months	5.5 - 7.0	2.6 - 3.6	2.9 - 3.4
> 1 year	5.7 - 8.5	3.5 - 4.5	2.2 - 4.0

Renin

Renin is a peptide hormone secreted by the kidneys. These are supine serum values.

Renin	
< 1 year	< 36 ng/mL/hr
1 - 3 years	< 12 ng/mL/hr
4 - 10 years	< 6 ng/mL/hr
> 10 years	< 4 ng/mL/hr

Thyroid Tests

Originating in the pituitary gland, thyroid stimulating hormone (TSH) activates the thyroid gland production of T4. The deiodination of T4 converts it into T3, chiefly in the periphery. Serum T4 is higher than T3, but T3 exhibits greater activity. T3 is the primary inhibitor of TSH. For TSH, some laboratories report normals 0.3-6 µU/mL, but the American Association of Clinical Endocrinologists revised the normal TSH range in 2003 to 0.3-3.0 µU/mL.

Thyroid Function Tests					
Age	TSH µU/mL	Total T4 µg/dL	Free T4 ng/dL	Total T3 ng/dL	Free T3 ng/dL
All ages	0.3 - 3.0		0.7 - 2.0		0.2 - 0.6
0 - 2 wks		9.8 - 22.6		100 - 470	
2 wks - 1 yr		5.6 - 16.6		90 - 245	
1 - 10 yrs		5.6 - 16.6		90 - 270	
> 10 yrs		4.6 - 13.0		100 - 200	

D - Laboratory Values

URINE ANALYSIS

Urinalysis Normal Values	
Color	Yellow
Appearance	Clear
Specific Gravity	1.001 - 1.035
pH	5.0 - 8.0
Protein	Negative
Glucose	Negative
Ketones	Negative
Blood	Negative
Leukocyte Esterase	Negative
Bilirubin	Negative
Nitrite	Negative
White Blood Cels (WBC)	≤ 5/hpf
Red Blood Cells (RBC)	≤ 3/hpf
Squamous Epithelial	≤ 5/hpf
Bacteria	None/hpf

Other Urine Tests

Urine amino & organic acids

➤ See reference 6 for Quest Diagnostics and Nichols Institute, their website has a list of urine organic acid tests.

Urine catecholamines

Metanephrine, homovanillic acid, and vanillylmandelic acid are metabolites of epinephrine and norepinephrine. In catecholamines secreting tumors, elevated levels of metanephrine, HVA, and VMA occur in the urine.

Metanephrine (total)

Age	Metanephrine (total) 24-hour urine collection
0 - 2 years	< 5.0 mcg/mg creatinine **or** < 3 mmol/mol creatinine
2 - 10 years	< 3.0 mcg/mg creatinine **or** < 2 mmol/mol creatinine
10 - 15 years	< 2.0 mcg/mg creatinine **or** < 1 mmol/mol creatinine

values vary by laboratory

D - Laboratory Values

Homovanillic acid (HVA) & Vanillylmandelic acid (VMA)

Homovanillic acid (HVA)		
Age	Spot	24 hr
All ages		< 7.0
0 - 2 yrs	10 - 40	
2 - 8 yrs	2.0 - 25	
> 8 yrs	1.0 - 15	

Spot is in mg/g of creatinine
24 hr is in mg without creatinine

Vanillylmandelic acid (VMA)		
Age	Spot	24 hr
0 - 6 months	5.0 - 25	
7 - 12 months	6.0 - 20	
1 - 2 yrs	2.5 - 20	
> 3 yrs	1.5 - 5.0	
3 - 8 yrs		< 2.5
9 - 12 yrs		< 3.5
> 12 yrs		< 4.0

Spot is in mg/gm of creatinine
24 hr is in mg without creatinine

D - Laboratory Values

REFERENCES

1 Westergren A. Diagnostic tests: the erythrocyte sedimentation rate range and limitations of the technique. Triangle 1957; 3: 20-25

2 McCann J, Schilling A. Nursing. Deciphering Diagnostic Tests. Ambler, Lippincott Williams & Wilkins, 2007

3 Avery GB, MacDonald MG, Seshia MMK, Mullett MD. Avery's Neonatology: Pathophysiology & Management of the Newborn. Philadelphia, Lippincott Williams & Wilkins, 2005

4 Nelson WE, Kliegman R. Nelson Essentials of Pediatrics. Philadelphia, Elsevier Saunders, 2006

5 Gomella TL, Cunningham MD, Eyal FG. Neonatology: Management, Procedures, On-call Problems, Disease, and Drugs. New York, McGraw-Hill Medical, 2009

6 Nichols Institute http://www.nicholsinstitute.com/TestList.aspx?List=Pediatrics

7 Mary L. Basic Skills in Interpreting Laboratory Data. Bethesda, American Society of Health-System Pharmacists, 2009

8 Koch A, Singer H. Normal values of B type natriuretic peptide in infants, children, and adolescents Heart 2003; 89: 875-878

9 Eisenhofer G, Lenders JWM, Linehan WM, Walther MM, Goldstein S, Keiser HR. Plasma normetanephrine and metanephrine for detecting pheochromocytoma in von Hippel–Lindau disease and multiple endocrine neoplasia type 2. N Engl J Med 1999; 340: 1872-1879

10 Genetic testing registry http://www.ncbi.nlm.nih.gov/gtr/

E - Eponyms

Alagille syndrome
Daniel Alagille is a pediatrician in France. He first described the clinical features in 1975. [1]

Axenfeld anomaly
Theodor Axenfeld was an ophthalmologist in Germany. He first described the corneal findings in 1920. [2]

Bazett formula
Henry Cuthbert Bazett was an English-American physiologist. He described the formula for measuring the QTc in 1920. [3]

Becker muscular dystrophy
Peter Becker was a geneticist in Germany. He first described the clinical features in the 1950s. [4]

Bernoulli equation
Daniel Bernoulli was an 18th century Dutch-Swiss mathematician. He was the first to describe the equation. [5]

Blalock-Taussig shunt
Alfred Blalock was a cardiac surgeon at Johns Hopkins who performed the first procedure in 1944, based on an idea inspired by Hopkins cardiologist Helen Taussig. [6, 7]

Brockenbrough needle
Edwin Brockenbrough was a cardiac surgeon at the NIH in 1962 when he first described his technique for atrial septal puncture to reach the left atrium. [8]

Brugada syndrome
Pedro and Josep Brugada are cardiologist brothers from Spain. They first described the condition while working in Belgium in 1992. [9]

Brushfield spots
Thomas Brushfield was a psychiatrist in England. He first described the iris findings in 1924. [10]

Chagas disease
Carlos Chagas was a physician in Brazil. He first described the disease characteristics in 1909. [11]

Cushing syndrome
Harvey Cushing was a neurosurgeon at Harvard. He first described the clinical features in 1932. [12]

Damus-Kaye-Stansel procedure
Paul Damus was a cardiac surgeon in training at UCLA; Michael Kaye was a cardiac surgeon at the Mayo Clinic, and Horace Stansel was a cardiac surgeon at Yale when all 3 independently described a hypothetical procedure for transposition of the great arteries in 1975. Surgeons later applied the DKS procedure for 1-functional ventricles with subaortic obstruction. [13-15]

DiGeorge syndrome
Angelo DiGeorge was a pediatric endocrinologist at Temple University. He first described the clinical features in 1968. [16]

Doppler effect
Christian Doppler was a 19th-century professor of mathematics. He discovered the frequency shift of waves (water, sound, or light) depended on whether the waves

approach or retreat from an observer. [17]

Down syndrome

John Langdon Down was a physician in England. He first described the clinical features in 1866. [18]

Duchenne muscular dystrophy

Guillaume Duchenne was a neurologist in France. He first described the clinical findings in 1861. [19]

Duke criteria

David Durack and colleagues at Duke University established clinical criteria for a diagnosis of endocarditis in 1994. [20]

Ebstein anomaly of the tricuspid valve

Wilhelm Ebstein was a physician in Germany. He first described the pathology in 1866. [21]

Edwards syndrome

John Edwards was a geneticist in England. He first described the features of trisomy 18 in 1960. [22]

Eisenmenger syndrome

Paul Wood adopted Austrian physician Victor Eisenmenger's name in 1950 to describe pulmonary hypertension with cardiac malformations. In 1897, Eisenmenger had described a VSD with aortic over-ride and no pulmonic stenosis. [23]

Fick cardiac output

Adolf Fick was a German physiologist. He described his theory for determining cardiac output in 1870. [24]

Foley catheter

Frederic Foley was an American urologist. He invented the catheter in 1929. [25]

Fontan procedure

Francis Fontan is a cardiac surgeon in France. He first published the results from his procedure for tricuspid atresia in 1971. [26]

Frank-Starling law of the heart

Otto Frank was an early 20th-century German physiologist and Ernest Starling was an early 20th-century British physiologist. The two independently described the cardiac physiological principle. [27, 28]

Fredrickson classification system

Donald Fredrickson was a scientist at the NIH in 1965 when he first described his dyslipidemia classification system. [29]

Friedewald equation

William Friedewald was a scientist at the NIH in 1972 when he first described his equation for calculating LDL-cholesterol. [30]

Glenn procedure

William Glenn was a cardiac surgeon at Yale. He described the procedure in 1958. [31]

Gorlin-Gorlin formula

Richard Gorlin was a cardiologist at Harvard, and his father, S.G. Gorlin, was a mechanical engineer. They first described the equation for valve area in 1951. [32]

Graves disease

Robert Graves was a physician from Ireland. He first described the clinical features in 1835. [33]

Hertz (frequency unit)

Named for 19th-century German physicist, Heinrich Rudolf Hertz. He was the great uncle of Carl Hertz, an inventor of cardiac ultrasound. [34]

His bundle
Wilhelm His Jr was a Swiss anatomist and internist. He described the microscopic anatomy in 1893. [35]

Hodgkin lymphoma
Thomas Hodgkin was British physician. He described the pathology in 1832. [36]

Holt-Oram syndrome
Mary Holt and Samuel Oram were cardiologists in England. They first described the clinical features in 1960. [37]

Holter monitor
Norman Holter was a biophysicist from Montana. He invented the monitor in 1949. [38]

Ivemark syndrome
Biörn Ivemark was a Swedish pediatrician and pathologist. He first described the association of cardiac malformations and asplenia in 1955. [39]

Janeway lesions
Edward G. Janeway was a physician in New York City. He described the findings in endocarditis in the late 19th century. [40]

Jatene procedure
Adib Jatene is a cardiac surgeon in Brazil. He performed the first successful arterial switch operation in 1975. [41]

Jervell & Lange-Nielsen
Anton Jervell and Fred Lange-Nielsen were pediatricians in Norway when they first described long QT syndrome and deafness in 1957. [42]

Jones criteria
T. Duckett Jones was a physician at Harvard. He first published his criteria for diagnosing acute rheumatic fever in 1944. [43]

Kartagener syndrome
Manes Kartagener was a Swiss internist. He described the syndrome as a distinct congenital entity in 1933. [44]

Kawasaki disease
Tomisaku Kawasaki is a physician in Japan. He described the clinical criteria in 1967. [45]

Kawashima procedure
Yasunaru Kawashima is a cardiac surgeon in Japan. He first described the procedure in 1984. [46]

Kerley lines (A, B, C)
Peter Kerley was a radiologist from Ireland. He first described the X-ray findings in the 1930s. [47]

Kommerell diverticulum
Burckhard Kommerell was a radiologist in Germany. He described the radiology findings of the diverticulum in 1936. [48]

Konno procedure
Soji Konno is a cardiac surgeon in Japan. He first described his procedure for complex subaortic and annular stenosis in 1975. [49]

Korotkoff (Korotkov) sounds
Nikolai Korotkov, a Russian vascular surgeon. He first described the auscultatory sounds for systolic and diastolic blood pressure in 1941. [50]

Kounis syndrome
Nicholas Kounis is a Greek cardiologist. He described the clinical features in 1991. [51]

Lugol solution
Jean Lugol was a physician in France who first suggested the iodine solution for treating TB in the 19th century. Lugol solution was later adapted for treating hyperthyroidism in the early 20th century by Mayo Clinic endocrinologist Henry Plummer. [52]

Marfan syndrome
Antoine Marfan was a pediatrician in France. He first described the clinical features in 1896. [53]

McGoon ratio
Dwight McGoon was a cardiac surgeon at the Mayo Clinic. He first described his method for assessing pulmonary artery sizes in 1975. [54]

Mobitz type I & II 2nd-degree heart block
Woldemar Mobitz was a Russian-German physician. He described the forms of 2nd degree heart block in 1924. [55]

Moyamoya disease
Moyamoya is Japanese for "puff of smoke," the angiographic appearance of certain cerebral vascular changes. [56]

Mustard procedure
William Mustard was an orthopedic and later a cardiac surgeon in Canada. He first described his version for an atrial switch procedure for transposition of the great arteries in 1964. [57]

Nakata index
Seisuke Nakata is a cardiac surgeon in Japan. He first described his method for assessing pulmonary artery sizes in 1984. [58]

Noonan syndrome
Jacqueline Noonan and Dorthy Ehmke first described the features of Noonan syndrome while working at the University of Iowa in 1963. [59]

Norwood procedure
William Norwood is a cardiac surgeon. While at the Children's Hospital of Philadelphia, he first applied the approach successfully in 1981. [60]

Osler nodes
William Osler was a physician at John Hopkins and later at Oxford in England. While at these locations, he recognized this finding in endocarditis in 1888 and reported the finding in 1909. [61]

Patau syndrome
Klaus Patau was a geneticist at the University of Wisconsin-Madison when he first described the clinical features of trisomy 13 in 1960. [62]

Pompe disease
Johannes Pompe was a physician from the Netherlands. He first described the disorder in 1932. [63]

Potter syndrome
Edith Potter was a pathologist at the University of Chicago. She first described the findings in 1946. [64]

Prader-Willi syndrome
Andrea Prader was a Swiss pediatric endocrinologist and

Heinrich Willi was a Swiss pediatrician. They first described the clinical features in 1956. [65]

Rashkind procedure
William Rashkind was a pediatric cardiologist at Children's Hospital of Philadelphia when he described his method for balloon atrial septostomy in 1966. [66]

Rastelli procedure
Giancarlo Rastelli was a cardiac surgeon at the Mayo Clinic. He first used the procedure for truncus arteriosus in 1967. [67]

Reye syndrome
R. Douglas Reye was an Australian pathologist. He described the clinical features in 1936. [68]

Romano-Ward
Cesarino Romano is an Italian pediatrician who described the long QT syndrome findings in 1963. Independently, Irish pediatrician, Owen Ward, described the same findings in 1964. [69, 70]

Ross procedure
Donald Ross was a London cardiac surgeon when he described his procedure for aortic valve disease in 1967. [71]

Roth spots
Moritz Roth was a Swiss pathologist. He described the findings in endocarditis in 1872. [72]

Sano procedure
Shunji Sano is a cardiac surgeon in Japan. He first applied his modification of the Norwood procedure for hypoplastic left heart in 2003. [73]

Senning procedure
Åke Senning was a cardiac surgeon in Sweden. He performed the first successful atrial switch procedure for transposition of the great arteries in 1959. [74]

Shone complex or syndrome
John Shone was a physician from England. While working with Jesse Edwards at University of Minnesota, Shone described the pathology in 1962. [75]

Shprintzen syndrome
Robert Shprintzen is a speech pathologist at Syracuse University. He first described the clinical features of velocardial facial syndrome in 1973. [76]

Sievert radiation unit
Named for Rolf Maximilian Sievert. He was an early 20th-century Swedish medical physicist. [77]

Sjögren syndrome
Henrik Sjögren was an ophthalmologist in Sweden. He first described the disorder in 1933. [78]

Starnes procedure
Vaughn Starnes is a cardiac surgeon. While at Stanford, he performed the first RV exclusion procedure for Ebstein anomaly in 1991. [79]

Steinberg thumb sign
Israel Steinberg was a radiologist at Cornell. He first described the finding in Marfan syndrome in the 1950s. [80]

E - Eponyms

Stevens-Johnson syndrome
Albert Mason Stevens and Frank Chambliss Johnson were American pediatricians. They described the clinical findings in 1922. [81]

Swan-Ganz catheter
Jeremy Swan and William Ganz were cardiologists at Cedars-Sinai in Los Angeles where they developed the flow-directed pulmonary artery catheter in 1970. [82]

Sydenham chorea
Thomas Sydenham, a 17th-century English physician, described chorea, but his name was not applied to rheumatic fever until the 20th century. [83]

Tetralogy of Fallot
Étienne-Louis Arthur Fallot was a physician in France. He was one of several descriptors of the anatomy, although Fallot enumerated the 4-point description in 1888. [84]

Todd units
Edgar William Todd was a physician and a researcher in England. He discovered antistreptolysin in the 1930s. [85]

Turner syndrome
Henry Turner was an endocrinologist at the University of Oklahoma. He first described the clinical features in 1938. [86]

Vaughan William classification
Edward Miles Vaughan Williams was Professor of Pharmacology at Oxford University in the 1970s when he developed his classification system for antiarrhythmic agents. [87]

Walker-Murdoch wrist sign
Bryan Walker and Lamont Murdoch were physicians at Johns Hopkins when they described this Marfan syndrome sign in 1970. [88]

Wenckebach rhythm
Karel Frederik Wenckebach was a Dutch anatomist. He described the rhythm in 1899, later called Mobitz type I 2nd-degree heart block. [89]

Williams syndrome
John Cyprian Phipps Williams is a cardiologist in New Zealand. He first described the clinical features in 1961. [90]

Wilms tumor
Carl Wilms was a surgeon and pathologist in Germany. He provided the first comprehensive review of renal tumors in 1899. [91]

Wolff-Parkinson-White (WPW) syndrome
Louis Wolff and Paul White were cardiologists in the US, and John Parkinson was a cardiologist in England. Together they first described the characteristic EKG findings in 1930. [92]

Wood units
Paul Wood was a cardiologist in England. He first described the method to calculate pulmonary vascular resistance in the 1950s. [23]

REFERENCES

1 Alagille D, Odievre M, Gautier M, Dommergues JP. Hepatic ductular hypoplasia associated with characteristic facies, vertebral malformations, retarded physical, mental, and sexual development, and cardiac murmur. J Pediatr 1975; 86: 63-71

2 Axenfeld T. "Embryotoxon cornea posterius". Berichte der Deutschen ophthalmologischen Gesellschaft 1930; 42: 301

3 Bazett HC. An analysis of the time-relations of electrocardiograms. Heart 1920; 7: 353-370

4 Becker PE, Kiener F. [A new x-chromosomal muscular dystrophy.] (article in German). Arch Psychiatr Nervenkr Z Gesamte Neurol Psychiatr 1955; 193: 427-448

5 Bernoulli D. Hydrodynamica, sive De Viribus et Motibus Fluidorum Commentarii. Opus Academicum. Strasbourg, JR Dulsecker, 1738

6 Blalock A, Taussig HB. The surgical treatment of malformations of the heart in which there is pulmonary stenosis or pulmonary atresia. JAMA 1945; 128: 189-202

7 Evans WN. The Blalock-Taussig shunt: the social history of an eponym. Cardiol Young 2009; 19: 119-128

8 Brockenbrough EC, Braunwald, E. A new technic for left ventricular angiocardiography and transseptal left heart catheterization. Amer. J Cardiol 1960; 6: 1062

9 Brugada P, Brugada J. Right bundle branch block, persistent ST segment elevation and sudden cardiac death: a distinct clinical and electrocardiographic syndrome. A multicenter report. J Am Coll Cardiol 1992; 20: 1391-1396

10 Brushfeld T. Mongolism. Brit J Child Dis 1924; 21: 241-258

11 Chagas C. Neue Trypanosomen. Vorläufige Mitteilung Arch Schiff Tropenhyg 1909; 13: 120-122

12 Cushing HW. The basophil adenomas of the pituitary body and their clinical manifestations (pituitary basophilism). Bulletin of the Johns Hopkins Hospital 1932; 50: 137-195

13 Damus PS. A proposed operation for transposition of the great vessels (correspondence) Ann Thorac Surg 1975; 20: 724-725

14 Kaye MP. Anatomic correction of transposition of great arteries. Mayo Clin Proc 1975; 50: 638-640

15 Stansel HC Jr. A new operation for d-loop transposition of the great vessels. Ann Thorac Surg 1975; 19: 565-567

16 DiGeorge AM. Congenital absence of the thymus and its immunologic consequences: concurrence with congenital hypoparathyroidism. White Plains, March of Dimes-Birth Defects Foundation 1968; IV: 116-121

17 Doppler JC. Ueber das farbige Licht der Doppelsterne und einiger anderer Gestirne des Himmels. Offprint from: Abhandlungen der k. böhm. Gesellschaft der Wissenschaften, 5th series, vol 2. Prague, Borrosch & Andrä, 1842

18 Down JLH. Observations on an ethnic classification of idiots. London Hospital Reports 1866; 3: 259-262

19 Duchenne GB. Recherches sur la paralysie musculaire pseudo-hypertrophique, ou paralysie myo-sclérosique. Archives Générales de Médecine, Paris, 6 sér, 1868; 11: 5-25, 179-209, 305-321, 421-443, 552-588

20 Durack DT, Lukes AS, Bright DK. New criteria for diagnosis of infective endocarditis: utilization of specific echocardiographic findings. Am J Med 1994; 96: 200-209

21 Ebstein W. Über einen sehr seltenen Fall von Insufficienz der Valvula tricuspidalis, bedingt durch eine angeborene hochgradige Missbildung derselben. Archiv für Anatomie, Physiologie und wissenschaftliche Medicin, Leipzig 1866: 238-254

22 Edwards J. A new trisomic syndrome. The Lancet 1960; 1: 787-790

23 Wood P. Congenital heart disease; a review of its clinical aspects in the light of experience gained by means of modern techniques II. Med J 1950; 2: 693-698

24 Fick A. Uber die messung des blutquantums in der herzventrikeln. Sits der Physik-Med ges Wurtzberg, 1870, p 16

25 Foley FEB. Cystoscopic prostatectomy: a new procedure: preliminary report. J Urol 1929; 21: 289-306

E - Eponyms

26 Fontan F, Baudet E. Surgical repair of tricuspid atresia. Thorax 1971; 26: 240-248

27 Frank O. Zur Dynamik des Herzmuskels. Zeitschrift für Biologie 1895; 32: 370

28 Starling EH. The Linacre lecture on the law of the heart. (Cambridge, 1915). London, 1918

29 Fredrickson DS, Lees RS. Editorial: A system for phenotyping hyperlipoproteinemia. Circulation 1965; 31: 321-327

30 Friedewald WT, Levy RI, Fredrickson DS. Estimation of the concentration of low-density lipoprotein cholesterol in plasma, without use of the preparative ultracentrifuge. Clinical Chemistry 1072; 18: 499-502

31 Glenn WWL. Circulatory bypass of the right side of the heart: IV. Shunt between superior vena cava and distal right pulmonary artery—report of clinical application. N Engl J Med 1958; 259: 117-120

32 Gorlin R, Gorlin SG. Hydraulic formula for calculation of area of stenotic mitral valves, other valves, and central circulatory shunts. Am. Heart J 1951; 41: 1-29

33 Graves R. Newly observed affection of the thyroid gland in females. (Clinical lectures). London Medical and Surgical Journal 1835; 7: 516-517

34 Hertz http://en.wikipedia.org/wiki/Heinrich_Rudolf_Hertz

35 His W Jr. Die Thätigkeit des embryonalen Herzens und deren Bedeutung für die Lehre von der Herzbewegung beim Erwachsenen. Arbeiten aus der medizinischen Klinik zu Leipzig, Jena, 1893: 14-50

36 Hodgkin T. On some morbid experiences of the absorbent glands and spleen. Med Chir Trans 1832: 17: 69-97.

37 Holt M, Oram S. Familial heart disease with skeletal malformations. Br Heart J 1960; 22: 236-242

38 Holter NJ, Generelli JA. Remote recording of physiological data by radio. Rocky Mt Med J 1949; 46: 747-751

39 Ivemark BI. Implications of agenesis of the spleen on the pathogenesis of conotruncus anomalies in childhood; an analysis of the heart malformations in the splenic agenesis syndrome, with fourteen new cases. Acta Paediatr Suppl. 1955; 44: 7-110

40 Janeway EG: Certain clinical observations upon heart disease. Med News 1899; 75: 257-262

41 Jatene AD, Fontes VF, Paulista PP, de Souza LC, Neger F, Galantier M, Souza JE. Successful anatomic correction of transposition of the great vessels. A preliminary report. Arq Bras Cardiol 1975; 28: 461-464

42 Jervell A, Lange-Nielsen F. Congenital deafmutism, functional heart disease with prolongation of the Q-T interval, and sudden death. Amer Heart J 1957; 54: 59

43 Jones TD. The diagnosis of rheumatic fever. JAMA 1944; 126: 481-484

44 Kartagener, M. Zur Frage der Bronchiektasen. Familiäres Vorkomen von Bronchiektasen. Beitr Klin Tbk 1933; 84: 73

45 Kawasaki T. [Acute febrile mucocutaneous syndrome with lymphoid involvement with specific desquamation of the fingers and toes in children] (article in Japanese). Arerugi 1967; 16: 178-222

46 Kawashima Y, Kitamura S, Matsuda H, Shimazaki Y, Nakano S, Hirose H. Total cavopulmonary shunt operation in complex cardiac anomalies. A new operation. J Thorac Cardiovasc Surg 1984; 87: 74-81

47 Kerley P. Radiology in heart disease. Br Med J. 1933; 2: 594-597, 612.3

48 Kommerell B. Verlagerung des Ösophagus durch eine abnorm verlaufende Arteria subclavia dextra (Arteria lusoria). Fortschr Geb Roentgenstrahlen 1936; 54: 590-595

49 Konno S, Imai Y, Iida Y, Nakajima M, Tatsuno K. A new method for prosthetic valve replacement in congenital aortic stenosis associated with hypoplasia of the aortic valve ring. J Thorac Cardiovasc Surg 1975; 70: 909-917

50 Shevchenko YL, Tsitlik JE. 90th Anniversary of the development by Nikolai S Korotkoff of the auscultatory method of measuring blood pressure. Circ 1996; 94: 116-118

51 Kounis NG, Zavras GM. Histamine-induced coronary artery spasm: the concept of allergic angina. Br J Clin Pract 1991; 45: 121-128

52 Lugol solution http://en.wikipedia.org/wiki/Jean_Guillaume_

Auguste_Lugol

53 Marfan A. Un cas de déformation congénitale des quatres membres, plus prononcée aux extremités, caractérisée par l'allongement des os avec un certain degré d'amincissiment. Bulletins et Memoires de la Société Medicale des Hôpitaux de Paris 1896; 13: 220-228

54 McGoon DC, Baird DK, Davis GD. Surgical management of large bronchial collateral arteries with pulmonary stenosis or atresia. Circulation 1975; 52: 109-118

55 Mobitz W. Über die unvollständige Störung der Erregungsüberleitung zwischen Vorhof und Kammer des menschlichen Herzens Exp Med 1924; 41: 180–237

56 Suzuki J, Takaku A. Cerebrovascular "moyamoya" disease. Disease showing abnormal net-like vessels in base of brain. Neurol 1969; 20: 288-299

57 Mustard WT. Successful two-stage correction of transposition of the great vessels. Surgery 1964; 55: 469-472

58 Nakata S, Imai Y, Takanashi Y, Kurosawa H, Tezuka K, Nakazawa M, Ando M, Takao A. A new method for the quantitative standardization of cross-sectional areas of the pulmonary arteries in congenital heart diseases with decreased pulmonary blood flow. J Thorac Cardiovasc Surg 1984; 88: 610-619

59 Noonan JA, Ehmke DA. Associated noncardiac malformations in children with congenital heart disease. [Abstract] Journal of Pediatrics 1963, 63: 468-470

60 Norwood WI, Lang P, Castaneda AR, Campbell DN. Experience with operations for hypoplastic left heart syndrome. J Thorac Cardiovasc Surg 1981; 82: 511-519

61 Osler W. Chronic infectious endocarditis. Quarterly Journal of Medicine Oxford 1908-1909; 2: 219-230

62 Patau K, Smith DW, Therman E, Inhorn SL, Wagner HP. Multiple congenital anomaly caused by an extra autosome. Lancet 1960; 1: 790-793

63 Pompe JC. Over idiopathische hypertrophie van het hart. Ned Tijdschr Geneeskd 1932: 76: 304-312

64 Potter EL. Bilateral renal agenesis. Journal of Pediatrics 1946; 29: 68-76

65 Prader A, Willi LH. Ein Syndrom von Adipositas, Kleinwuchs, Kryptorchismus und Oligophrenie nach myatonieartigem Zustand im Neugeborenenalter. Schweizerische Medizinische Wochenschrift, Basel 1956; 86: 1260-1261

66 Rashkind WJ, Miller WW. Creation of an atrial septal defect without thoracotomy. A palliative approach to complete transposition of the great arteries. JAMA 1966; 196: 991-992

67 Rastelli GC, Titus JL, McGoon DC. Homograft of ascending aorta and aortic valve as a right ventricular outflow. An experimental approach to the repair of truncus arteriosus. Arch Surgery 1967; 95: 698-708

68 Reye RD, Morgan G, Baral J. Encephalopathy and fatty degeneration of the viscera. A disease entity in childhood. Lancet 1963; 2: 749-752

69 Romano C, Gemme G, Pongiglione R. Aritmie cardiache rare dell' etá pediatrica. II. Accessi sincopali per fibrillazione ventricolare parossistica. Clinica pediatrica, Bologna, 1963; 45: 656-683

70 Ward OC. A new familial cardiac syndrome in children. J Ir Med Assoc 1964; 54: 103-106

71 Ross, D.N. Replacement of aortic and mitral valves with a pulmonary autograft. Lancet 1967; 2: 956-958

72 Roth M. Über Netzhautaffectionen bei Wundfiebern. I. Die embolische Panophthalmitis. Deutsche Zeitschrift für Chirurgie Leipzig 1872; 1: 471-484

73 Sano S, Ishino K, Kawada M, Honjo O. Right ventricle-pulmonary artery shunt in first-stage palliation of hypoplastic left heart syndrome. J Thorac Cardiovasc Surg 2003; 126: 504-509

74 Senning A. Surgical correction of transposition of the great vessels. Surgery 1959; 45: 966-980

75 Shone JD, Sellers RD, Anderson RC, Adams P Jr, Lillehei CW, Edwards JE. The developmental complex of "parachute mitral valve," supravalvular ring of left atrium, subaortic stenosis, and coarctation of aorta. Am J Cardiol 1963; 11:714-725

76 Shprintzen RJ, Goldberg RB, Lewin ML Sidoti EJ, Berkman MD, Argamaso RV, Young D. A new syndrome involving cleft palate, cardiac anomalies, typical facies and learning disabilities. Velo-cardio-facial syndrome. Cleft Palate 1978; 15: 56-62

77 Sievert http://en.wikipedia.org/wiki/Rolf_Maximilian_Sievert

78 Sjögren H. Zur Kenntnis der keratoconjunctivitis sicca. Doctoral thesis, 1933

79 Starnes VA, Pitlick PT, Bernstein D, Griffin ML, Choy M, Shumway NE. Ebstein's anomaly appearing in the neonate. A new surgical approach. J Thorac Cardiovasc Surg 1991; 101: 1082-1087

80 Steinberg I. A simple screening test for the Marfan syndrome. Am J Roentgenol Radium Ther Nucl Med 1966; 97: 118-124

81 Stevens AM, Johnson FC. A new eruptive fever associated with stomatitis and ophthalmia; report of two cases in children. Am J Dis Child 1922; 24: 526-533

82 Swan HJC, Ganz W, Forrester J, Marcus H, Diamond G, Chonette D. Catheterization of the heart in man using a flow directed balloon tipped catheter. N Engl J Med. 1970; 238: 447-451

83 Walker K, Lawrenson J, Wilmshurst JM. Sydenham's Chorea- clinical and therapeutic update 320 years down the line. SAMJ 2006; 96: 906-912

84 Evans WN. "Tetralogy of Fallot" and Etienne-Louis Arthur Fallot. Pediatr Cardiol 2008; 29: 637-640

85 Todd EW. Antigenic streptococcal hemolysin. J Exper Med 1932; 55: 267-280

86 Turner HH. A syndrome of infantilism, congenital webbed neck, and cubitus valgus. Endocrinology 1938; 23: 566-574

87 Vaughan Williams EM. Classification of antidysrhythmic drugs. Pharmacol Ther B 1975; 1: 115-138

88 Walker BA, Murdoch JL The wrist sign. A useful physical finding in the Marfan syndrome. Arch Intern Med 1970; 126: 276-277

89 Wenckebach KF. Zur Analyse des unregelmässigen Pulses. Klin Med 1899; 36: 181-199.

90 Williams JCP, Barratt-Boyes BG, Lowe JB. Supravalvular aortic stenosis. Circulation 1961; 24: 1311-1318

91 Wilms M. Die Mischgeschwülste der Niere. Leipzig, Verlag von Arthur Georgi, 1899

92 Wolff L, Parkinson J, White PD. Bundle-branch block with short PR interval in healthy young people prone to paroxysmal tachycardia. Am Heart J 1930; 5: 685-699

F - Abbreviations

A_2	Aortic component of the 2nd heart sound	BNP	B - natriuretic peptide
AAo	Ascending aorta	BP	Blood pressure
ABG	Arterial blood gas	BPD	Bronchopulmonary dysplasia
ACE	Angiotensin-converting enzyme	bpm	Beats per minute
ACT	Activated coagulation time	BSA	Body surface area
ADD	Attention deficit disorder	BUN	Blood urea nitrogen
AET	Atrial ectopic tachycardia	C-CAM	Congenital cystic adenomatoid malformation
AF	Atrial flutter	CAH	Congenital adrenal hyperplasia
AGN	Acute glomerulonephritis	CBC	Complete blood count
AIDS	Acquired immunodeficiency syndrome	CHB	Complete heart block
AIVR	Accelerated idioventricular rhythm	CHD	Congenital heart disease
ALCAPA	Anomalous left coronary artery from the pulmonary artery	CHF	Congestive heart failure
		CPK-MB	Creatine phosphokinase-myocardial band
ALT/SGPT	Alanine transaminase / serum glutamic pyruvic transaminase	CMV	Cytomegalic virus
		CNS	Central nervous system
ALTE	Aborted life threatening event	CO	Cardiac output
AR	Aortic regurgitation	CoA	Coarctation of the aorta
ARB	Angiotensin II receptor blocker	CP	Chest pain (not cerebral palsy in this text)
ARF	Acute rheumatic fever	CPB	Cardiopulmonary bypass
ARVC	Arrhythmogenic right ventricular cardiomyopathy	CPVT	Catecholaminergic polymorphic ventricular tachycardia
AS	Aortic stenosis		
ASD	Atrial septal defect	CRP	C-reactive protein
ASO	Arterial switch operation (surgery)	CRYO	Cryothermal
ASO	Antistreptolysin (strep antibody)	CT	Computed tomography
AST/SGOT	Aspartate transaminase / serum glutamic oxaloacetic transaminase	CWD	Continuous wave Doppler
		CXR	Chest X-ray
ATN	Acute tubular necrosis	DA	Ductus arteriosus
AV	Aortic valve	DAo	Descending aorta
AV	Atrioventricular	DCM	Dilated cardiomyopathy
AVN	Atrioventricular node	DH	Diaphragmatic hernia
AVSD	Atrioventricular septal defect	DKS	Damus-Kaye-Stansel
BAS	Balloon atrial septostomy	DORV	Double outlet right ventricle
BMI	Body mass index	EBV	Epstein-Barr virus
		Echo	Echocardiography

F - Abbreviations

ECMO	Extracorporeal membrane oxygenation	**LV**	Left ventricle
EF	Ejection fraction	**LVEDD**	Left ventricular end-diastolic dimension
EKG	Electrocardiogram	**LVEDV**	Left ventricular end-diastolic volume
ELISA	Enzyme-linked immunosorbent assay	**LVESD**	Left ventricular end systolic dimension
EP	Electrophysiology	**LVESV**	Left ventricular end systolic volume
ESR	Erythrocyte sedimentation rate	**LVH**	Left ventricular hypertrophy
ET	Endotracheal tube	**MAP**	Mean arterial pressure
FISH	Fluorescent in situ hybridization	**MAPCA**	Major aortopulmonary collateral artery
FTT	Failure-to-thrive	**MAS**	Meconium aspiration syndrome
GI	Gastrointestinal	**MAT**	Multifocal atrial tachycardia
HbA1C	Glycosylated hemoglobin	**MHz**	Mega Hertz
HCM	Hypertrophic cardiomyopathy	**MPA**	Main pulmonary artery
HDL	High density lipoprotein	**MR**	Mitral regurgitation
HIV	Human immunodeficiency virus	**MRI**	Magnetic resonance imaging
HLHS	Hypoplastic left heart syndrome	**MTHFR**	Methylene-tetra-hydro-folate-reductase
HMD	Hyaline membrane disease	**MV**	Mitral valve
HR	Heart rate	**NCS**	Neurocardiogenic syncope
HSM	Hepatosplenomegaly	**NEC**	Necrotizing enterocolitis
HTN	Hypertension	**NSAID**	Nonsteroidal anti-inflammatory drug
HUT	Head-up tilt	**P$_2$**	Pulmonary component of the 2nd heart sound
HVA	Homovanillic acid	**PA**	Pulmonary artery
IAA	Interrupted aortic arch	**PAB**	Pulmonary artery band
ICD	Implantable cardioverter defibrillator	**PAC**	Premature atrial contraction
ICE	Intracardiac echocardiography	**PAP**	Pulmonary arterial pressure
IDM	Infant of diabetic mother	**PAPVR**	Partial anomalous pulmonary venous return
IEM	Inborn error of metabolism	**PAVM**	Pulmonary arteriovenous malformation
IM	Intramuscular	**PD**	Pulsed Doppler
IV	Intravenous	**PDA**	Patent ductus arteriosus
IVIG	Intravenous immune globulin	**PFO**	Patent foramen ovale
IVUS	Intravascular ultrasound	**PFV**	Peak flow velocity
JET	Junctional ectopic tachycardia	**PGE1**	Prostaglandin E1
KD	Kawasaki disease	**PICC**	Peripherally inserted central catheter
LA	Left atrium	**PIH**	Pregnancy induced hypertension
LBBB	Left bundle branch block	**PJRT**	Permanent junctional reciprocating tachycardia
LDL	Low density lipoprotein	**POTS**	Postural orthostatic tachycardia syndrome
LPA	Left pulmonary artery	**PPH**	Primary pulmonary hypertension
LQTS	Long QT syndrome	**PPHN**	Persistent pulmonary hypertension of the newborn

F - Abbreviations

PPS	Peripheral pulmonic stenosis		**SVT**	Supraventricular tachycardia
PR	Pulmonary regurgitation		**T3**	Triiodothyronine
PS	Pulmonic stenosis		**T4**	Thyroxine
PT	Prothrombin time		**TAPVR**	Total anomalous pulmonary venous return
PTT	Partial thromboplastin time		**TAR**	Thrombocytopenia-absent radius
PVC	Premature ventricular contraction		**TC**	Total cholesterol
PVR	Pulmonary vascular resistance		**TEE**	Transesophageal echocardiography
QP	Pulmonary blood flow		**TGA**	Transposition of the great arteries
QS	Systemic blood flow		**TNF**	Tissue necrosis factor
RA	Right atrium		**ToF**	Tetralogy of Fallot
RAS	Renal artery stenosis		**TPN**	Total parenteral nutrition
RBBB	Right bundle branch block		**TR**	Tricuspid regurgitation
RCM	Restrictive cardiomyopathy		**TSH**	Thyroid stimulating hormone
RDS	Respiratory distress syndrome		**TTE**	Transthoracic echocardiography
RF	Radio frequency		**TV**	Tricuspid valve
RNP	Ribonucleic protein		**UA**	Urine analysis
RPA	Right pulmonary artery		**UAC**	Umbilical artery catheter
RSV	Respiratory syncitial virus		**UPJ**	Ureteropelvic junction
RV	Right ventricle		**UVC**	Umbilical venous catheter
RVDAI	Right ventricular diastolic area index		**VCF**	Velocity of circumferential fiber shortening
RVEDD	Right ventricular end-diastolic dimension		**VCUG**	Voiding cystourethrogram
RVEDV	Right ventricular end-diastolic volume		**VF**	Ventricular fibrillation
RVH	Right ventricular hypertrophy		**VLDL**	Very low density lipoprotein
℞	Treatment		**VMA**	Vanillylmandelic acid
S$_1$	The 1st heart sound		**VSD**	Ventricular septal defect
S$_2$	The 2nd heart sound		**VT**	Ventricular tachycardia
SBE	Subacute bacterial endocarditis		**VTI**	Velocity time integral
SC	Subcutaneous		**WPW**	Wolff-Parkinson-White
SCD	Sudden cardiac death			
SF	Shortening fraction			
SLE	Systemic lupus erythematosus			
SLV	Semilunar valve (pulmonary or aortic valve)			
SSA or B	Sjögren syndrome antigen A or B			
SV	Stroke volume			
SVAS	Supravalvular aortic stenosis			
SVC	Superior vena cava			
SVR	Systemic vascular resistance			

ANSWERS TO THE CLINICAL VIGNETTES

1. c
2. d
3. b
4. a
5. c
6. b
7. b
8. c
9. b
10. a
11. b
12. c
13. d
14. a
15. c
16. b
17. a
18. d
19. d
20. b
21. a
22. c
23. b
24. a
25. c
26. b
27. d
28. c
29. d
30. a

Index

References pages followed by **E** denotes equation, **F** denotes figure, and **T** denotes table

— A —

A-wave spectral Doppler 363**F**
A'-wave spectral tissue Doppler 364**F**
a-wave atrial pressure 400, 401**F**
a-wave fetal echocardiography 379-380**F**
Abdomen 4, 98, 169, 371, 421
Abdominal
    aorta (fetal) 386
    mass 181
    pain 71, 80, 142, 268
    situs 219, 220, 222, 225, 226, 309, 313, 371, 384
    trauma 116
    view for fetal Echo 371, 372, 375
    wall defect 113, 180
    X-ray 111
Aberrant left subclavian artery 212, 300
ABG (arterial blood gas) 97, 515
Ablation (EP) 54-58, 60, 64, 79, 417, 419-420**F**
Abbreviations 515-517
Aborted life threatening event (ALTE) 123
Acanthosis 190, 196
Accelerated idioventricular rhythm 58
Accessory pathway 52, 53, 420
ACE (angiotensin-converting enzyme)
    inhibitors 77-79, 182, 183, 260, 515
    specific agent dosing 468, 473, 475, 479, 487
Acetaminophen 144, 450
    dosing 469, 476, 478
Acidosis
    keto 117, 159, 497
    metabolic/lactic 18, 60, 73, 101, 104, 115, 284, 452, 469, 475, 476, 486, 497
    respiratory 449
Acquired heart block 62, 73, 76, 114, 116, 124, 146, 169, 410, 419, 423
    EKG tracings 61**F**, 332**F**
Acquired heart disease
    endocarditis 8, 12, 80, 135, 137, 141, 147-149, 150, 152, 257, 260, 506, 507, 508, 509
    endocarditis prophylaxis 12, 136, 457-458**T**
    Kawasaki disease 72, 73, 124, 141-144, 152, 507
    myocarditis 49, 56, 58, 62-64, 72, 74, 76, 78, 80, 112, 114, 125, 128, 145-146, 150, 152, 383, 412
    myopericarditis 3, 141, 145, 152, 159, 169
    pericarditis 10, 72, 173, 76, 79, 80, 141, 145-146, 150, 152, 159, 162, 169, 339
    rheumatic fever 71, 72, 73, 80, 141, 145, 148, 150-151, 257, 507, 509
Acquired immunodeficiency syndrome (AIDS) 72, 145
Acrocyanosis 95, 97
Acute glomerulonephritis (AGN) 72, 150, 180
Acute phase reactants 76, 135, 146, 151, 160, 489, 490
Acute rheumatic fever 150-151, 507
Acute tubular necrosis (ATN) 180, 453
ADD (attention deficit disorder) 12, 461
Adenosine (Adenocard) 54-55
    dose 466
Adenovirus 72, 145
Adrenergic agents
    α_1 agonists
        midodrine (ProAmatine) 171
        dose 480
        norepinephrine (Levophed) 449
        dose 482
        phenylephrine (Neosynephrine) 104
        dose 483
    α_2 agonists
        dexmedetomidine (Precedex) 57
        dose 469
    β_1 agonists
        dobutamine (dobutrex) 78, 104, 449
        dose 472
        levalbuterol (Xopenex)
        dose 478
    β_1 antagonists
        bisoprolol (Zebeta)
        dose 467
        esmolol (Brevibloc) 55, 56, 104, 117, 181, 268

Index

A

dose 473
metoprolol (Lopressor)
   dose 480
β₁ & α₁ agonists
   dopamine (Intropin) 78, 104, 449
   dose 472, 473T
Nonselective α & β agonists
   epinephrine 78, 104, 111, 117, 450
   dose 473
Nonselective β agonists
   albuterol (Proventyl, Ventolin)
   dose 60T, 466
   isoproteronol (Isuprel) 62, 79, 170
   dose 478
Nonselective β antagonists
   nadolol (Corgard)
   dose 481
   propranolol (Inderal) 55, 56, 64, 79, 117
   dose 484
   sotalol (Betapace) 56, 57, 58
   dose 486
Nonselective β & selective α₁ antagonists
   carvedilol (Coreg) 79
   dose 468
   labetolol (Trandate)
   dose 478
AET (Atrial ectopic tachycardia) 54-56, 73, 79, 469
AF (atrial flutter) 54-56, 112, 124, 515
   tracings 54F, 56F
Afterload 78, 253, 360, 449-450, 452

AGN (acute glomerulonephritis) 72, 150, 180
AICD (also ICD) 60, 128, 129, 268, 269, 421F-424
Alagille syndrome 27, 42, 493, 505
Albuterol (Proventyl, Ventolin)
   dose for hyperkalemia 60T, 466
ALCAPA (Anomalous left coronary artery from the pulmonary artery) 73, 74, 75T, 76, 78, 159, 268
Alcohol (ethanol)
   fetal alcohol syndrome 27, 31
   toxin 73, 145
Aldactone (spironolactone) 475
   dose 486
Aldosterone 181
   normal levels 497
Alpha-1 antitrypsin
   normal levels 497
Alpha-agonists
   nonselective
      epinephrine 78, 104, 111, 117, 450
      dose 473
   selective (α₁)
      midodrine (ProAmatine) 171
      dose 480
      norepinephrine (Levophed)
      dose 482
      phenylephrine (Neosynephrine)
      dose 483
Alpha-blockers
   selective (α₁)
      carvedilol (Coreg) 79

dose 468
labetolol (Trandate)
   dose 478
ALTE (aborted life threatening event) 123
Ambiguous genitalia 181
Aminocaproic acid (Amicar) 451
   dose 466
Amiodarone (Cordarone) 55-58, 60, 64,
   dose 466
Amlodipine (Norvasc) 182
   dose 466
Ammonia 115
   normal levels 497
Ammonul (sodium benzoate + sodium phenylacetate) 117
   dose 486
Amphetamines 60, 159
Amphotericin B 145
Ampicillin for endocarditis prophylaxis
   dose 458T
Amoxicillin for endocarditis prophylaxis
   dose 458T
Amyloidosis 73
Anabolic steroids & hypertension 180, 183
Anal atresia 35
Anaphylaxis 111, 113, 115, 117, 473
Anemia
   general 8, 20, 52, 7, 73, 111, 113, 115, 116, 143, 151, 169, 328, 402, 485
   fetal 382-383

A

sickle cell 490
Anesthesia 98, 104, 365, 391, 392, 399, 418
Aneurysm
    atrial septal (ASA) 63, 244, 375, 384
    ductus arteriosus 246
    coronary artery 73, 142, 143**F**, 144
    left ventricular 266
    pulmonary artery 406
    systemic arterial 42, 148, 405, 408
Angiography 76, 102, 105, 219, 231, 279, 292, 298, 361, 391, 397, 398, 399, 404, 406, 407**F**, 409**F**, 508
Angioplasty
    coarctation 77, 264, 408, 409**F**, 453
Angiotensin-converting enzyme inhibitors (ACE inhibitors) 77-79, 182, 183, 260
    specific agent dosing 468, 473, 475, 479, 487
Angiotensin II-receptor blockers (ARB) 78, 182, 183, 260
    specific agent dosing 479, 487
Anion gap
    normal levels 497
Anomalous left coronary artery from the pulmonary artery (ALCAPA) 73, 74, 75**T**, 76, 78, 159, 268
Anomalous pulmonary venous drainage
    partial 254, 255**F**, 313
    total 10, 96, 103, 105, 112, 135, 276, 282, 283**F**, 316, 431

Anthracyclines 73, 145
Anti-arrhythmic agents dosing
    <u>Vaughan Williams Classification</u>
    Class I (sodium-channel blockers)
        Norpace-disopyramide 472
        Tambocor-flecainide 474
    Class II (beta-blockers)
        Brevibloc-esmolol 473
        Corgard-nadolol 481
        Inderal-propranolol 484
        Lopressor-metoprolol 480
        Tenormin-atenolol 467
        Trandate-labetolol 478
        Zebeta-bisoprolol 467
    Class III (potassium-channel blockers)
        Betapace-sotalol 486
        Cordarone-amiodarone 466
    Class IV (calcium-channel blockers)
        Cardene-nicardipine 482
        Norvasc-amlodipine 466
        Procardia-nifedipine 482
    Class V (multiple mechanisms)
        Adenocard-adenosine 466
        Lanoxin-digoxin 470
Antibiotic prophylaxis
    bacterial endocarditis 457-458**T**
    rheumatic fever 151
Antibodies
    SSA/SSB 61, 62, 269, 469, 477, 491
    streptococcal 76, 151, 491, 509
Antidromic tachycardia 53

tracing 53**F**
Anti-hypertensive agents dosing
    ACE inhibitors
        Capoten-captopril 468
        Monopril-fosinopril 475
        Vasotec-enalapril 473
        Zestril-lisinopril 479
    ARBs
        Benicar-olmesartan 483
        Cozaar-losartan 479
        Diovan-valsartan 487
    Beta-blockers
        Brevibloc-esmolol 473
        Coreg-carvedilol 468
        Corgard-nadolol 481
        Inderal-propranolol 484
        Lopressor-metoprolol 480
        Tenormin-atenolol 467
        Trandate-lobetolol 478
        Zebeta-bisoprolol 467
    Calcium-channel blockers
        Cardene-nicardipine 482
        Norvasc-amlodipine 466
        Procardia-nifedipine 482
    Direct vasodilators
        Apresoline-hydralazine 476
        Nipride-nitroprusside 482
    Diuretics
        Aldactone-spironolactone 486
        Diuril-chlorothiazide 469
        Hydrodiuril-hydrochlorothiazide 476
        Lasix-furosimide 475

Index

A

Anti-inflammatories use in
    Kawasaki disease 143-144
    myopericarditis 72
    post-pericardiotomy 135
    rheumatic fever 151

Antiplatelet agents
    Aspirin
        dose 467
        for: Kawasaki disease 143-144,
        rheumatic fever 151
    Dipyridamole (Persantine)
        dose 469
        for: Kawasaki disease 144

Aorta
    general 5, 87-89, 99, 100, 219, 226, 243, 246, 257, 270, 277, 279, 281, 282, 290, 316, 354, 355F, 391, 399, 404, 408, 436, 438, 446
    coarctation of the 4, 28, 72, 74, 75T 77, 87, 125, 147, 169, 180, 212, 241, 245, 262, 264-265F, 268, 269, 318, 358, 392, 393F 400, 402, 429, 430, 453
    coarctation angioplasty/stent 136, 264, 408, 409F
    coarctation with VSD 114, 272-273F, 290
    fetal 355, 371F, 372F, 375F-378F, 382F, 386F

Aortic annulus 248, 364

Aortic arch
    general 114, 210, 212, 243, 314 358F, 360, 391, 398
    embryology 210-212
    fetal 378F, 379F
    interrupted 34, 114, 210, 212, 274-275F, 288, 413, 431, 442
    obstruction 39, 101, 102, 412
    repair 290, 413, 444
    right 35
    vascular ring 300F-301F

Aortic atresia 270

Aortic cross-clamp 446

Aortic override 277F, 506

Aortic oxygen saturation 403

Aortic pressure 100, 272, 402-404

Aortic regurgitation (AR) 10, 36, 143, 145, 146, 159, 249, 251F, 252, 253, 260, 262, 263, 402, 408

Aortic root
    cardioplegia 446
    dilation 33, 36, 125, 357, 262
    dissection 33, 36, 125, 159

Aortic stenosis
    general 4, 6, 8, 9T, 10, 33, 39, 72, 73, 78, 114, 124, 169, 243, 245, 258, 260, 261F-263, 268, 269, 404, 430, 457
    Shone syndrome 260, 264, 509
    subvalvular 249, 252, 260-263, 266, 505, 507
    supravalvular 27, 39, 260-263
    valvular 77, 260T, 260-263, 356, 364
    valvular balloon valvuloplasty 134, 260, 262, 399, 408, 408F

Aortic valve
    general 4, 5, 150, 243, 252, 243, 249, 252, 257, 280, 282, 352, 354, 355F, 356, 357F, 364
    bicuspid 10, 33, 125, 147, 222, 242, 260, 262, 264, 270, 356
    fetal 355, 357, 376
    regurgitation 6, 10, 36, 72, 143, 145, 146, 159, 249, 251, 252, 257, 408

Aortopulmonary
    collaterals/connections 360, 410
    window 210

AP projection for chest X-ray 310, 311F, 316

Apresoline (hydralazine) 78, 182, 183
    dose 476

ARB (angiotensin II-receptor blockers) 78, 182, 183, 260
    specific agent dosing 479, 487

Arrhythmias
    general 49-64, 71, 74, 76, 99, 145, 146, 147, 159, 160, 168, 169, 171, 255, 405, 410, 470, 472, 473, 475, 478, 481, 483, 484
    brady 61-62
    cardiomyopathy associated 266, 268, 269
    EKG interpretation 327-334
    electrophysiology 417-424
    extremis cause 112-117, 241, 242, 270-274, 296
    fetal 384-386

A

heart failure cause 73, 77**T**, 79
heterotaxy associated 224
irregular 63-64
post-procedure 134, 451, 452
sinus 49, 63, 327, 328**F**
sudden cardiac death (SCD) 124-128
tachy 52-60
Arrhythmogenic right ventricular cardiomyopathy (ARVC) 58, 64, 76, 124, 126, 128, 269
Arsenic 73, 145
Arterial
    blood gases 97, 99, 111, 159, 446, 451
    markings on chest X-ray 317
    oxygen saturation 104, 246
    PaO_2 97, 99, 104, 234, 236
    plaques 192
Arterial pressure
    pulmonary 5, 10, 96, 100, 244, 45, 398, 402, 432, 442
    systemic 236, 244, 245, 402, 516
Arterial pulses
    general 4, 20, 71, 160, 167, 170, 177, 178, 449
    bounding 247
    diminished 74, 126, 169, 164, 181, 183, 270, 272, 274, 432
Arterial switch operations 102, 134, 280, 290, 431, 436, 437**F**, 507
Arteriovenous malformations
    pulmonary 97, 103, 105, 298, 299**F**, 431
    systemic 72, 382, 383**F**, 405
Arthralgias 147, 150, 485
Arthritis 150, 183
ARVC (arrhythmogenic right ventricular cardiomyopathy) 58, 64, 76, 124, 126, 128, 269
ASA (atrial septal aneurysm) 63, 244, 373, 384
Ascaris 72, 145
ASH (asymmetric septal hypertrophy) 266
ASO titer 151, 491
Aspergillus 72, 145
Aspirin
    dose 467
    Kawasaki disease 143-144
    poisoning 116
    rheumatic fever 151
Asplenia syndrome 222, 223**F**, 224**T**
Asthma 103, 168, 300, 309
Atenolol (Tenormin)
    dose 467
Atherosclerosis 178, 196, 429
Athletic screening 12, 122, 461**F**
ATN (acute tubular necrosis) 180, 453
Atorvastatin (Lipitor) 198
    dose 467
Atrial appendage 317, 385
Atrial ectopic tachycardia (AET) 54-56, 73, 79, 469
Atrial enlargement 56, 254, 317
Atrial fibrillation 56, 124
Atrial flutter (AF) 54-56, 112, 124
    tracings 54**F**, 56**F**
Atrial pacemaker (intrinsic)
    low atrial 224, 330
    sinus 49, 327
Atrial pressure 236, 400, 401**F**, 403**E**
Atrial septal aneurysm (ASA) 63, 244, 375, 384
Atrial septal defect (ASD)
    general 3, 4, 5, 6, 9**T** 4, 28, 72, 136, 208, 226, 241, 244, 245, 250, 254**T**, 255**F**, 358, 375, 392, 398, 399, 406, 430
    atrial septal restriction 205, 270, 284, 285, 292, 412
    device closure 256, 294, 399, 410, 411**F**, 412
    syndromes 29, 30, 32, 35, 38, 40, 41, 42
Atrial septation 208-209**F**
Atrial septectomy 406
Atrial septostomy
    balloon (BAS) 102, 279, 280**F**, 285, 397, 406, 413, 505
Atrial septum
    echocardiogram view 358, 359**F**
    embryology-primum 208, 209**F**
    embryology-secundum 208, 209**F**
    foramen ovale 96, 205, 208, 222, 231, 232, 236, 254, 260, 375, 412
    intact 113, 406
Atrial switch (Mustard or Senning) 436,

Index

A – B

437**F**
Atrial tachycardia 55-57, 73
Atrioventricular block
    acquired 62, 124, 134, 452
    congenital 61, 124
    EKG tracings
        1st-degree 335**F**
        2nd-degree 332**F**
        3rd-degree 61**F**, 332**F**
    pacing indications 423
Atrioventricular canal 250
Atrioventricular conduction 386
Atrioventricular connections 219, 222, 282, 358, 360
Atrioventricular dissociation 57
Atrioventricular nodal reentrant tachycardia (AVNRT) 52
Atrioventricular node 52, 53**F**, 54, 418**F**, 419, 420
Atrioventricular orifices 208, 209**F**
Atrioventricular reentrant tachycardia (AVRT) 52-53**F**
Atrioventricular septal defect (AVSD) 28, 97, 250, 341, 373**F**
Atrioventricular valve regurgitation 268 281, 282, 452
Atrioventricular valves 205, 208, 294, 295**F**, 296, 400, 402, 451
Atropine
    dose 467
Attention deficit disorder (ADD) 12, 461
Atypical Kawasaki disease 142
Auscultation
    cardiac 1-12, 147, 252, 262
    for blood pressure 177-178, 507
Autoimmune disorders 34, 135, 142, 145, 150, 268
Autonomic nervous system 167, 236
Autosomal dominant inheritance
    Alagille syndrome 42, 493, 505
    ARVC (arrhythmogenic right ventricular cardiomyopathy) 58, 64, 76, 124, 126, 128, 269
    Brugada syndrome 59, 64, 124, 126, 127, 128, 493, 494, 505
    CHARGE syndrome 38, 493
    chromosome 22q11 deletion 21, 34, 210, 274, 288, 300, 316, 452, 493
    CPVT (catecholaminergic polymorphous ventricular tachycardia) 59, 124, 128, 493, 494
    Holt-Oram syndrome 40, 493, 507
    Long QTS Romano-Ward 58, 509
    Marfan syndrome 36, 125, 126, 159, 257, 493, 508, 509, 510
    Noonan syndrome 32, 73, 180, 181, 258, 262, 268, 406, 493, 508
    Polycystic kidney disease 180, 181, 182
    SVAS syndrome 39, 260, 493
    Tuberous sclerosis 37, 180, 181, 493
    Williams syndrome 39, 258, 260, 262, 263, 493, 510
Autosomal recessive inheritance
    CPVT (catecholaminergic polymorphous ventricular tachycardia) 59, 124, 128, 493, 494
    Kartagener syndrome 222, 313, 507
    Long QTS Jervell Lange-Nielsen 58, 507
    Polycystic kidney disease 180, 181, 182
    TAR syndrome 41
AVNRT (atrioventricular nodal reentrant tachycardia) 52
AVRT (atrioventricular reentrant tachycardia) 52-53**F**
AVSD (atrioventricular septal defect) 28, 97, 250, 341, 373**F**
Azithromycin for endocarditis prophylaxis
    dose 458**T**
Azygos vein 222, 223**F**, 442

– B –

B-natriuretic peptide (BNP) 21, 74, 76, 99, 103, 146, 160, 269, 379, 489, 496**T**
Bacterial endotoxin 145
Bacterial etiology 72, 112, 114, 135, 145, 147**T**, 159, 268, 517
Balloon angioplasty 77, 265, 406, 408, 409**F**, 453
Balloon atrial septostomy (BAS) 102, 279, 280**F**, 285, 397, 406, 413, 505

B

Balloon valvuloplasty
    aortic valve 134, 260, 262, 399, 408, 409**F**
    pulmonic valve 102, 134, 258, 278, 406, 407**F**
Banding pulmonary artery/arteries 253, 432-433**F**, 444
Baroreceptors 167, 235
Bazett formula 338, 505**EF**
Becker muscular dystrophy 73, 505
Benadryl (diphenhydramine) 143, 144
    dose 472
    dose with infliximab 478
Benicar (olmesartan)
    dose 483
Bernoulli equation 362**EF**, 505
Beta-agonists
    nonselective
        albuterol (Proventyl, Ventolin)
        dose 60**T**, 466
        epinephrine 78, 104, 111, 117, 450
        dose 473
        isoproterenol (Isuprel) 62, 79, 170
        dose 478
    selective (β_1)
        dobutamine (Dobutrex) 78, 104, 449
        dose 469
        dopamine (Intropin) 78, 104, 449
        dose 472, 473**T**
        levalbuterol (Xopenex)
        dose 478
Beta-blockers
    general 55, 56, 60, 61, 64, 79, 104, 117, 128, 171, 182, 183, 197, 260, 263, 268
    nonselective agents
        carvedilol (Coreg) 79
        dose 468
        labetolol (Trandate)
        dose 478
        nadolol (Corgard)
        dose 481
        propranolol (Inderal) 55, 56, 79, 117
        dose 484
        sotalol (Betapace) 56, 57, 58d
        dose 486
    selective (β_1) agents
        biosprolol (Zebeta)
        dose 467
        esmolol (Brevibloc) 55, 56, 104, 117, 181, 268
        dose 473
        metoprolol (Lopressor)
        dose 480
Betapace (sotalol) 56, 57, 58
    dose 486
Bicarbonate 104, 117
    dose 486
Bicuspid aortic valve 10, 33, 125, 147, 222, 242, 260, 262, 264, 270, 356
Bilateral left- & right-sidedness 222, 223-224**T**
Bile acid sequestrants 198
    dose 469
Bisoprolol (Zebeta)
    dose 467
Biventricular pacing (cardiac resynchronization) 79, 423
Blalock-Taussig shunt (BT shunt) 399, 408, 429, 432, 433**F**, 505
Blocked PACs bradycardia
    EKG tracing 61**F**
Blood pressure (BP) 74, 99, 101, 167, 168-171, 177, 178, 179**FT**, 183, 190, 196, 264, 449, 452, 507
BMI (body mass index) 98, 183, 189, 190, 196, 197
BNP (B-natriuretic peptide) 21, 74, 76, 99, 103, 146, 160, 269, 379, 489, 496**T**
BPD (bronchopulmonary dysplasia) 21, 85, 86, 180
Boot-shaped heart 278, 318
Bradyarrhythmias (bradycardias) 49, 50 61**F**-62, 134, 169, 171, 235, 282, 332**F**, 384, 423, 450, 466, 467, 468, 469, 470, 474, 476, 478, 480, 481, 485, 486
Branch pulmonary arteries 39, 205, 243, 258, 259, 277, 278, 284, 288, 292, 386, 391, 404, 406, 412, 434
Brevibloc (esmolol) 55, 56, 79, 104, 117, 181, 268
    dose 473
Brockenbrough needle 406, 505
Bronchiolitis 114, 158
Bronchomalacia 96
Bronchopulmonary dysplasia (BPD) 21, 85, 86, 180

B – C

Bronchospasm 466, 367, 468, 474, 478, 480, 481, 485, 486
Brugada syndrome 59, 64, 124, 126, 127, 128, 493, 494, 505
Bundle branch block (LBBB or RBBB) 5, 126, 269, 337, 451
   EKG tracing 337**F**
Bypass, cardiopulmonary

– C –

Cafe au lait spots 181
Calcium channel 493-494
Calcium-channel blockers 55, 79, 182, 183, 263,
   specific agent dosing 466, 472, 482, 483
Calcium chloride 78, 452
   dose 468
Cancer (anthracyclines) 73, 145
Candida 72, 113, 145
Captopril (Capoten) 78, 182
   dose 468
Carbohydrates 189, 192, 195, 197, 198**T**
Cardene (nicardipine)
   dose 482
Cardiac catheterization
   diagnostic 397-404
   interventional 405-413
Cardiac output (CO)
   general 4, 8, 77, 97, 111, 245, 264, 266, 284, 292, 364**E**, 397, 399, 423, 500
   fetal 234-235, 382
   Fick principle 402-403**E**, 404**E**, 506
   postoperative 449-452
Cardiac tumors 37, 53, 58
Cardiogenic shock 112, 114, 116, 264, 270, 272, 274,
Cardiomegaly
   chest X-ray 74, 135, 146, 247, 252, 256, 257, 262, 264, 268, 269, 270, 272, 274, 284, 288, 294, 309, 310, 316, 317
   fetal echocardiography 374, 382
Cardiomyopathy
   general 76, 123, 124, 128, 160, 266, 267**F**, 268-269, 412
   dilated (DCM) 21, 56, 58, 64, 73, 74, 112, 267**F**, 268, 383
   hypertrophic (HCM) 32, 73, 79, 116, 126, 159, 168, 169, 260, 262, 263, 266, 267**T**, 493
   infant diabetic mother (IDM) 73, 79, 260, 262, 266, 268
   restrictive (RCM) 73, 76, 79, 267**F**, 269, 400
Cardiopulmonary bypass
   102, 412, 430, 446, 447**F**, 448
Cardiothoracic ratio
   chest X-ray 316
   fetal echocardiography 374, 382-383
Cardiovascular exam 4-10
Cardiovascular malformations
   general 239-304
   1-functional ventricles 73, 285, 296, 297**F**, 430, 431, 440, 441**F**, 442, 443**F**, 444, 445**F**
   Aortic stenosis (AS)
      general 4, 6, 8, 9**T**, 10, 33, 39, 72, 73, 78, 114, 124, 169, 243, 245, 258, 260, 261**F**-263, 268, 269, 404, 430, 457
      Shone syndrome 260, 264, 509
      subvalvular 249, 252, 260-263, 266, 505, 507
      supravalvular 27, 39, 260-263
      valvular 77, 260**T**, 260-263, 356, 364
      valvular balloon valvuloplasty 134, 260, 262, 399, 408, 408**F**
   Atrial septal defect (ASD)
      general 3, 4, 5, 6, 9**T** 4, 21, 28, 72, 136, 208, 226, 241, 244, 245, 250, 254**T**, 255**F**, 256, 358, 375, 392, 398, 399, 406, 430
      atrial septal restriction 205, 270, 284, 285, 292, 412
      device closure 256, 294, 399, 410, 411**F**, 412
      syndromes 29, 30, 32, 35, 38, 40, 41, 42
   Cardiomyopathies
      general 76, 123, 124, 128, 160, 266, 267**F**, 268-269, 412
      dilated (DCM) 21, 56, 58, 64, 73,

Index

C

74, 112, 267**F**, 268, 383
hypertrophic (HCM) 32, 73, 79, 116, 126, 159, 168, 169, 260, 262, 263, 266, 267**F**, 493
infant diabetic mother (IDM) 73, 79, 260, 262, 266, 268
restrictive (RCM) 73, 76, 79, 267**F**, 269, 400

Coarctation of the aorta (CoA)
general 4, 9**T** 28, 72, 74, 75**T**,77, 87, 125, 147, 169, 180, 212, 241, 245, 262, 264-265**F**, 268, 269, 318, 358, 392, 393**F**, 400, 402, 429, 430, 453
coarctation angioplasty/stent 136, 264, 408, 409**F**

Coarctation of the aorta with VSD 114, 272-273**F**, 290

Double outlet right ventricle (DORV) 30, 34, 35, 97, 210, 276, 290, 291**F**, 431, 438-439**F**

Ebstein anomaly 53, 97, 112, 114, 276, 294, 295**F**, 431, 506, 509

Hypoplastic left heart syndrome (HLHS)
general 29, 97, 111, 112, 114, 205, 270, 271**F**, 406, 509
hybrid palliation 102, 270, 443**F**, 444
Norwood/Sano 102, 270, 443, 444, 445**F**

Interrupted aortic arch (IAA) 114, 210, 212, 274, 275**F**, 288, 413, 431

Partial anomalous pulmonary venous return 254, 255**F**, 313

Patent ductus arteriosus (PDA)
general 4, 6, 8, 9**T**, 21, 28, 29, 30, 42, 72, 100, 147, 226, 241, 244**F**, 245, 246, 247, 363, 398, 400, 402, 405, 429, 430, 453, 477
device closure 136, 410, 411**F**, 430
premature infant 85-89
with other malformations 101, 102, 112, 116, 262, 264, 272, 274, 285, 292, 300, 392, 406, 412, 434, 444

Pulmonary atresia with intact ventricular septum 97, 114, 276, 292, 293**F**, 296, 398, 406

Pulmonary arteriovenous malformations (PAVM) 97, 103, 105, 298, 299**F**, 431

Pulmonic stenosis (PS) all forms 4, 8, 9**T**, 32, 39, 72, 77, 100, 103, 124, 245, 258, 259**F**, 260, 262, 277, 285, 290, 318, 400, 406, 407**F**, 429, 434, 436, 440

Tetralogy of Fallot (ToF)/pulmonary atresia with ventricular septal defect 10, 28, 29, 30, 34, 35, 38, 41, 42, 60, 96, 103, 112, 114, 134, 135, 210, 242, 276, 277**F**, 278, 318, 404, 429, 431, 432, 433**F**, 434, 509

Total anomalous pulmonary venous return (TAPVR) 10, 96, 103, 105, 112, 135, 276, 282, 283**F**, 316, 431

Transposition of the great arteries
D-TGA 10, 28, 96, 102, 112, 134, 135, 159, 210, 242, 276, 279**F**, 280**F**, 282, 316, 397, 406, 431, 436, 437**F**, 507, 508, 509, 517
L-TGA 281**F**, 282

Tricuspid atresia 10, 114, 276, 284, 285**F**-287**F**, 292, 296, 341, 400, 406, 440, 4401**F**, 442, 443**F**, 506

Truncus arteriosus 10, 34, 97, 102, 114, 205, 209, 211, 276, 288, 289**F**, 431, 438, 439**F**, 509

Valvular regurgitation
general 6, 7**F**, 8, 72, 143, 148, 150, 245, 257**F**, 392, 430, 452
aortic (AR) 10, 36, 143, 145, 146, 159, 249, 251**F**, 252, 253, 260, 262, 263, 402, 408
fetal 381, 382, 383**F**
left-sided AV valve 281
mitral (MR) 21, 36, 143, 145, 250**F**, 254, 256, 266, 268
pulmonic (PR) 252, 262, 317, 318, 361, 402, 403, 408
tricuspid (TR) 100, 112, 270, 292, 294, 295**F**, 361, 362, 363, 403, 444
truncal valve 114, 288

Vascular rings 18, 34, 35, 96, 212, 242, 300**F**, 301**F**, 302, 378, 392, 393**F**, 429, 431

Ventricular septal defects (VSD) 4, 6, 8, 9**T**, 10, 21, 28, 29, 30, 31, 34, 35,

527

Index

C

38, 40, 41, 42, 72, 95, 97, 100, 103, 104, 114, 134, 136, 208, 226, 241, 244-245, 248F-253, 257, 272, 274, 277, 284, 290, 341, 363, 373, 375, 398, 400, 410, 430, 457

Cardiotoxic drugs 73, 145

Cardioversion
    electrical 55, 56, 60, 79, 116
    adenosine (Adenocard) 54, 55
        dose 466

Carditis in acute rheumatic fever 150-151

Cardizem (diltiazem)
    dose 472

Carnitine (Carnitor) 71, 73, 74, 76, 79, 117
    dose 468
    normal values 498T

Carnitine deficiency 71, 73, 74, 76, 79

Carvedilol (Coreg) 79
    dose 468

Catecholaminergic polymorphous ventricular tachycardia (CPVT) 59, 124, 493, 494

Catecholamines
    general 21, 52, 64, 71, 104
    testing 127, 181, 183, 452, 499, 502, 503

Catheterization
    diagnostic 397-404
    interventional 405-413

Causes/etiologies
    acrocyanosis 97
    cardiovascular malformations 205, 242

chest pain cardiac 159
chest pain noncardiac 158
complete heart block 61-62
congestive heart failure 71, 72, 74, 75T
cyanosis (desaturation) newborn 96-97
cyanosis (desaturation) infant & older child 103-105
dyslipidemia 196-197
ectopic beats 64
extremis 111-113
failure-to-thrive (FTT) 18
fetal CHF 382-383
heart murmurs 6-9
hypertension 180
Kawasaki disease 142
methemoglobinemia 97
multi-focal atrial tachycardia 57
myopericarditis 145
post-pericardiotomy syndrome 135
post-procedure problems 449-453
sinus bradycardia 61
sinus tachycardia 52
sudden cardiac death (SCD) 124-125
ventricular tachycardia 58-59

CBC 20, 76, 146, 169, 181, 451
    normal values 495

Cefazollin for endocarditis prophylaxis
    dose 458T

Ceftriaxone for endocarditis prophylaxis
    dose 458T

Channelopathies 58-59, 124, 128, 493-494

Chagas disease 72, 145, 505

Chaotic atrial rhythm (multi-focal atrial tachycardia) 57

CHARGE syndrome 38, 493

Chest pain
    48, 127, 135, 145, 147, 157-161, 262

Chest X-ray
    general 20, 74, 96, 99, 105, 111, 112, 135, 136, 146, 160, 181, 214, 219, 225, 242, 309-319, 451
    1-functional ventricle 296
    aortic stenosis 262
    atrial septal defects 256
    cardiomyopathies 268-269
    coarctation of the aorta 264
    coarctation with VSD 272
    double outlet right ventricle 290
    Ebstein anomaly 294
    hypoplastic left heart syndrome 270
    interrupted aortic arch 274
    patent ductus arteriosus 247
    pulmonary atresia intact ventricular septum 292
    pulmonary arteriovenous malformations 298
    pulmonic stenosis 258
    tetralogy of Fallot 278
    total anomalous pulmonary venous return 283

C

D-transposition of the GA 280
L-transposition of the GA 282
tricuspid atresia 285
truncus arteriosus 288
valvular regurgitation 257
vascular rings 300
ventricular septal defects 252

CHF (congestive heart failure)
general 4, 19-21, 49, 52, 71-76, 85, 103, 141, 147, 151, 169, 177, 178, 180, 245, 247, 256, 257, 262, 264, 266, 288, 328, 432, 490
fetal 382-383
treatment 77-79

Childhood obesity 177, 180, 183, 189-191, 195, 196, 197

Chlorothiazide (Diuril) 77
dose 468

Choanal atresia 96

Cholesterol
general 42, 192, 193**F**, 194**F**, 196**E**, 197, 198, 469, 476, 482, 506
normal values 500**T**
R agents 467, 474

Cholestyramine resin (Questran) 198
dose 468

Chorea, Sydenham 151, 510

Chromosome 22q11 deletion 21, 34, 210, 274, 288, 300, 316, 452, 493

Chromosome anomalies
Gene deletion syndromes
chromosome 22q11 21, 34, 210, 274, 288, 300, 316, 452, 493
TAR 41
Williams 39, 258, 260, 262, 263, 493, 510

Gene mutation syndromes
Alagille 42, 493, 505
Brugada 59, 64, 124, 126, 127, 128, 493, 494, 505
CHARGE 38, 493
CPVT 124, 128, 494 59, 493, 494
DCM 268 (see cardiomyopathy)
HCM 266, 493 (see cardiomyopathy)
long QT 58-59, 124, 126, 128, 493
Marfan 36, 125, 126, 159, 257, 493, 508, 509, 510
MTHFR 492
neurofibromatosis 180, 181, 493
Noonan 32, 73, 180, 181, 258, 262, 268, 406, 493, 508
Holt-Oram 40, 493, 507
Tuberous sclerosis 37, 180, 181, 493

Other chromosomal syndromes
Turner (XO) 33, 159, 205, 262, 264, 493, 509

Trisomies
13 (Patau syndrome) 30
18 (Edwards syndrome) 29, 506
21 (Down syndrome) 17, 21, 28, 220, 250, 243, 452, 506

Chylomicrons 192, 193**F**, 197
Chylothorax 89, 451, 452, 483
Cisticercosis 72, 145
Clicks (auscultatory) 10-11**F**, 160, 258, 262, 264, 288

Clubbing 105, 278, 298**F**
CMV 72, 145
CO (cardiac output)
general 4, 8, 77, 97, 111, 245, 264, 266, 284, 292, 364**E**, 397, 399, 423, 500
fetal 234-235, 382
Fick principle 402-403**E**, 404**E**, 506
postoperative 449-452

Coarctation of the aorta
general 4, 9**T**, 28, 72, 74, 75**T**, 77, 87, 125, 147, 169, 180, 212, 241, 245, 262, 264-265**F**, 268, 269, 318, 358, 392, 393**F**, 400, 402, 429, 430, 453
coarctation angioplasty/stent 136, 264, 408, 409**F**
coarctation with VSD 114, 272-273**F**, 290

Cocaine 60, 64, 73, 124, 159, 180
Codeine 450
dose 469

Coil embolization 136, 247, 410, 412
Collagen vascular disease (systemic connective tissue disease) 62, 72, 73, 74, 145, 159

Coloboma 30, 37, 38**F**
Color flow Doppler 87, 100, 361-362**F**, 365, 375, 382

Commotio cordis 125, 127
Complete heart block
Acquired 62, 73, 76, 114, 116, 124,

C

144, 169, 332, 410, 419, 423
congenital 61-62, 73, 79, 114, 116, 169, 281, 282, 332, 423, 469
EKG tracings 61F, 332F
Computed tomography scan (CT scan) 391-393, 397, 398
Concealed accessory pathway 52
Conduction 40, 52, 54, 62, 124, 281, 386, 418-419
Congenial adrenal hyperplasia (CAH) 114, 117, 180
Congenital accessory pathway 52, 336
Congenital junctional ectopic tachycardia
    EKG tracing 57F
Congenital methemoglobinemia 97, 102
Congenital renal disease 180
Congenitally corrected transposition 281
Congestive heart failure
    general 4, 19-21, 49, 52, 71-76, 85, 103, 141, 147, 151, 169, 177, 178, 180, 245, 247, 256, 257, 262, 264, 266, 288, 328, 432, 490
    fetal 382-383
    treatment 77-79
Constrictive pericarditis 73, 76, 79
Continuous murmur 6-7F, 247, 292
Continuous-wave Doppler (CWD) 362
Conversion of tachyarrhythmias
    supraventricular tachycardia 54-56, 73, 79
    ventricular tachycardia 60
Cordarone (amiodarone) 55-58, 60, 64,
    dose 466

Coreg (carvedilol) 79
    dose 468
Corgard (nadolol)
    dose 481
Coronary arteries
    general 123, 124, 128, 159, 232, 243, 384, 391, 398, 446
    atherosclerosis 178, 197, 429
    congenital abnormalities 12, 39, 73, 74, 75T, 91, 92, 94, 96, 126, 128, 168, 177, 268, 279, 291, 398, 436, 444
    Kawasaki disease 73, 142-144
Coronary artery aneurysm 73, 142, 143F, 144
Cor triatriatum 318
Corticosteroids, therapeutic
    Glucocorticoids
        agents & dosing:
            hydrocortisone (Solu-Cortef) 476
            methylprednisolone (Solu-Medrol) 480
            prednisolone (Prelone) 484
            prednisone 484
        for:
            congenital adrenal hyperplasia 117
            fetal heart block 62
            Kawasaki disease 142-144
            myopericarditis 78
            post-pericardiotomy syndrome 135
            rheumatic fever 151
            thyrotoxicosis 117
        side effects:

            hypertension cause 180
            hypertrophic cardiomyopathy 73
            lipid disorder 197
    Mineralocorticoids
        agents & dosing:
            fludrocortisone (Florinef)
                dose 474
        for:
            syncope 171
        side effects:
            hypertension180
Cortisol 181
    normal values 499
Costochondritis 158, 160
Coumadin (warfarin) 144
    dose 487
Coxsackie A & B 72, 145
Cozaar (losartan)
    dose 479
CPK (creatine phosphokinase)
    general 467, 475
    myocardial band (MB) 76, 135, 146,
    levels 496
CPVT (Catecholaminergic polymorphous ventricular tachycardia) 59, 124, 493, 494
CRP (C-reactive protein) 20, 76, 135, 143, 146, 150, 160
    normal levels 490
Cryoablation 420
CT-scan (computed tomography scan) 391-393F, 397, 398
Cushing syndrome 183

C – D

Cyanosis (desaturation)
    general 95, 97, 102
    cardiac 10, 21, 96-97, 102-105, 112, 114, 134, 210, 241-242, 276-298, 317, 369, 432-445, 457
    pulmonary 96, 103, 112-114
    methemoglobinemia 95, 97, 102, 480, 482
Cyanotic spell 103, 104, 114, 116, 278

– D –

D-dimer 160
    normal levels 492
D-transposition of the great arteries 10, 28, 96, 102, 112, 134, 135, 159, 210, 242, 276, 279F, 280F, 282, 316, 397, 406, 431, 436, 437F, 507, 508, 509
Damus-Kaye-Stansel procedure 505
DCM (dilated cardiomyopathy) 21, 56, 58, 64, 73, 74, 112, 267F, 268, 383
Decadron (dexamethasone)
    dose 469
Defibrillator
    electrical cardioversion 55, 78
    implantable 60, 128, 267, 417, 421F
Deletion syndromes
    chromosome 22q11 21, 34, 210, 274, 288, 300, 316, 452, 493
    TAR 41

Williams 39, 258, 260, 262, 263, 493, 510
Delta-wave
    EKG tracings 52F, 336F
Desaturation (cyanosis)
    general 95, 97, 102
    cardiac 10, 21, 96-97, 102-105, 112, 114, 134, 210, 241-242, 276-298, 317, 369, 432-445, 457
    methemoglobinemia 95, 97, 102, 480, 482
    pulmonary 96, 103, 112-114
Development of the heart 205F-215F, 225, 277, 279, 288, 313
Device closure 256, 294, 399, 410, 411F, 412, 430
    atrial septal defect 256, 294, 399, 410, 411F, 412, 430
    patent ductus arteriosus 4410, 411F, 430
    ventricular septal defect 253, 399, 410, 430
Dexamethasone (Decadron)
    dose 469
Dexmedetomidine (Precedex) 57
    dose 469
Dextrocardia 29, 30, 35, 95, 206, 222, 225F, 242, 313, 373, 440
Dextro (D) looping of the embryonic heart tube 206, 207F, 279
Dextrose with insulin for hyperkalemia
    dose 60T, 470
Diabetes

    maternal 98, 262, 266
    type I 18, 38, 197
    type II 190, 191, 197
Diaphragmatic hernia 96, 98, 101, 113, 225, 312, 372, 377
Diaphragmatic paralysis 451
Diastole 4, 6, 360, 363, 379, 380, 400, 404, 440
Diastolic dysfunction 71, 73, 74, 79, 266, 363F, 364, 379, 450
Diastolic murmurs 6, 7F, 10, 252, 256, 257, 262, 288
Diazepam (Valium) 151
    dose 470
Dicrotic notch 402
DiGeorge syndrome 34, 493, 505
Digibind/DigiFab (digoxin immune Fab)
    dose 470. 471T
Digoxin (Lanoxin) 55-57, 60, 64, 79, 384, 466
    dose 470, 471T
Dilated cardiomyopathy (DCM) 21, 56, 58, 64, 73, 74, 112, 267F, 268, 383
Dilation
    aortic 125, 260-261F, 262
    balloon 397, 406-407F, 408-409F
    pulmonary artery 36, 258-259F, 262
    ventricular 245, 268, 361
Diltiazem (Cardizem)
    dose 472
Diovan (valsartan) 78, 182, 183
    dose 487
Diphenhydramine (Benadryl) 143, 155

D – E

dose 472
dose with infliximab 478
Diphtheria 72, 145
Dipyridamole (Persantine) 144
dose 472
Disopyrimide (Norpace) 171
dose 472
Diuretics
cause lipid disorders 197
for congestive heart failure 78, 79, 116, 253
for hypertension 182
medication dosing
Aldactone-spironolactone 486
Diuril-chlorothiazide 469
Hydrodiuril-hydrochlorothiazide 476
Lasix-furosimide 475
Diuril (chlorothiazide) 77
dose 468
Dobutrex (dobutamine) 78, 104, 449
dose 472
Dopamine (Intropin) 78, 104, 449
dose 472, 473T
Doppler blood pressure 176, 178
Doppler echocardiography
color flow 87, 100, 361-362F, 365, 375, 382
spectral 100, 257, 258, 260, 264, 266, 361-363F, 365, 379F-381F, 382, 386
tissue 365F
DORV (double outlet right ventricle) 30, 34, 35, 97, 210, 290-291F, 438-439F
Double aortic arch 212, 213F, 300, 300F
Down syndrome 17, 21, 28, 220, 250, 253, 452, 506
Duchenne muscular dystrophy 73, 506
Ductal dependent heart disease 101, 116, 246, 258, 262, 264, 270, 272, 274, 278, 280, 285, 290, 292, 296
Ductus arteriosus 231-236, 377-378
Ductus arteriosus aneurysm 246
Ductus venosus 232-236, 282, 379-380, 382-283
Duke criteria for endocarditis 148, 506
Dyslipidemia 42, 192, 193F, 194F, 196E, 197, 198, 469, 476, 482, 506
normal values 500T
R agents 467, 474
Dysplastic valvular pulmonic stenosis 32, 258, 259, 262, 406

— E —

E-wave spectral Doppler 363F, 386
E'-wave spectral tissue Doppler 364F
Ebstein anomaly 53, 97, 112, 114, 257, 276, 294, 295F, 431, 506, 509
EBV (Epstein-Barr virus) 72, 145
Echocardiography (Echo)
General/transthoracic 3, 10, 12, 21, 27, 54, 56, 74, 76, 77, 85, 87-88, 99, 100, 101, 105, 111, 123, 126, 128, 135, 143, 144, 146, 150, 160, 169, 181, 183, 219, 225, 244, 313, 351-365, 298, 450
Cardiovascular malformations
1-functional ventricle 296
Aortic stenosis 260T, 262
Atrial septal defects & PAPVR 254
Cardiomyopathies 266, 268-269
Coarctation of the aorta (CoA) 264
CoA with VSD 272
Double outlet right ventricle 290
Ebstein anomaly 294
Hypoplastic left heart syndrome 270
Interrupted aortic arch 274
Patent ductus arteriosus 246-247
Pulmonary arteriovenous malformation 298
Pulmonary atresia intact ventricular septum 292
Pulmonic stenosis 258T
Tetralogy of Fallot 278
Total anomalous pulmonary venous return 282
D-transposition 279
L-transposition 281
Tricuspid atresia 284
Truncus arteriosus 288
Valvular regurgitation 257
Vascular rings 300
Ventricular septal defects 248, 252
Doppler

E

color flow 87, 100, 361-362**F**, 365, 375, 382
spectral 100, 257, 258, 260, 264, 266, 361-363**F**, 365, 379**F**-381**F**, 382, 386
tissue 365**F**
Endocarditis 148**F**
Fetal 27, 241, 242, 369-386
Kawasaki disease 143**F**-144
Pre/postoperative 450-451
Transesophageal 365, 410, 446, 450
Echovirus 72, 145
ECMO (extracorporeal membrane oxygenation) 78, 101, 399, 452
Ectopics 63**F**-64, 73, 134, 159, 333**F**, 452
Edwards syndrome 29, 506
EFE (endocardial fibroelastosis) 269
Eisenmenger syndrome 72, 103, 244, 253, 506
Ejection click 10-11**F**, 160, 258, 262, 264, 288
Ejection fraction (EF) 360**E**-361, 404
Ejection murmur 5, 6, 7**F**, 8, 9**F**, 10, 245, 262, 264, 278
EKG (electrocardiogram)
general 3, 12, 49-50, 52, 54, 55-57, 59, 73-74, 99, 111, 126, 127, 150, 160, 169, 170, 224, 242, 243, 250, 256, 269, 285, 449, 451, 510
interpretation 323**F**-346**F**
Electrical cardioversion 55, 56, 79, 116
Electrocution 145

Electrolytes
general 57, 60, 64, 76, 99, 125, 127, 146, 171, 181, 446, 451, 452
normal values 499**T**
Electrophysiology (EP) study 49, 52, 55-58, 60, 76, 77, 79, 161, 269, 365, 417-424
ELISA (enzyme-linked immunosorbent assay 491
Embolization procedures 105, 247, 298, 410, 412
Embryology of the heart 205**F**-215**F**, 225, 277, 279, 288, 313
Enalapril (Vasotec) 77-79, 182-183
dose 473
Endocardial cushion defect (or AVSD) 28, 97, 250, 341, 373**F**
Endocardial fibroelastosis (EFE) 269
Endocarditis
general 8, 12, 80, 135, 137, 141, 147-150, 152, 257, 260, 506, 508
Duke criteria 148, 507
empiric R 473
prophylaxis 457-458**T**
Endocrine problems 4, 18, 111, 113, 115, 116, 177, 180, 268
Endomyocardial biopsy 76, 128, 146, 269, 405, 412
Enoxaparin (Lovenox)
dose 473
Ephedrine 124
Epinephrine 78, 104, 111, 117, 450
dose 473

Eponyms 505-510
Epstein-Barr virus (EBV) 72, 147
Erythema marginatum 150
Esmolol (Brevibloc) 55, 56, 79, 104, 117, 181, 268
dose 473
Esophageal atresia 35, 365
ESR (erythrocyte sedimentation rate) 20, 76, 135, 143, 146, 150, 151, 160
normal values 490
Ethanol (alcohol)
fetal alcohol syndrome 27, 31
toxin 73, 145
Etiologies/causes
acrocyanosis 97
cardiovascular malformations 205, 242
chest pain cardiac 159
chest pain noncardiac 158
complete heart block 61-62
congestive heart failure 71, 72, 74, 75**T**
cyanosis (desaturation) newborn 96-97
cyanosis (desaturation) infant & older child 103-105
dyslipidemia 196-197
ectopic beats 64
extremis 111-113
failure-to-thrive (FTT) 18
fetal CHF 382-383
heart murmurs 6-9
hypertension 180

E – F

    Kawasaki disease 142
    methemoglobinemia 97
    multi-focal atrial tachycardia 57
    myopericarditis 145
    post-pericardiotomy syndrome 135
    post-procedure problems 449-453
    sinus bradycardia 61
    sinus tachycardia 52
    sudden cardiac death (SCD) 124-125
    ventricular tachycardia 58-59

Event monitor 49-51**F**, 127, 161, 171
Exercise-induced asthma 168, 300
Exercise testing 12, 49, 128
Extracorporeal membrane oxygenation (ECMO) 78, 101, 399, 452
Extremis 112-117, 241, 242, 270-274, 296
Ezetimibe (Zetia) 198
    dose 474

– F –

Failure to thrive (FTT) 17-21
Fainting (syncope) 49, 50, 127, 167-171, 258, 262, 423
Fallot, tetralogy of 10, 28, 29, 30, 34, 35, 38, 41, 42, 60, 96, 103, 112, 114, 134, 135, 205, 210, 242, 276, 277**F**, 278, 318, 404, 429, 431, 432, 433**F**, 434, 509
Familial cardiomyopathy 73, 262, 268, 269, 493
Familial hypercholesterolemia 196-197
Family history
    clearance ADD drugs & sports 12, 461
    hypertension 177, 181, 183
    obesity/lipids disorders 189, 190, 196-197
    sudden cardiac death 126
    syncope 168
    syndromes 36
Fatty acids 192, 468, 482, 498
Fatty acid oxidation abnormalities 73, 115
Fatty liver 189
Fenestration for Fontan procedure 410-411
Fer-In-Sol (ferrous sulfate)
    dose 474
Fetal alcohol syndrome 27, 31
Fetal anemia
Fetal arrhythmias 384**F**, 385**F**, 386**F**
Fetal circulation 232, 233**F**, 234-235
Fetal congestive heart failure 382-383
Fetal echocardiography 241, 369-386
Fetal/neonatal cardiovascular physiology 231-236, 379
Fever
    general 8, 71, 72, 73, 98, 103, 160, 257
    postoperative 135, 452

prolonged 141-151, 257
    prostaglandin E1 102
Fibroelastosis 269
Fibrillation
    atrial 56, 124
    ventricular 55, 56, 59, 123, 124, 423, 446
Fick principle 402-403**E**, 404**E**, 506
First (1st)-degree AV block 62
    EKG tracing 335**F**
First (1st)-heart sound (S$_1$) 4-7
FISH (fluorescence in situ hybridization) probe 34, 39, 493
Fish oil 198
    dose 474
Fixed splitting of S$_2$ 5**F**, 256
Flecainide (Tambocor) 56, 57, 58
    dose 474
Florinef (fludrocortisone) 171
    dose 474
Fluids, postoperative 450
Fluids, syncope 171
Fontan procedure 135, 270, 285, 292, 294, 296, 398, 410, 413-413, 440, 442, 443**F**, 444, 445**F**, 506
Fosinopril (Monopril)
    dose 474
Foramen ovale
    embryology 205, 208, 209**F**
    fetal 231, 232, 236, 375
    postnatal & older (PFO) 96, 222, 254, 256
    restricted 270, 284, 292, 413

F – H

Fosinopril (Monopril)
    dose 475
Frank-Starling law of the heart 234, 235, 245, 506
Friction rub 10, 135, 135, 160, 449
Friedewald formula 196E, 506
Fredrickson classification 196, 506
Fungal 72, 113, 145
Furosemide (Lasix) 77, 78, 450
    dose 475

— G —

Gallbladder
    hydrops in Kawasaki disease 142
    fetal echocardiogram 371
Gallop rhythm 10, 74, 145, 160
Gammaglobulin
    intravenous immune (IVIG) ℞ 62, 78, 116, 142-144
    dose 477
    normal levels 500T
Gastroesophageal reflux 18, 96, 123, 157, 158
Gastroschisis 113
Gemfibrozil (Lopid) 198
    dose 475
Gene deletion syndromes
    chromosome 22q11 21, 34, 210, 274, 288, 300, 316, 452, 493
    TAR 41

Williams 39, 258, 260, 262, 263, 493, 510
Gene mutation syndromes
    Alagille 42, 493, 505
    Brugada 59, 64, 124, 126, 127, 128, 493, 494, 505
    CHARGE 38, 493
    CPVT 124, 128, 494 59, 493, 494
    DCM 268 (see cardiomyopathy)
    HCM 266, 493 (see cardiomyopathy)
    long QT 58-59, 124, 126, 128, 493
    Marfan 36, 125, 126, 159, 257, 493, 508, 509, 510
    MTHFR 492
    neurofibromatosis 180, 181, 493
    Noonan 32, 73, 180, 181, 258, 262, 268, 406, 493, 508
    Holt-Oram 40, 493, 507
    Tuberous sclerosis 37, 180, 181, 493
Genetic conditions
    cardiomyopathies 76, 266, 493
    cardiovascular malformations 205, 242
    channelopathies 58, 59, 124, 493, 494
    lipid disorders 196-197
    sudden cardiac death 126, 138, 493
    syndromes 27-42, 493
Glenn procedure 135, 270, 285, 287F, 292, 296, 398, 413, 432, 440, 442-443F, 444-445F, 506
Glomerulonephritis 72, 147, 148, 150, 180

Glomerulosclerosis 42
Glucophage (metformin) 191
    dose 479
Glycogen storage disease 53, 73, 113, 266
Glycosylated hemoglobin (HbA1C)
    levels 495
Gore-Tex® 432
Gorlin-Gorlin formula 404E, 506
Grading murmurs 6
Graves disease 113, 506
Great arteries (transposition)
    D-TGA 10, 28, 96, 102, 112, 134, 135, 159, 210, 242, 276, 279F, 280F, 282, 316, 397, 406, 431, 436, 437F, 507, 508, 509, 517
    L-TGA 281F, 282
Growth charts 17
Growth failure 17-21

— H —

Hair grooming syncope 167, 168
Haloperidol (Haldol) 151
    dose 475
HbA1C (glycosylated hemoglobin) 495
HCM (hypertrophic cardiomyopathy) 32, 73, 79, 116, 126, 159, 168, 169, 260, 262, 263, 266, 267F, 493
HDL (high-density lipoprotein) 192, 196E

Index

H

Head-up tilt (HUT) table test 169-170
Heart block 61, 62, 64, 73, 76, 79, 114, 116, 146, 169, 281, 282, 332, 410, 420, 423
    EKG tracings 61**F**, 332**F**, 337**F** 397-413
Heart chest X-ray 311-319
Heart embryology 2-5-215
Heart electrophysiology 417-422
Heart failure
    general 4, 19-21, 49, 52, 71-76, 85, 103, 141, 147, 151, 169, 177, 178, 180, 245, 247, 256, 257, 262, 264, 266, 288, 328, 432, 490
    fetal 382-383
    treatment 77-79
Heart fetus 232-236, 369-386
Heart malformations 241-302
Heart malposition 99, 225
Heart MRI/CT-scan 12, 21, 76, 101, 102, 105, 128, 136, 150, 181, 219, 254, 266, 269, 279, 282, 298, 300, 361, 391-393, 397, 398, 424
Heart murmurs general 3-11
Heart rate & rhythm abnormalities 49-54
Heart size 99, 112
Heart sounds 3-7, 10, 126, 127, 145, 160, 169, 280, 282, 288
Heart surgery 134-136, 429-453
Heart transplantation 73, 77, 78, 79, 268, 269, 292, 412, 430, 444, 457
Heavy metals 72, 145
Hematology 495

Hemochromatosis 73, 76
Hemodynamics
    fetal 234-235, 372
    other 52, 54, 64, 87, 98, 266, 410, 412, 413, 452
Hemoglobin
    fetal 234, 382
    other 93, 97, 101, 402-403
Hemolytic uremic syndrome 180
Hemophilus influenza 72, 145
Heparin 446, 451
    dose 475, 476**T**
Hepatitis 72, 142, 145
HERG gene 494
Herpes 72, 113, 115, 145
Hertz 31, 506
Heterotaxy 220, 222, 223**F**
High-density lipoprotein (HDL) 192, 196**E**
His bundle 417, 418, 507
Histoplasmosis 72, 145
HIV (human immunodeficiency virus) 72, 145
HLHS (hypoplastic left heart syndrome)
    general 29, 97, 111, 112, 114, 205, 270, 271**F**, 406, 509
    hybrid palliation 102, 270, 443, 444
    Norwood/Sano 102, 270, 443, 444, 445**F**
HMG-CoA reductase inhibitors (statins) 194, 198
    dose atorvastatin (Lipitor) 467

Holosystolic murmurs 6, 8, 252, 256, 257, 292
Holt-Oram syndrome 40, 493, 507
Holter monitoring 12, 49, 50, 51**F**, 64, 126, 127, 128, 161, 169, 171, 507
Homeobox genes 205
Homovanillic acid (HVA) 52, 53**T**
Hybrid palliation general 102, 270, 272, 74, 290, 296, 405, 412, 413**F**, 430, 444
Hydralazine (Apresoline) 78, 182, 183
    dose 476
Hydrocodone+acetaminophen (Lortab) 450
    dose 476
Hydrocortisone (Solu-Cortef) 117
    dose 476
Hydrodiuril (hydrochlorothiazide) 77
    dose 476
Hydrops 111, 112-113, 116, 268, 294, 372, 382
Hydrops of the gallbladder 142
Hypercholesterolemia 196-198
Hypercyanotic spells (Tet spells) 103, 104, 114, 116, 278
Hyperdynamic precordium 4, 8, 10, 71, 74, 99, 247, 252, 256, 257, 270, 272, 274, 280, 284, 288, 290, 296
Hypereosinophilic syndrome 73, 76, 159
Hyperkalemia
    general 60, 61, 88, 117, 182, 337
    EKG effect 60**F**
    ℞ 60**T**

H – I

Hyperpyrexia 145
Hypertension, systemic
    177-183, 189, 190, 197, 264, 268,
    400, 450, 451, 453
Hyperthyroidism 8, 52, 64, 72, 113, 115,
    116-117, 180, 181, 183, 328
Hypertriglyceridemia 196-198
Hypertrophic cardiomyopathy (HCM)
    32, 73, 79, 116, 126, 159, 168, 169,
    260, 262, 263, 266, 267**F**, 493
Hypertrophy
    left ventricular 124, 126, 128, 159,
    178, 245, 266, 346
    right ventricular 169, 245, 277, 278,
    317, 343, 344, 345
Hypocalcemia 34, 274, 288, 452
Hypoplastic left heart syndrome (HLHS)
    general 29, 97, 111, 112, 114, 205,
    270, 271**F**, 406, 509
    hybrid palliation 102, 270, 443,
    444
    Norwood/Sano 102, 270, 443, 444,
    445**F**
Hypothermia in cardiac surgery 446, 448
Hypothyroidism 28, 39, 61, 73, 197, 328
Hypoxia
    fetal 234-235
    other 60-61, 73, 96, 98, 168, 452,
    500

— I —

IAA (interrupted aortic arch) 34, 114,
    210, 212, 274-275**F**, 288, 413, 431,
    442
Ibuprofen (Motrin & NeoProfen) 85, 88
    dose 477
ICD (implantable cardioverter
    defibrillator) 55, 60, 128, 268, 417,
    421**F**
ICE (intracardiac echocardiography) 365
Idiopathic
    arrhythmias 63, 125
    cardiomyopathy 73-74, 112
    chest pain 158
    hydrops 113
    hypertension systemic 177, 180
    left ventricular hypertrophy 124
IDL (intermediate-density lipoprotein)
    192-193**F**
IDM (infant of diabetic mother) 73, 79,
    260, 262, 266, 268
Immune globulin (IVIG) 62, 78, 116,
    142-144
    dose 477
Immunizations 136, 144
Implantable cardioverter defibrillator
    (ICD) 55, 60, 128, 268, 417, 421**F**
Inborn error of metabolism (IEM) 18,
    111, 113, 115
Incessant tachycardia 56, 57, 58, 73
Incidence of conditions
    cardiac malformations 222,
    242, 313, 373, 375
    familial hypercholesterolemia 197
    Kawasaki disease 142
    rheumatic fever 150
    sudden cardiac death 123
    syncope 167
    syndromes 27-42
Inderal (propranolol) 5, 56, 64, 79, 117
    dose 484
Indomethacin (Indocin) 85, 88
    dose 477
Infant of diabetic mother (IDM) 73, 79,
    260, 262, 266, 268
Infarction 159, 196, 197, 420, 496
Infective endocarditis 8, 12, 135, 137,
    141, 147-149, 150, 152, 257, 260,
    506-509
    prophylaxis 457-458**T**
Inferior vena cava
    general 260, 269
    Fontan 285, 440, 442-443**F**
    fetal 232, 233**F**, 371, 379, 380, 386
    interrupted 214 220,, 222, 223**F**, 226
    partial/total anomalous pulmonary
    venous return to IVC 256, 282,
    283**F**
Inflammation
    general 490
    heart 58, 73, 74, 112, 114, 116, 124
Infliximab (Remicade) 144
    dose 478
Influenza 72, 145
Infundibulum 243, 277

Index

I

Inheritance
  Autosomal dominant inheritance
    Alagille syndrome 42, 493, 505
    ARVC (arrhythmogenic right ventricular cardiomyopathy) 58, 64, 76, 124, 126, 128, 269
    Brugada syndrome 59, 64, 124, 126, 127, 128, 493, 494, 505
    CHARGE syndrome 38, 493
    chromosome 22q11 deletion 21, 34, 210, 274, 288, 300, 316, 452, 493
    CPVT (catecholaminergic polymorphous ventricular tachycardia) 59, 124, 128, 493, 494
    Holt-Oram syndrome 40, 493, 507
    Long QTS Romano-Ward 58, 509
    Marfan syndrome 36, 125, 126, 159, 257, 493, 508, 509, 510
    Noonan syndrome 32, 73, 180, 181, 258, 262, 268, 406, 493, 508
    Polycystic kidney disease 180, 181, 182
    SVAS syndrome 39, 260, 493
    Tuberous sclerosis 37, 180, 181, 493
    Williams syndrome 39, 258, 260, 262, 263, 493, 510
  Autosomal recessive inheritance
    CPVT (catecholaminergic polymorphous ventricular tachycardia) 59, 124, 128, 493, 494
    Kartagener syndrome 222, 313, 507
    Long QTS Jervell Lange-Nielsen 58, 507
    Polycystic kidney disease 180, 181, 182
    TAR syndrome 41
Inlet VSD 248, 250**F**, 253, 410
Innocent murmurs 3, 6, 8, 9**F**
INR (international normalized ratio) 144, 487, 492
Insulin
  fasting 190, 196
  infant diabetic mother 262, 266
  normal levels 499
  resistance 189, 197
  with dextrose for hyperkalemia dose 60**T**, 469
Intermediate-density lipoprotein (IDL) 192-193**F**
Interrupted aortic arch (IAA) 34, 114, 210, 212, 274-275**F**, 288, 413, 431, 442
Interrupted inferior vena cava 214, 222, 223**F**
Intervals EKG (PR, QRS, QTc) 49, 52, 57, 60, 124, 150, 325**F**, 332**F**, 335**F**-338**F**, 470
Interventional cardiac catheterization 397-398, 405-413, 432, 434, 438, 452, 457
Intracardiac clots/vegetations 56, 148-149
Intracardiac echocardiography (ICE) 365
Intracardiac electrical pathways 52, 53**F**, 336, 417-420
Intracardiac indwelling lines 147, 451
Intracardiac patch 134, 430-431, 434-435**F**, 438, 439**F**
Intracardiac pressures 397, 399**F**-402**F**
Intracardiac shunts
  left-to-right 2, 77, 87, 88, 95, 244-245, 246-247, 252, 254, 272, 278, 309, 317-318, 361, 398, 399, 403**E**, 452
  right-to-left 87-88, 95**F**, 96-97, 99-100, 102, 103-105, 135, 236, 241, 276**F**-299**F**, 399, 403, 452
Intrauterine/ in utero 27, 96, 113, 205, 46, 254, 255, 379, 382
Intravascular ultrasound (IVUS) 365
Intravenous gammaglobulin (IVIG) 62, 78, 116, 142-144
  dose 477
Intropin (dopamine) 78, 104. 449
  dose 472, 473**T**
Ion channelopathies 58-59, 124, 128, 493-494
Irregular rhythm
  EKG tracings 63**F**, 332**F**, 328**F**, 333**F**
Ischemia, myocardial 74, 124, 127, 159, 245, 446, 448, 449, 452
Isoproterenol (Isuprel) 62, 79, 170
  dose 478
Isthmus of the aorta 379
Ivemark syndrome 222, 507

Index

I – L

IVIG (intravenous gammaglobulin) 62, 78, 116, 142-144
  dose 477
IVUS (intravascular ultrasound) 365

— J —

Janeway lesions 147, 148, 507
Jatene procedure 436, 507
Jervell & Lang-Nielsen 58, 507
Jones criteria 150, 507
Junctional ectopic tachycardia (JET) 55, 57, 73, 452
  EKG tracing 57F
Junctional rhythm 54, 134, 400

— K —

K-Dur (potassium supplementation)
  dose 483
Kartagener syndrome 222, 313, 507
Kawasaki disease 72, 73, 124, 141-144, 152, 507 507
Kawashima procedure 442, 507
Kayexalate
  dose 60
Kerley lines 318, 507
Ketoacidosis 117, 159, 497
Kidney/renal disease
  general 18, 29, 30, 33, 34, 35, 37, 39, 41, 42, 88, 177, 178, 180-183, 268, 399, 405, 450, 453, 510
  renin levels 501T
  urine analysis 502T
  urine catecholamines 502T, 503T
Kommerell diverticulum 300, 507
Konno procedure 263, 507
Korotkoff (Korotkov) sounds 178, 507
Kounis syndrome 159, 508

— L —

L-transposition of the great arteries (L-TGA) 281F, 282
Labetolol (Trandate)
  dose 478
Laboratory values 489-503
Lactate 451, 500
Lanoxin (digoxin) 55-57, 60, 64, 79, 384, 466
  dose 470, 471T
Large for gestational age (LGA) 98, 268
Lasix (furosemide) 77, 78, 450
  dose 475
Leads for EKG 58, 324F, 339, 343, 346
Left-sidedness 222, 223F, 224T
Left-to-right shunts 72, 77, 87, 88, 95, 244-245, 246-247, 252, 254, 272, 278, 309, 317-318, 361, 398, 399, 403E, 452
Left ventricle 8, 97, 100, 210, 226, 232, 270, 279, 281, 284, 290, 314, 354, 355F, 356, 357F, 375F, 376F, 400, 401F, 408, 410, 436, 437F, 438, 439F
Levalbuterol (Xopenex)
  dose 478
Levocardia 219, 221, 225F, 242, 313, 373
Levo (L)-looping of the embryonic heart tube 206
levo (L)-transposition of the great arteries 281F, 282
Levophed (norepinephrine) 449
  dose 482
LDL (low-density lipoproteins) 192-193F, 197, 506
Lidocaine 56, 60, 64, 79, 97
  dose 478
Ligation of PDA 85, 88, 89, 247, 429, 430
Lipids 192-198, 500
Lipitor (atorvastatin) 198
  dose 467
Lipoproteins 192-193F, 196, 197
Listeria 72, 115, 145
Lisinopril (Zestril)
  dose 479
Liver
  general 105, 113, 192, 193F, 194F, 236, 282, 298, 382, 452
  situs 99, 220, 222, 223F
Liver function tests
  disease 20, 76, 115, 143, 146,

539

L – M

190-191, 196, 197, 198, 451
normal values 492, 497, 500
Long QT syndrome (LQTS)
general 3, 12, 58-59, 60, 61, 123, 124, 127, 128, 169, 328, 338-339, 384, 423, 493**T**-494, 507, 509
Bazett formula 338**F**
Jervell & Lange-Nielsen (deaf) 58, 507
medications to avoid 60, 124
Romano-Ward 58, 509
Looping of the embryonic heart tube 206-207**F**, 279, 281
Lopid (gemfibrozil) 198
dose 475
Lopressor (metoprolol)
dose 480
Lortab (hydrocodone+acetaminophen) 450
dose 476
Losartan (Cozaar)
dose 479
Lovenox (enoxaparin)
dose 473
Low atrial pacemaker 224, 330
Low-density lipoproteins (LDL) 192-193**F**, 197, 506
Lung
chest X-ray 312, 317-318
disease 18, 20, 21, 37, 89, 96, 101, 105, 113, 114, 181, 256, 284, 410
situs 220, 222, 223**F**
Lupus 61-62

LVEDD 360-361
LVEDP 400
LVEDV 360-361
LVESV 360-361
LVH (left ventricular hypertrophy) 124, 126, 128, 159, 178, 245, 266, 346
Lyme disease 72, 76, 145, 146
lymph node 142

— M —

M-mode echocardiography 351, 360-361, 384, 385
Machinery murmur 6, 247
Magnesium sulfate 101
dose 479
Magnetic resonance imaging (MRI) 2, 21, 76, 101, 102, 105, 128, 136, 150, 181, 219, 254, 266, 269, 279, 282, 298, 300, 361, 391-393, 397, 398, 424
Malposition of the heart 99, 225
Marfan syndrome 36, 125, 126, 159, 257, 493, 508, 509, 510
MAT (multifocal atrial tachycardia)
EKG tracing 57**F**
Maternal age, advanced 27-30, 98
Maternal autoantibodies 62
Maternal diabetes 98, 262, 266
Maternal graves 113
Maternal lupus 61-62

Maternal prenatal factors 98, 113, 180, 205, 232, 234
Maternal steroids 62
McGoon ratio 508
MCLNS (mucocutaneous lymph node syndrome or Kawasaki disease) 72, 73, 124, 141-144, 152, 507 507
Measles 141
Meconium aspiration 96, 98, 99, 113
Mediastinum 158, 280, 284, 316, 319
Mesocardia 225**F**, 242, 313
Metabolic disorders 18, 19, 76, 111, 115, 180, 192, 268, 339, 451
Metabolic syndrome 189, 191
Metanephrine 499, 502
Metformin (Glucophage) 191
dose 479
Methemoglobinemia9 5, 97, 102, 480, 82
Methimazole (Tapazole) 117
dose 479
Methylene blue 102
dose 480
Methylprednisolone (Solu-Medrol) 144
dose 480
Metoprolol (Lopressor)
dose 480
Midazolam (Versed)
dose 480
Midodrine (ProAmatine) 171
dose 480
Midsystolic click 10, 11**F**
Milrinone (Primacor) 78, 104, 449

M – N

dose 481
Mitral valve, normal anatomy 243**F**, 354, 355F, 356, 357**F**
Mitral valve atresia 270, 271**F**
Mitral valve cleft 250, 254, 256
Mitral valve prolapse 10, 36, 147, 159, 257
Mitral valve regurgitation (MR) 21, 36, 143, 145, 250**F**, 254, 256, 266, 268
Mitral valve rheumatic fever 150
Mitral valve stenosis 318
Mobitz type I & II 2nd-degree heart block 332, 508
   EKG tracing type II 332**F**
Monitor
   bedside 54, 111, 399, 449
   event 49-51**F**, 127, 161, 171
   Holter 12, 49, 50, 51**F**, 64, 126, 127, 128, 161, 169, 171, 507
Monopril (fosinopril)
   dose 474
Morphine 104, 450
   dose 481
Moyamoya disease 508
MPI (myocardial performance index) 364
MRI (magnetic resonance imaging) 2, 21, 76, 101, 102, 105, 128, 136, 150, 181, 219, 254, 266, 269, 279, 282, 298, 300, 361, 391-393 397, 398, 424
MTHFR 492
Mucocutaneous lymph node syndrome (MCLNS or Kawasaki disease) 72, 73, 124, 141-144, 152, 507 507
Multifocal atrial tachycardia (MAT)
   EKG tracing 57**F**
Mumps virus 72, 145
Murmurs
   General 3-11
   Continuous murmur 6-7**F**, 247, 292
   Diastolic murmurs 6, 7**F**, 10, 252, 256, 257, 262, 288
   Ejection murmur 5, 6, 7**F**, 8, 9**F**, 10, 245, 262, 264, 278
   Holosystolic murmurs 6, 8, 252, 256, 257, 292
   Innocent murmurs 3, 6, 8, 9**F**
   Machinery murmur 6, 247
   Still's murmur 6, 8
   Systolic murmurs 5-7**F**, 8-9**F**, 10, 134
     aortic stenosis 262
     atrial septal defect 256
     coarctation 264
     coarctation & VSD 272
     hypertrophic cardiomyopathy 268
     patent ductus arteriosus 247
     pulmonary atresia & intact ventricular septum 292
     tetralogy of Fallot 278
     tricuspid atresia 285
     truncus arteriosus 288
     valvular regurgitation 257
     VSD 252
Muscular dystrophy 71, 73, 268, 496, 505, 506
Muscular VSD 249**F**

Mustard procedure 436, 437**F**, 508
Myocardial biopsy 76, 128, 146, 269, 405, 412
Myocardial infarction 159, 196, 197, 420, 496
Myocarditis 49, 56, 58, 62-64, 72, 74, 76, 78, 80, 112, 114, 125, 128, 145-146, 150, 152, 383, 412
Myopericarditis 3, 141, 145, 152, 159, 169

— N —

Nadolol (Corgard)
   dose 481
Nakata index 508
Naprosyn (naproxen) 151
   dose 481
Natrecor (nesiritide) 77
   dose 481
NEC (necrotising entercolitis) 86, 88, 114
Neonatal cardiovascular physiology 231, 234, 294
Neonatal coarctation 264
Neonatal extremis 112-117, 270-275
Neonatal hypertrophic cardiomyopathy 266
NeoProfen (ibuprofen lysine) 85, 88
   dose 477
Neosynephrine (phenylephrine) 104
   dose 483

N – P

Nephrotic syndrome 180, 197

Nesiritide (Natrecor) 77
    dose 481

Neurodevelopment
    Premature PDA ligation 89
    syndromes 28-42

Neurofibromatosis 180, 181, 493

Nicardipine (Cardene)
    dose 482

Niaspan (niacin) 198
    dose 481

Nifedipine (Procardia) 79, 183
    dose 482

Nipride (nitroprusside) 78, 181, 450, 453
    dose 482

Nitric oxide (NO) 101, 116, 453
    dose 482

Nitroglycerine
    dose 482

Noncompaction 124, 269, 384

Nondisjunction 27

Nonsinus low atrial rhythm
    EKG tracing 330**F**

Noonan syndrome 32, 73, 181, 258, 262, 268, 406, 508

Norepinephrine (Levophed) 449
    dose 482

Norpace (amlodipine) 171
    dose 472

Norvasc (amlodipine)
    dose 466

Norwood procedure 102, 270, 443-444, 445**F**

NSAIDs (nonsteroidal anti-inflammatory drugs) 135

– O –

Obesity 177, 180, 183, 189-191, 195-197

Obstructive apnea 183, 190

Obstructive uropathy 181

Occluders 136, 410-411**F**

Octreotide (Sandostatin) 452
    dose 483

Olmesartan (Benicar)
    dose 483

One (1)-functional ventricle 73, 285, 296, 297**F**, 430, 431, 440, 441**F**, 442, 443**F**, 444, 445**F**

Orthodromic SVT
    EKG tracings 52**F**, 53**F**, 331**F**

Orthostatic vital sign changes 168

Osler nodes 147, 148, 508

Outflows, ventricular
    general 102, 243**F**, 361, 364, 400
    embryology 210-211**F**
    fetal echo 369, 376**F**-377**F**, 386**F**
    LV-hypertrophic cardiomyopathy 266-267**F**, 268
    LV-Rastelli repair 438-439**F**
    RV-interventional cath 408
    RV-tetralogy of Fallot 104, 277**F**, 278, 434-435**F**

Outlet septum 10, 205, 208, 210-211**F**, 277

Outlet VSD 10, 248, 251**F**, 252-253, 410

Overactive precordium (hyperdynamic precordium) 4, 8, 10, 71, 74, 99, 247, 252, 256, 257, 270, 272, 274, 280, 284, 288, 290, 296

Oximetry 241-242, 264, 398

Oxygen consumption 397, 403**E**

Oxygen saturation 98-99, 102, 104, 112-113, 242, 276, 278, 398, 399**F**-400**F**, 403**E**

– P –

P-wave 49, 52, 54, 57, 58, 134, 324, 331, 334, 336
    EKG tracings 325**F**, 332**F**, 330**F**, 340**F**, 341**F**

PACs (premature atrial contractions)
    EKG tracings 63**F**, 333**F**

PA projection for chest X-ray 310, 311**F**

Pacemakers
    EKG tracing 334**F**
    indications 423

Pain
    abdominal 71, 80, 142, 268
    chest 157-161, 262
    hypertension 180, 181
    postoperative 450, 452
    syncope from 167, 168
    tachycardia from 328

P

Palivizumab (Synagis) 103
   dose 483
Palliation of cardiac malformations 102, 135, 270, 278, 294, 296, 412-413**F**, 430, 431, 440-441**F**, 442-443**F**
Palpation 4, 10, 160, 17, 178
Palpitations 49, 50, 54, 127, 160, 168, 268
Paradoxic pulse 74, 77, 105, 145, 160, 452
Parasternal views Echo 352-353**F**, 354-355**F**, 356-357**F**
Partial anomalous pulmonary venous return 254, 255**F**, 313
Parvovirus 72, 145
Patau syndrome 508
Patent ductus arteriosus (PDA)
   general 4, 6, 8, 9**T**, 21, 28, 29, 30, 42, 72, 100, 147, 226, 241, 244**F**, 245, 246, 247, 363, 398, 400, 402, 405, 429, 430, 453, 477
   device closure 136, 410, 411**F**, 430
   premature infant 85-89
   with other malformations 101, 102, 112, 116, 262, 264, 272, 274, 285, 292, 300, 392, 406, 412, 434, 444
Patent foramen ovale (PFO) 96, 222, 254, 256
Pectus 32, 36, 160
Pericardial
   effusions 10, 71, 72, 74, 75**T**, 77, 112, 114, 123, 135, 143, 145, 146, 150, 160, 169, 269, 316, 356, 451, 452
   stripping 79
   thickening 76
Pericardiocentesis 77, 116, 135, 398, 452
Pericarditis 10, 72, 173, 76, 79, 80, 141, 145-146, 150, 152, 159, 162, 169, 339
Perimembranous VSD 248-249**F**, 252, 253
Perinatal
   asphyxia 8, 96, 112, 268
   atrial flutter 156
   outcome 379
Persantine (dipyridamole) 144
   dose 472
PFC (persistent fetal circulation) 96
PFO (patent foramen ovale) 96, 222, 254, 256
PGE1 (prostaglandin E1) 101-102, 116, 246, 258, 262, 264, 270, 272, 274, 278, 280, 285, 290, 292, 296
   dose 485
Phenylephrine (Neosynephrine) 104
   dose 483
Pharyngitis, streptococcal 150
Pheochromocytoma 125, 180, 181, 183
PJRT (permanent junctional reciprocating tachycardia)
   EKG tracing 58**F**
Plasma proteins 500
Platelets 34, 41, 88, 143, 451
Pleural
   effusions 74, 96, 116, 135, 146, 309, 313, 318, 372, 382, 451
   space 318
Pneumonia 96, 101, 103, 105, 114, 135, 158, 242, 309, 318
Pneumothorax 36, 89, 96, 101, 114, 116, 158, 225, 313, 318, 319, 451
Polycystic kidney disease 180, 181, 182
Polysplenia 222, 223**T**
Pompe disease 266, 508
Postoperative care 449-453
Post-pericardiotomy syndrome 72, 134, 135-136, 159, 451
Potassium chloride (K-Dur)
   dose 483
Potassium iodide (SSKI) 117
   dose 484
POTS (postural orthostatic tachycardia syndrome) 168-169, 170, 171
Potter syndrome 180, 508
PPHN (persistent pulmonary hypertension of the newborn) 72, 95, 96, 98-101, 114
PPS (peripheral pulmonic stenosis) 8
PR interval 49, 52, 150, 332
   EKG tracings 335**F**, 336**F**
Prader-Willi syndrome 508
Precedex (dexmedetomidine) 57
   dose 469
Precordial overactivity (hyperdynamic precordium) 4, 8, 10, 71, 74, 99, 247, 52, 256, 257, 270, 272, 274, 280, 284, 288, 290, 296

543

P – Q

Prednisone 78, 117, 135, 142-144, 151
    dose 484
Preexcitation 3, 12, 42, 52-53F, 55, 126, 169, 294, 336F
Prelone (prednisolone) 78, 117, 135, 142-144, 151
    dose 484
Premature atrial contractions (PACs)
    EKG tracings 64F, 333F
Premature infants 85-89, 180, 246, 397
Premature rupture of membranes 98, 113
Premature ventricular contractions (PVCs) 49, 64, 73, 337
    EKG tracings 63F, 333F
Prenatal care/evaluation
    general 61, 62, 98, 112, 180, 181, 219, 231, 241, 242, 268, 276, 369
    echocardiogram 369-386
Pressure data from cardiac catheterization 399F-402F, 403E
Pressure overload 71, 72, 74, 75T, 77, 99, 245, 258F-265F, 278,
Preventive cardiology 192F-198T
Primacor (milrinone) 78, 104, 449
    dose 481
Primum ASD 208, 250, 254-255F, 256
ProAmatine (midodrine) 171
    dose 480
Procardia (nifedipine) 79, 183
    dose 482
Prophylaxis
    endocarditis 457-458T
    rheumatic fever 151

asplenia antibiotic 222
Propranolol (Inderal) 5, 56, 64, 79, 117
    dose 484
Propylthiouracil (PTU) 117
    dose 485
Prosthetic material/valves 148, 149, 457
Prostin (prostaglandin E1) 101-102, 116, 246, 258, 262, 264, 270, 272, 274, 278, 280, 285, 290, 292, 296
    dose 485
Protamine 446, 451
    dose 485
Proventyl (albuterol)
    dose for hyperkalemia 60T, 466
Pseudocoarctation 264
PT (prothrombin time) 451, 492T
PTT (partial thromboplastin time) 451, 492
PTU (propylthiouracil) 117
    dose 485
Pulmonary arteriovenous malformation 97, 103, 105, 298F, 299F, 431
Pulmonary arterial pressure 5, 10, 96, 100, 236, 244, 245E, 398, 402F, 403E, 432, 442
Pulmonary atresia with intact ventricular septum 97, 114, 276, 292, 293F, 296, 398, 406
Pulmonary hypertension 5, 8, 21, 72, 74, 75T, 77, 88, 95, 96, 103, 125, 159, 160, 169, 244, 247, 252, 254, 270, 272, 317, 318, 398, 400, 408, 432, 449, 451, 452, 453

Pulmonary vascular resistance 10, 76, 96, 236, 244-245E, 246, 252. 294, 403E, 442, 449, 510
Pulmonic regurgitation (PR) 252, 262, 317, 318, 361, 402, 403, 408
Pulmonic stenosis all forms 8, 9T, 32, 39, 72, 77, 100, 103, 124, 245, 258, 259F, 260, 262, 277, 285, 290, 318, 400, 406, 407F, 429, 434, 436, 440
Pulmonic valvuloplasty 102, 134, 258, 278, 406, 407F
Pulsed Doppler 362, 363, 385
Pulses
    general 4, 20, 71, 160, 167, 170, 177, 178, 449
    bounding 247
    diminished 74, 126, 169, 164, 181, 183, 270, 272, 274, 432
Pulsus paradoxus 74, 77, 105, 145, 160, 452
PVCs (premature ventricular contractions) 49, 64, 73, 337
    EKG tracings 63F, 333F
PVR (pulmonary vascular resistance) 10, 76, 96, 236, 244-245E, 246, 252, 294, 403E, 442, 449, 510

– Q –

Qp (pulmonary flow) 245E, 403E
Qp:Qs ratio (pulmonary to systemic flow ratio) 392, 403E

Q – S

QRS frontal axis
    EKG tracings 340**F**, 341**F**
QRS interval 49, 52-55, 57, 59, 60, 63, 78-79, 134, 250, 285, 325**F**. 331**F**, 333**F**, 334**F**, 337**F**, 340**F**-342**F**, 423
Qs (systemic flow) 245**E**, 403**E**
QT/QTc interval 58, 61, 126, 127, 128, 338**F**, 505
Questran (cholestyramine resin) 198
    dose 468

– R –

R-wave 344
    EKG tracings 345**F**, 346**F**
Radiation dose 392**T**
Radiofrequency ablation 54-58, 60, 64, 79, 417, 419-420**F**
Ranitidine (Zantac)
    dose 484
Rashkind procedure 509
Rastelli procedure 509
RBBB (right bundle branch block) 5, 126, 269
RCM (restrictive cardiomyopathy) 73, 76, 79, 267**F**, 269, 400
RDS (respiratory distress syndrome) 85, 86, 88
Reentry 52-53**F**, 54, 419
Remicade (infliximab) 144
    dose 478

Renal/kidney disease
    general 18, 29, 30, 33, 34, 35, 37, 39, 41, 42, 88, 177, 178, 180-183, 268, 399, 405, 450, 453, 510
    renin levels 501**T**
    urine analysis 502**T**
    urine catecholamines 502**T**, 503**T**
Renin 180, 181
    normal serum levels 501**T**
Resistance, vascular
    Pulmonary vascular resistance 10, 76, 96, 236, 244-245**E**, 246, 252. 294, 403**E**, 442, 449, 510
    systemic vascular 104, 236, 244-245**E**, 246, 379, 403**E**, 450, 496
Respiratory distress syndrome (RDS) 85, 86, 88
Restrictive cardiomyopathy (RCM) 73, 76, 79, 267**F**, 269, 400
Resynchronization 79, 423
Revatio (sildenafil) 78, 101
    dose 486
RF ablation (radiofrequency) 54-58, 60, 64, 79, 417, 419-420**F**
Rhabdomyoma 79, 423
Rheumatic fever 150-151
Rheumatic fever prophylaxis 151
Rheumatoid arthritis 141
Rib notching 264, 318
Rickettsia 72, 145
Right-sidedness 222, 223**F**, 224**T**
Right-to-left shunts 87-88, 95**F**, 96-97, 99-100, 102, 103-105, 135, 236, 241, 276**F**-299**F**, 399, 403, 452
Right ventricle 5, 8, 10, 97, 100, 104, 126, 208, 210, 211**F**, 226, 232, 254, 277, 278, 279, 281, 284, 314, 354, 355**F**, 356, 357**F**, 360, 361**F**, 372, 373**F**, 374**F**, 375**F**, 400, 401**F**, 403, 408, 410, 412, 424, 435**F**, 436, 437**F**
Romano-Ward 58, 509
Ross procedure 509
Roth spots 147, 148, 509
RSV (respiratory syncitial virus) 103
Rubella 205
Rubs 10, 135, 135, 160, 449
Rumble 6, 252, 256
RVDAI (right ventricular diastolic area index) 361**E**
RVEDD (right ventricular end-diastolic dimension) 361**E**
RVEDV (right ventricular end-diastolic volume) 361

– S –

S_1 (1st heart sound) 4-7
S_2 (2nd heart sound) 4-7
S'-wave spectral tissue Doppler 364**F**
Saint Vitus dance 150
Salmonella 72, 145
Sandostatin (octreotide) 452
    dose 483
Sano procedure 509

Index

S

SBE (subacute bacterial endocarditis) 8, 12, 135, 137, 141, 147-149, 150, 152, 257, 260, 506-509
    prophylaxis 457-458T
Scimitar syndrome 256, 313
SCD (sudden cardiac death) 12, 55, 123-128, 160, 168, 266, 269, 336
Schistosoma 72, 145
Scleroderma 73
Second (2nd) degree AV block
    EKG tracing 332F
Second heart sound (S_2) 3F-7F, 160, 169, 280, 282, 288
Secundum ASD 208, 254-255F, 256, 392, 430
Seizures 28, 37, 97, 102, 104, 123, 136, 168, 177, 180, 405
Semilunar valves 4, 159, 205, 210, 288, 400, 402, 452
Senning procedure 436, 437F, 509
Septation
    atria & ventricles 208-209F
    conotruncus 210-211F, 288
Septostomy/septectomy 102, 279, 397, 406, 412, 509
Sertraline (Zoloft) 171
    dose 485
Serum proteins 500
Shock 111-117, 264, 270-275, 453
Shone syndrome 260, 264, 509
Shprintzen syndrome 34, 509
Shunts
    left-to-right shunts 72, 77, 87, 88, 95, 244-245, 246-247, 252, 254, 272, 278, 309, 317-318, 361, 398, 399, 403E, 452
    right-to-left shunts 87-88, 95F, 96-97, 99-100, 102, 103-105, 135, 236, 241, 276F-299F, 399, 403, 452
Sick sinus syndrome 418
SIDS (sudden infant death syndrome) 269
Sidenafil (Revatio, Viagra) 78, 101
    dose 486
Single ventricle (1-functional ventricle) 73, 285, 296, 297F, 430, 431, 440, 441F, 442, 443F, 444, 445F
Sinus arrhythmia 49, 63, 327
    EKG tracing 328F
Sinus bradycardia
    EKG tracing 61F, 329F
Sinus node 134, 224, 418F, 452
Sinus rhythm 49, 50, 54-55, 60, 169, 423
    EKG tracing 49F, 327F
Sinus tachycardia
    EKG tracing 329F
Situs ambiguus 220-221T, 222-223F
Situs inversus 220-221T, 222-223F, 313
Situs solitus 220-221T, 222-223F, 313, 371F
Sjögren syndrome 62, 509
SLE (systemic lupus erythematosus) 61-62
Snake venom 145
Snowman 284
Sodium benzoate + sodium phenylacetate (Ammonul) 117
    dose 486
Sodium bicarbonate 104, 117
    dose 486
Solu-Cortef (hydrocortisone) 117
    dose 476
Solu-Medrol (methylprednisolone) 144
    dose 480
Sotalol (Betapace) 56, 57, 58
    dose 486
Spectral Doppler 362, 365, 382
Spironolactone (Aldactone) 475
    dose 486
Splenic syndromes 222-223F, 224T, 507
Splenomegaly 42, 145, 147, 160, 169
Split S_1 (1st heart sound) 5
Split S_2 (2nd heart sound) 5
Squatting 278
SSA/SSB autoantibodies 61, 62, 269, 469, 477, 491
SSKI (potassium iodide) 117
    dose 484
ST-T waves 74, 99, 146, 169, 243, 335, 338
    EKG tracings 339F
Starnes procedure 294, 509
Statins 194, 198
    dose atorvastatin (Lipitor) 467
Steinberg thumb sign 509
Stents 102, 134, 136, 284, 285, 292, 399, 406, 407, 409F, 412, 432, 434, 438, 444
Steroids, anabolic 180, 183

S

Steroids, therapeutic
  Glucocorticoids
    agents & dosing:
      hydrocortisone (Solu-Cortef) 476
      methylprednisolone (Solu-Medrol) 480
      prednisolone (Prelone) 484
      prednisone 484
    for:
      congenital adrenal hyperplasia 117
      fetal heart block 62
      Kawasaki disease 142-144
      myopericarditis 78
      post-pericardiotomy syndrome 135
      rheumatic fever 151
      thyrotoxicosis 117
    side effects:
      hypertension cause 180
      hypertrophic cardiomyopathy 73
      lipid disorder 197
  Mineralocorticoids
    agents & dosing:
      fludrocortisone (Florinef) 171
      dose 474
    for:
      syncope 171
    side effects:
      hypertension 180
Stevens Johnson syndrome 141, 510
Still's murmur 6, 8
Stomach decompression 449
Stomach in situs 99, 220, 222, 242, 313, 371, 372

Streptococcal antibodies 76, 151, 491, 509
Stress testing (exercise/treadmill) 12, 49, 126, 127, 128, 161
Stridor 98, 242, 300, 301**F**
Subacute bacterial endocarditis (SBE) 8, 12, 135, 137, 141, 147-149, 150, 152, 257, 260, 506-509
  prophylaxis 457-458**T**
Subclavian artery
  aberrant 212-213**F**, 300-301**F**
  Blalock-Taussig shunt (BT shunt) 399, 408, 429, 432, 433**F**, 505
Subvalvular aortic stenosis 249, 252, 260-263, 266, 505, 507
Subvalvular pulmonic stenosis 258-259, 434
Sudden cardiac death (SCD) 12, 55, 123-128, 160, 168, 266, 269, 336
Sulfonamides 145
Supraventricular tachycardia (SVT) 52-55, 57, 63, 73, 79, 112, 134, 159, 257, 294, 336, 420
  EKG tracings 52**F**, 329**F**
Surgery for cardiovascular malformations 429-453
Supravalvular pulmonic stenosis 39, 258-259, 434
SVAS (supravalvular aortic stenosis syndrome) 27, 39, 260-263
SVR (systemic vascular resistance) 104, 236, 244-245**E**, 246, 379, 403**E**, 450, 496

Swan-Ganz catheter 402, 510
Swiss cheese VSD 249, 253
Sydenham chorea 150-151, 510
Synagis (palivizumab) 103
  dose 483
Syncope 167-171, 258, 262, 263, 423
Syndromes
  general 27-42, 493-494
  Alagille 42, 505
  Asplenia 222-223**F**, 224
  Brugada 59, 64, 124, 126-128, 494, 505
  CHARGE 38
  chromosome 22q11 21, 34 210
  Cushing 183
  DiGeorge 34, 493, 505
  Down 17, 21, 28, 250, 253, 452, 506
  Edwards (trisomy 18) 29, 506
  Eisenmenger 72, 103, 344, 253, 506
  Fetal alcohol 31
  hemolytic uremic 180
  Holt-Oram 40, 507
  Hypereosinophilic 73, 76, 159
  Hypoplastic left heart 29, 30, 33, 97, 102, 111, 112, 114, 205, 270-271**F**, 406, 444-445**F**
  Ivemark 222, 507
  Jervell & Lange-Nielsen 58, 507
  Kartagener 222, 313, 507
  Kounis 159, 508
  Long QT 58-60, 123, 124, 328, 338, 339, 384, 423
  Marfan 36, 125, 126, 159, 257, 508

547

S – T

meconium aspiration 96, 113
metabolic 189, 191
mucocutaneous lymph node (Kawasaki disease) 142-144
nephrotic 180, 197
Noonan 32, 73, 181, 258, 262, 268, 406, 508
Patau (trisomy 13) 30, 5-8
Polysplenia 222-223F, 224
postural orthostatic 168-169
post-pericardiotomy 72, 134, 135, 159, 451
Potter 180, 508
Prader Willi 190, 508
respiratory distress 85
Romano Ward 58
scimitar 256-257F, 313
Shone 260, 264, 509
Shprintzen 34, 509
sick sinus syndrome 418
Sjögren 62, 509
Stevens-Johnson 141, 510
sudden infant death 269
supravalvular aortic stenosis 39
TAR 41
tuberous sclerosis 37, 181
Turner 33, 159, 181, 262, 264, 510
VACTERL 35
velocardial facial 34
Williams 39, 181, 258, 260, 262, 263, 510
WPW 3, 42, 123, 336, 510
Systemic-to-pulmonary artery shunts 102, 104, 135, 278, 285, 294, 391, 429, 431, 432-433F, 440-441F, 442-443F
Systemic arteriovenous malformation 72, 382
Systemic arterial pressure 244, 245E, 402F, 403E
Systemic blood flow (Qs) 245E, 403E
Systemic connective tissue disease (or collagen vascular disease) 62, 72, 73, 74, 145, 159
Systemic diseases in failure-to-thrive 18
Systemic vascular resistance 104, 236, 244-245E, 246, 379, 403E, 450, 496
Systole 4, 6, 360, 363, 379, 380, 385, 400, 404
Systolic murmurs 5-7F, 8-9F, 10, 134
    aortic stenosis 262
    atrial septal defect 256
    coarctation 264
    coarctation & VSD 272
    hypertrophic cardiomyopathy 268
    patent ductus arteriosus 247
    pulmonary atresia & intact ventricular septum 292
    tetralogy of Fallot 278
    tricuspid atresia 285
    truncus arteriosus 288
    valvular regurgitation 257
    VSD 252
Systolic dysfunction 71, 72, 74, 78, 245, 268, 450

– T –

T-wave 60, 126, 127, 146, 339,
    EKG tracings 325F, 344F
Tachyarrhythmias (tachycardias) all forms 49, 50, 52-60, 123, 124, 134, 135, 145, 171, 268, 331, 384, 417, 421, 423, 452, 493-494
Tachycardia induced cardiomyopathy 7, 73, 112, 114, 116
Tachypnea 21, 71, 145, 181, 268
Tambocor (flecainide) 56, 57, 58
    dose 474
Tamponade 71-72, 74, 75T, 77, 114, 116, 135, 146, 451, 452
Tapazole (methimazole) 117
    dose 479
TAPVR (total anomalous pulmonary venous return) 10, 96, 103, 105, 112, 135, 276, 282, 283F, 316, 431
TAR syndrome 41
TEE (transesophageal echocardiogram) 148, 365, 410, 446, 450
Tenormin (atenolol)
    dose 467
Tet spells 103, 104, 114, 116, 278
Tetracycline 143, 158, 160
Tetralogy of Fallot (ToF) 10, 28, 29, 30, 34, 35, 38, 41, 42, 60, 96, 103, 112, 114, 134, 135, 205, 210, 242, 276, 277F, 278, 318, 404, 429, 431, 432, 433F, 434, 509
Thermodilution cardiac output 403

Index

T

Third (3rd)-degree AV block
  EKG tracings 61F, 332F
Thoracoabdominal situs 206, 219-224, 242, 313, 359, 371F, 384, 440
Thoracotomy
Thrills 4, 262
Thrombocytopenia absent radius (TAR) 41
Thymus 316
Thyroid hormones
Tilt table (head up tilt) 169-170
Tissue Doppler 361, 364F
Torsades de pointes 58, 59
  EKG tracing 59F
Total anomalous pulmonary venous return (TAPVR) 10, 96, 103, 105, 112, 135, 276, 282, 283F, 316, 431
Toxins 27, 73, 97, 111, 113, 115, 116, 145, 205, 269
Trandate (labetolol)
  dose 478
Transducer 351, 352, 361, 362, 365, 371
Transesophageal echocardiogram (TEE) 148, 365, 410, 446, 450
Transesophageal electrophysiology 417
Transesophageal overdrive pacing 56
Transplant, heart 73, 77, 78, 79, 268, 269, 292, 412, 430, 444, 457
Transposition of the great arteries
  D-TGA 10, 28, 96, 102, 112, 134, 135, 159, 210, 242, 276, 279F, 280F, 282, 316, 397, 406, 431, 436, 437F, 507, 508, 509, 517

L-TGA 281F, 282
Tricuspid atresia 10, 114, 276, 284, 285F-287F, 292, 296, 341, 400, 406, 440, 4401F, 442, 443F, 506
Tricuspid valve
  Ebstein anomaly 294-295F, 506
  L-TGA 281
  normal 243F
  perimembranous VSD 249
  rumble 6
  S_1 (1st heart sound) 4
Tricuspid valve regurgitation (TR) 100, 112, 270, 292, 294, 295F, 361, 362, 363, 403, 444
Trisomies
  13 (Patau syndrome) 30
  18 (Edwards syndrome) 29
  21 (Down syndrome) 17, 21, 28, 220, 250, 243, 452, 506
Troponin I 76, 135, 146, 160, 496
Treadmill 126, 127, 161
Triglycerides 196E -198, 475
Truncal valve 114, 288
Truncus arteriosus 10, 34, 97, 102, 114, 205, 209, 211, 276, 288, 289F, 431, 438, 439F, 509
Trypanosoma cruzi (Chagas disease) 72, 145
Tuberous sclerosis 37, 180, 181, 493
Turner (XO) 33, 159, 205, 262, 264, 493, 510
Two (2)-dimensional echocardiography

General/transthoracic 3, 10, 12, 21, 27, 54, 56, 74, 76, 77, 85, 87-88, 99, 100, 101, 105, 111, 123, 126, 128, 135, 143, 144, 146, 150, 160, 169, 181, 183, 219, 225, 244, 313, 351-365, 298, 450
Cardiovascular malformations
  1-functional ventricle 296
  Aortic stenosis 260T, 262
  Atrial septal defects & PAPVR 254
  Cardiomyopathies 266, 268-269
  Coarctation of the aorta (CoA) 264
  CoA with VSD 272
  Double outlet right ventricle 290
  Ebstein anomaly 294
  Hypoplastic left heart syndrome 270
  Interrupted aortic arch 274
  Patent ductus arteriosus 246-247
  Pulmonary arteriovenous malformation 298
  Pulmonary atresia intact ventricular septum 292
  Pulmonic stenosis 258T
  Tetralogy of Fallot 278
  Total anomalous pulmonary venous return 282
  D-transposition 279
  L-transposition 281
  Tricuspid atresia 284
  Truncus arteriosus 288
  Valvular regurgitation 257
  Vascular rings 300
  Ventricular septal defects 248, 252

T – V

Doppler
  color flow 87, 100, 361-362F, 365, 375, 382
  spectral 100, 257, 258, 260, 264, 266, 361-363F, 365, 379F-381F, 382, 386
  tissue 365F

– U –

U-wave
  EKG tracing 339
UAC (umbilical artery catheter) 72, 98, 180, 181, 268
Umbilical artery 35, 232, 233F, 379F, 382
Umbilical vein 232, 233F, 371F, 379, 381F, 383, 383
Umbrella devices 410, 411F, 412
Univentricle (1-functional ventricle) 73, 285, 296, 297F, 430, 431, 440, 441F, 442, 443F, 444, 445F
Urine testing
  urine analysis 502T
  urine catecholamines 502T, 503T
UVC (umbilical venous catheter) 98, 180, 181, 236

– V –

v-wave atrial pressure 400, 401F
VACTERL association 35
Vagal maneuvers for converting SVT 54
Valium (diazepam) 151
  dose 470
Valsartan (Diovan) 78, 182, 183
  dose 487
Valvular regurgitation
  general 6, 7F, 8, 72, 143, 148, 150, 245, 257F, 392, 430, 452
  aortic (AR) 10, 36, 143, 145, 146, 159, 249, 251F, 252, 253, 260, 262, 263, 402, 408
  fetal 381, 382, 383F
  left-sided AV valve 281
  mitral (MR) 21, 36, 143, 145, 250F, 254, 256, 266, 268
  pulmonic (PR) 252, 262, 317, 318, 361, 402, 403, 408
  tricuspid (TR) 100, 112, 270, 292, 294, 295F, 361, 362, 363, 403, 444
  truncal valve 114, 288
Valvular aortic stenosis 4, 77, 260, 261F, 262-263, 404, 408, 409F, 430
Valvular pulmonic stenosis 10, 32, 77, 258, 259F, 318, 406, 407F, 430
Valvuloplasty
  aortic 134, 260, 262, 399, 408, 409F
  pulmonic 102, 134, 258, 278, 406, 407F
Vanillylmandelic acid (VMA) 502, 503T

Varicella 72, 145
Vasodilation 77, 103, 168, 449, 450
Vasodilators
  pulmonary 78, 101, 236, 398, 452
  systemic 103, 449, 450, 476, 479, 481, 482
Vasotec (enalapril) 77-79, 182-183
  dose 473
Vasovagal syncope 167
Vascular access 399
Vascular resistance
  general 244-245E, 398, 403E, 446
  pulmonary 10, 76, 96, 236, 244-245E, 246, 252, 294, 403E, 442, 449, 510
  systemic 104, 236, 244-245E, 246, 379, 403E, 450, 496
Vascular ring 18, 34, 35, 96, 212, 313F, 242, 300F, 301F, 378, 392, 393F, 429, 431
Vegetation 148F
Velocardial facial syndrome 34, 509
Vena cavas
  general 214-215, 219, 220, 222-223F, 226, 232-233F, 358
  anomalous pulmonary venous return to superior or inferior vena cava 254-255F, 282, 283F
  bilateral superior vena cavas 222-223F
  chest X-ray 314
  fetal 371F, 377F, 380F, 386F

V – W

Fontan/Glenn 285-286, 287F, 432, 440, 441F-445F
inferior vena cava (IVC) 260
interrupted inferior vena cava 214, 222-223F
left SVC to coronary sinus 214-215F
superior vena cava (SVC) 403, 408
Venous hum 8
Ventolin (albuterol)
   dose for hyperkalemia 60T, 466
Ventricles
   1-functional 73, 285, 296, 297F, 430, 431, 440, 441F, 442, 443F, 444, 445F
   left 8, 97, 100, 210, 226, 232, 270, 279, 281, 284, 290, 314, 354, 355F, 356, 357F, 375F, 376F, 400, 401F, 408, 410, 436, 437F, 438, 439F
   right 5, 8, 10, 97, 100, 104, 126, 208, 210, 211F, 226, 232, 254, 277, 278, 279, 281, 284, 314, 354, 355F, 356, 357F, 360, 361F, 372, 373F, 374F, 375F, 400, 401F, 403, 408, 410, 412, 424, 435F, 436, 437F
Ventricular arrhythmias
   ectopics (PVCs) 49, 64, 73, 337
   EKG tracing 333F
   tachycardia 52, 58-60, 124, 134, 423
   EKG tracing 58F, 331F
Ventricular end-diastolic pressures 364, 398, 400, 440
Ventricular function
Ventricular outflows
   general 102, 243F, 361, 364, 400
   embryology 210-211F
   fetal echo 369, 376F-377F, 386F
   LV-hypertrophic cardiomyopathy 266-267F, 268
   LV-Rastelli repair 438-439F
   RV-interventional cath 408
   RV-tetralogy of Fallot 104, 277F, 278, 434-435F
Ventricular pressures
   general 10, 400F, 401F
   left 104, 272
   right 278
Ventricular tachycardia (VT) 52, 58-60, 124, 125, 134, 423
   EKG tracing 58F, 331F
Verapamil 55
Versed (midazolam)
   dose 480
Viagra (sildenafil) 78, 101
   dose 486
Vibratory murmur 6, 8
Visceral larva migrans 72, 145
Visceral situs 206, 219-224, 242, 313, 359, 371F, 384, 440
VLDL (very-low density lipoprotein) 192, 193F, 197
VMA (Vanillylmandelic acid) 503T
Volume overload 71, 72, 77, 246-257
VSD (ventricular septal defect) 4, 6, 8, 9T, 10, 21, 28, 29, 30, 31, 34, 35, 38, 40, 41, 42, 72, 95, 97, 100, 103, 104, 114, 134, 136, 208, 226, 241, 244-245, 248F-251F, 252, 253, 257, 272, 274 277, 284, 290, 341, 363, 373, 375, 398, 400, 410, 430, 457
VT (ventricular tachycardia) 52, 58-60, 124, 134, 423
   EKG tracings 58F, 331F
VTI (velocity time integral) 362, 363, 364E

— W —

Walker-Murdock wrist sign 36, 510
Warfarin (Coumadin) 144
   dose 487
Weight 4, 17, 19F, 21, 178, 179F, 183, 189-191, 252, 268, 412
Wenckebach rhythm 510
Wide QRS supraventricular tachycardia
   EKG tracing 53F
Widely split second heart sound S_2 3, 5F, 256
Williams syndrome 39, 258, 260, 262, 263, 493, 510
Wilms tumor 180, 510
Wolff-Parkinson-White (WPW) 3, 52, 123, 336F, 510
   EKG tracings 53F, 336F
Wood units 244-245E, 403, 510

X – Z

— X —

X-ray 20, 74, 96, 99, 105, 111, 12, 134, 136, 146, 160, 181, 214, 219, 225, 242, 309-319, 392

Xanthomas 42, 196

Xopenex (levalbuterol)
 dose 478

XO (Turner syndrome) 33, 159, 205, 262, 264, 493, 509

Xylocaine (lidocaine)
 dose 478

— Y —

Yeast (candida) 72, 113, 145

— Z —

Zantac (ranitidine)
 dose 484

Zebeta (bisoprolol)
 dose 467

Zestril (lisinopril)
 dose 479

Zetia (ezetimibe) 198
 dose 474

Zoloft (sertraline) 171
 dose 485